Ill Composed

Ill Composed

Sickness, Gender, and Belief
in Early Modern England

Olivia Weisser

Yale

UNIVERSITY PRESS

NEW HAVEN AND LONDON

Published with assistance from the Annie Burr Lewis Fund.

Yale University Press books may be purchased in quantity for educational,
business, or promotional use. For information, please e-mail sales.press@yale.edu
(U.S. office) or sales@yaleup.co.uk (U.K. office).

Set in Fournier MT Regular type by Westchester Book Group.
Printed in the United States of America.

Library of Congress Control Number: 2015931442
ISBN: 978-0-300-20070-6 (cloth : alk. paper)

A catalogue record for this book is available from the British Library.

This paper meets the requirements of ANSI/NISO Z39.48-1992
(Permanence of Paper).

10 9 8 7 6 5 4 3 2 1

Contents

Acknowledgments   vii

Introduction   1

1. Curing and Caring for the
   Early Modern Body   16

2. Learning How to Be Ill   46

3. Emotional Causes of Illness   81

4. Suffering on the Sickbed   104

5. Perceptions of Pain   129

6. Illness Narratives by the Poor   159

Conclusions   180

List of Abbreviations   187

Appendixes   189

Notes   203

Bibliography   243

Index   273

Acknowledgments

A few words here cannot fully express my immense gratitude to Mary Fissell, who has supported this project in so many ways. I first spoke to Mary on the phone as an undergraduate student, and in the fourteen years since that phone call she has transformed my thinking and writing. I am deeply indebted to Mary for her attentive, critical reading of my work, for her good humor and sage advice, and for her unflagging encouragement. A student could not ask for a more generous mentor. Several others at Johns Hopkins University have given feedback and guidance that have deeply informed this book and my growth as a historian. I am incredibly grateful to John Marshall for all that he has taught me about early modern England and for his enthusiastic support over the years. Gianna Pomata and Toby Ditz read every chapter of this book long before it was a book, and their advice has been invaluable. This project has also greatly benefited from perceptive feedback by Randy Packard, whose mentorship means so much to me. Harry Marks was one of my chief advocates at Hopkins, as well as one of my toughest critics. I miss him, and I can only imagine how he would have helped me make this book stronger.

I first learned the joys of history long before graduate school. Judy Pittenger instilled in me a passion for studying the past, and she modeled how to do so with inquisitiveness and zeal. While I was an undergraduate student at Wesleyan University, Richard Buel, Stewart Gillmor, Gary Shaw, Suzy Taraba, and Jennifer Tucker taught me the thrill of archival research. Under their guidance, I made my first trip to the archives and discovered the history of medicine. A number of additional mentors, colleagues, and friends have helped with this project over the years in a range of ways. Versions of individual chapters benefited from insightful comments by Chris Close,

Sana Haroon, Ben Johnson, Lauren Kassell, Laura Knoppers, and Seth LeJacq. David Hunt read numerous chapters of the manuscript, and his thoughtful observations helped direct my revisions. Lynn Botelho and Craig Horner generously shared transcriptions of primary sources with me, and Laura Gowing pointed me toward sources at the British Library and the London Metropolitan Archives, a few of which became central to the project. I owe thanks to many more who have shared wisdom, feedback, a shoulder to lean on, or tips about sources, or have supported my work in other ways: Wendy Belcher, Sandra Eder, Marta Hanson, Amanda Herbert, Abby Markoe, Liza McCahill, Ruth Miller, Margaret Pelling, Massimo Petrozzi, Christine Ruggere, Jimmy Schafer, Dan Todes, Amanda Irwin Wilkins, and Mara Willard. I am especially grateful to my writing partner, Rachel Galvin, who continually inspires me to keep writing, even if I can only manage a few minutes a day. Tova Goodman graciously made the map in chapter 6 and offered helpful edits on the introduction. I also thank the two anonymous reviewers for their incredibly useful feedback, Juliana Froggatt for her careful copy edits, as well as Chris Rogers, Christina Tucker, Ann-Marie Imbornoni, and Erica Hanson at Yale University Press. Many thanks also to my colleagues at the University of Massachusetts Boston for creating such a warm and collegial work environment as I completed the book.

I am indebted to participants at a number of institutions where I gave talks or presented material from this project. While I cannot thank everyone individually, I would like to acknowledge the illuminating questions and advice I received at the University of Oxford, Swarthmore College, the University of Minnesota, Wesleyan University, the Princeton Writing Program works-in-progress seminar, the Johns Hopkins University gender history seminar, and the "Vernacular Health and Healing" and "Forms of Religious Experience in the Atlantic World" colloquia at the Folger Shakespeare Library in Washington DC. I was able to travel to England to undertake preliminary research thanks to a generous Mellon Fellowship from the Institute of Historical Research. I returned for longer stints with support from a Bernadotte E. Schmitt Grant from the American Historical Association, the Theodora Bosanquet Bursary, a Sheldon Hanft Travel Award from the Southern Council on British Studies, and a research grant from the Program for the Study of Women, Gender, and Sexuality at Johns Hopkins University. The Princeton University Tuck Fund enabled me to return to England to conduct research on paupers in provincial record offices, and the

Huntington Library provided a beautiful and intellectually stimulating environment for subsequent research and writing. I am deeply appreciative of the curators, librarians, and staff at all of the archives I consulted, most especially those at the British Library, Folger Library, and Huntington Library. Portions of chapter 3 are reprinted from my article "Grieved and Disordered: Gender and Emotion in Early Modern Patient Narratives" in the *Journal of Medieval and Early Modern Studies* by kind permission of Duke University Press.

Finally, a hearty thanks to my family and to my dearest friends, who have cheered successes and softened letdowns—most especially Rehanna Chaudhri, who has hosted me on countless trips to the United Kingdom. I hold the warmest appreciation for Christopher Willard, for his patience, encouragement, thorough edits, and cooking. After a long day immersed in the past, there is no one I would rather have welcome me back to the present.

Introduction

On her wedding day in 1651, Alice Thornton fell suddenly, dreadfully ill. Violent pains in her head and stomach caused vomiting and what Thornton called "sicknesse at my heart" for eight continuous hours. She did not know the source of the trouble, though she suspected it had developed from cold feet in a very literal sense: "I might have brought itt upon me by cold taken the night before, when I satt up late in preparing for the next day, and washing my feete at that time of the yeare." In seventeenth-century England, individuals were believed to possess a unique balance of internal bodily fluids, or humors. A variety of external forces—from sudden changes in weather to extreme emotions, diet, sleep, exercise, and even cold water in a washbasin— could alter the movement and emission of humors and cause ill health. According to this theory, Thornton's sudden exposure to cold water created an internal obstruction or corruption of humors, resulting in illness on the day of her wedding.[1]

Thornton recorded the episode as a divine portent, or what she called "a sad omen to my future comfort." She searched regularly for divine messages in life events—both trivial day-to-day accidents and significant occurrences like sudden sickness on her wedding day. She was particularly anxious about marriage, a fear encapsulated in her description of "sicknesse at my heart." Marriage signified full female adulthood in this period and marked a crucial turning point at which women relinquished legal and civic identity to their husbands. What is more, Thornton professed not to love her husband. She had only agreed to marry him out of duty to her family, as he would be able to restore the family's perilous financial status. Thornton explained that she entered marriage with "feare and caution," forgoing her own happiness to make herself "a more publick instrument of good to those severall relations." Attributing her illness to cold enabled her to present herself as a paragon of female virtue. She modeled obedience toward her family and acceptance of her new situation even as her words revealed glimpses of fear and doubt.[2]

Like Thornton, most men and women in early modern England viewed their bodies according to an overarching humoral framework. Yet an underlying logic accounting for patients' explanations of sickness is often elusive. Why did the famous diarist Samuel Pepys associate his good health with a lucky hare's foot but link his eye problems six months later to a lack of sleep and "strange" beer?[3] Patients' perceptions in this period were informed by a broad range of factors beyond the humors, including particular circumstances, such as an imminent marriage, but also prior ailments, age, spiritual beliefs, and geographical locations. This book analyzes these multiple influences by recovering illness from the perspectives of patients like Pepys and Thornton. Such stories of sickness matter because patients played important roles in defining medical care in the early modern period. Prior to the end of the eighteenth century, patients shared an understanding of medicine and the body with practitioners and maintained an advantage as consumers in a competitive medical marketplace. Ordinary sufferers further wielded authority because their accounts of illness and decisions to withhold or divulge personal information could determine healers' diagnoses and treatments. In short, the voices and choices of ordinary patients were integral to structuring medical practice.[4] Yet we know few details of those words and actions—the actual expressions, beliefs, and behaviors that were so crucial to this patient-driven system of medical care. *Ill Composed* recovers that history and, in doing so, reveals how the multiple influences shaping patients' perceptions were mediated by a significant, often overlooked factor: gender.

Illness, then as now, is not only a sequence of biological processes but also a complex social event defined by prevailing norms and behaviors. Writing in the 1950s, Talcott Parsons was one of the first scholars to view illness in these terms—as a learned and patterned cultural exchange. More recently, medical anthropologists and sociologists have analyzed the impact of gender on this exchange and the complex dynamics between patients and practitioners.[5] As men and women, we unknowingly adhere to culturally defined roles, norms, and ideals that are propagated by our society and performed on the body. Gender implicitly shapes the ways we comport ourselves and communicate with others, as well as the ways we perceive corporeal experiences such as sickness and wellness. *Ill Composed* examines the historical significance of these insights. A close examination of a collection of voices from the seventeenth century uncovers the building blocks patients relied upon to make sense of illness and how men and women arranged those building blocks differently.

This book argues that, despite key overlaps, seventeenth-century English men and women perceived illness in gendered ways. Women commonly looked to others as models of suffering and attributed their own illness and recovery to negative or positive affective relations: the ailing health of a loved one could cause illness, while the compassion and pity of a visitor aided recovery. Men tended to privilege their own bodily experiences over the words and opinions of others. While these men recognized that social interactions could affect health, they commonly articulated this process within the context of occupational and financial concerns. Each chapter offers evidence of this pattern from a different perspective: from the stories patients told to conceptualize illness through their explanations of illness onset to their articulations of suffering, time, and pain. Of course, individual patients told more complicated stories. Sufferers from varying backgrounds or those who documented their experiences in particular genres of writing might express diverging concerns or possess varying priorities. The distinctions outlined here fall along a spectrum of difference rather than any strict male-female binary. That is, as opposed to indicating essentially different views of illness, writing by seventeenth-century patients reveals varying emphases. The central aim of this book is to locate and explain those accentuations in order to make sense of men's and women's perceptions relative to one another.[6] The middle areas within this spectrum are just as telling as the extremes, reflecting where gender mattered and where it did not.

Patients' perceptions were shaped by gender, but not gender alone. A host of beliefs, expectations, and experiences influenced sufferers' thoughts and actions, including medical knowledge, personal relationships, spirituality, daily work, and writing practices. Thornton's account of sickness on her wedding day illustrates a few of these influences. She linked her illness to anxiety surrounding a gendered life event, but she also believed that her disorder resulted from a physical cause (washing her feet with cold water), as well as a spiritual one (God's punishment). Thornton demonstrates how a patient in this period could draw on coexisting humoral, emotional, and religious explanations of illness, and how a nexus of concerns could determine resulting interpretations of the body. The following chapters analyze the range of beliefs and behaviors that intersected with gender to inform patients' views, particularly writing practices, religious beliefs, and economic status.

By the phrase *writing practices*, I refer to the norms and objectives that structured various forms of writing in early modern England. The daily, terse entries of an account book, the introspective meditations in a spiritual journal, and the clinical observations of a medical case each reflect a particular set of concerns and customs. This book examines how the conventions and intentions of texts determined the kinds of stories recorded in those texts. Illness was performed on the sickbed, and it was also performed in writing. Alice Thornton, for instance, composed her narrative retrospectively, in part to defend her reputation against nasty rumors. Her resulting account is organized around significant episodes and events rather than the details of daily life. Thornton's particular goals as an autobiographer dictated what she included and how she chose to present herself. The following chapters show how, in some instances, patterns that seem to break down along gendered lines reflect, in part, the nature of the sources themselves. While writing practices could be crucial to shaping articulations of illness, they can by no means explain all of the patterns outlined in this book. In many instances, men and women employed overlapping genres and conventions but revealed diverging perceptions of similar bodily processes. And writing practices themselves could be shaped by gendered ways of knowing and thinking. Jane Shakerley responded to news of her son's illness in 1701 by claiming to suffer in tandem with him: "Your illness Gaue me as Grett a torment as you paine."[7] Such assertions of sympathetic suffering were a common approach to conveying compassion in correspondence. Yet, as chapter 3 discusses, the trope resurfaces in the self-writing of a significant number of women, informing their explanations of disease causation in much more evident ways than was the case for men.

While patients' accounts reveal certain material realities about the past, we can never fully comprehend what it was like to be sick in the 1600s. Historical sources provide only linguistic renderings of what it was like to be sick. Following Joan Scott, I do not approach firsthand accounts as clear reflections of experience but instead analyze the role of writing in constructing that experience.[8] In other words, self-writing is perhaps most valuable for reveal-ing how gender operated in individuals' written constructions of their lives. After all, the nuanced ways patients chose to articulate their experiences on the page—the metaphors they employed and the scripts they appropriated—expose the impact of gender on bodily perceptions most clearly. Viewing writ-ing as a process of self-actualization and self-constitution rather than as a transparent window onto lived experience enables us to see gender more fully.

Like writing, religious beliefs deeply influenced patients' expressions of suffering. Religion offered early modern men and women a shared reper-toire for making sense of the body, suffering, and the world. Spiritual mod-els such as Christ on the cross and martyrs at the stake taught believers how to understand and respond to pain piously. Spiritual beliefs could also structure private writing, which was central to the Protestant goal of self-examination. Like the Catholic confession, personal writing provided a means of monitoring spiritual health and enforcing self-discipline.[9] Some of the discussions in the following chapters concentrate solely on religion in order to capture the complex influences of devotional texts, practices, and beliefs on the bodily perceptions of men and women alike. Other discussions, such as that of pain in chapter 5, explore how concerns about spirituality over-lapped with gendered scripts to form the patterns in patients' writing.

My approach to recovering the intersections between spirituality and illness addresses two imbalances in the history of early modern religion and medicine. First, our image of patients in seventeenth-century England has been skewed by the disproportionate number of extant diaries written by the zealous Protestants known as Puritans. "Puritan" remains a vexed category, but this kind of writing is generally associated with self-examination, self-discipline, and the documentation of divine providence in the most trivial de-tails of daily life. For instance, an apprentice was convinced that a woman named Mary Naylor was his destined wife upon finding an N and half of an M divinely formed in the wrinkles of his breeches. Others recorded the mi-nutiae of their bodily processes, as the body housed the soul and was thought to display important signs from heaven. These believers documented each sniffle and sneeze as evidence of God's mercy—a "morbid self-absorption," according to the historian Alexandra Walsham, but a treasure trove for his-torians of the patient.[10] This emphasis on writing, self-scrutiny, and bodily maintenance certainly influenced how fervent Protestants understood and wrote about health, and their resulting accounts inform much of what we know about patients in the early modern period.[11] Yet many men and women did not hold these beliefs and so perhaps understood illness in other ways. This book offers a more balanced view by examining writing by patients who held a range of beliefs, including Anglicans, Quakers, and Catholics.

Rather than delineate doctrinal differences among these denominations and confessional affiliations, *Ill Composed* analyzes religion as it was lived and embodied. This approach redresses a second imbalance in our understanding of religion and medicine. Because historians have relied so heavily on fervent Protestants' writing, they have tended to focus on providential theology—the conviction that God sent ill health to convey some sort of message.[12] Providence offered a principal framework for making sense of natural phenomena, most especially illness, yet religion also influenced patients' perceptions in other significant ways. Piety was enacted and displayed on the body. Men and women expressed their anxiety about salvation and felt the reception of God's grace as physical sensations. And embodied spiritual practices could be integral to the ways devout men and women understood and responded to ill health. For instance, comportment in church and daily devotional exercises such as praying and meditating were corporeal practices that taught believers how to view shifting physical sensations in spiritual terms. Examining the lived experience of religion opens up a fuller view of how beliefs influenced bodily perceptions.[13]

Finally, economic status is a key factor that ordered early modern bodily concerns. The men we meet in the following pages worked in a range of fields—from merchants and ministers to shopkeepers, apothecaries, and book traders. Their varying occupational responsibilities, educational backgrounds, and aspirations could color their perceptions of infirmity and determine the modes they used to record those perceptions. Although most of the women in this book represented the upper strata of society, we have two rare, firsthand accounts by middling-status women. Katherine Austen was the daughter of a cloth trader, and Lydia Dugard came from a family of teachers and printers. Mostly middling- and upper-status individuals compiled the diaries and letters that have survived from the period.[14] Only a small percentage of the population in the seventeenth century was literate, and only a portion of that group felt moved to document their lives. To capture the voices of the poor, chapter 6 examines terse legal documents compiled by clerks on behalf of impoverished men and women seeking financial support. These petitions provide valuable, if indirect, accounts of debility by the very poorest, often illiterate members of English society. Economic circumstances compelled these petitioners to construct stories of sickness in different terms than those of their wealthier counterparts, by highlighting nonhumoral sources of illness and defining resulting disorders in terms of incapacity and industry. Such distinctions demonstrate how concerns about suffering could be refracted through a broad range of priorities and anxieties, including not only piety and gender but also economic security, duty, and community.

This study covers 1630 to 1730, a time span that stops short of the mid-eighteenth century, when a new framework for explaining illness began to take shape. According to this emerging vision of the body, ill health resulted from irritable or slackened nerves rather than obstructed or imbalanced humors. To limit the scope of the project, *Ill Composed* ends before this conceptual shift. Yet the seventeenth century too was a time of considerable change. In England, civil war, regicide, and growing secularization marked the century. Expanding trade across the British empire led to an influx of foreign products, some of which became important remedies and medicinal ingredients. Competing medical theories challenged traditional understandings of the body and how to treat it. These movements advocated for medicines made from metals and minerals rather than plants and herbs and looked to practical training and firsthand observations to define a treatment's efficacy rather than blindly trusting ancient authority.[15] Despite such profound transformations, this book tells a story of continuities. Religious beliefs and practices continued to inform the ways early modern men and women made sense of their bodies. And patients' explanations of bodily processes, such as the physiological effects of emotions, or the nature of pain remained fairly static throughout the period. The words of ordinary men and women reveal the enduring power of particular models and scripts for thinking and writing about the body over the course of the 1600s.[16]

Ill Composed opens with an introduction to the early modern body from the perspective of patients, as well as the medical remedies available to sufferers within a diverse and vibrant marketplace of healers. This initial chapter focuses on interactions between patients and their practitioners to assess the extent to which gendered beliefs and behaviors structured medical encounters. Subsequent chapters loosely trace the progression of illness from the patient's point of view—from the models that individuals relied upon to diagnose and gauge the severity of their ailments to explanations of the causes of illness, expressions of pity, and responses to pain and recovery. The final chapter uses petitions by the sick poor to examine the impact of economic status on narratives of illness. Rather than analyze sex-specific diseases, the book concentrates on ailments that afflicted men and women alike. This approach allows for the development of a rich comparative framework that does not stress bodily explanations of one sex over those of the other. This is not to say sex is insignificant. In fact, sex-specific physiology could be crucial to patients' views of bodily processes. Some women were almost continually pregnant or recovering from pregnancy-related health issues, making it difficult to distinguish reproductive disorders from nonreproductive ones. Yet few of the sufferers here associated day-to-day infirmities with their generative functions. And even fewer female authors compared the physical anguish of illness to the pain of giving birth, perhaps because they viewed childbirth to be as much a social event as a medical one.[17]

This exploration of gendered perceptions of illness contributes to three broad fields of study: the history of the patient, women's and gender history, and scholarship on constructions of the self. Until the 1970s, we knew relatively little about what it was like to be a patient in the past. Scholars then began criticizing older histories of medicine that extolled the progress of science and promoted the innovations of doctors. These scholars were concerned with the patient's role in the development of modern medicine, specifically the shifting nature of the patient-healer relationship and the decline of patient authority by the nineteenth century.[18] Subsequent work by Roy Porter, Dorothy Porter, Lucinda Beier, and others attempted to recover patients' experiences preceding this loss of authority.[19] *Ill Composed* builds on this pioneering scholarship in a number of ways. Rather than examining medical encounters to show that patients wielded power, I examine patients' views and voices to recover the defining features of that power—the actual utterances that structured the patient-driven system of early modern medical care. My analysis centers on firsthand accounts recorded in more than forty diaries and over fifty collections of correspondence, a significantly larger source base than those of previous studies. This substantial collection of voices deepens our understanding of early modern illness, which until now has developed largely from studies based on a single or a small handful of patients. Bringing gender into the picture is perhaps the most significant departure from previous scholarship, which has largely overlooked or underemphasized it.[20] Barbara

Duden's work on the patients of an eighteenth-century German physician, for example, has been pivotal in establishing "the body" as a historical subject. But Duden focused solely on female patients, and as a result she was less attentive to gender differences and the ways gender informed the patient-healer interactions at the center of her rich and important book. A few historians have even argued that gender had no impact on early modern experiences of illness.[21] By examining disorders that afflicted men and women alike, this book illuminates the significant ways that gender shaped patients' perceptions and, by extension, how ordinary individuals managed health and navigated life more broadly.

Just as scholarship on early modern illness has underemphasized gender, women's and gender historians have overlooked the ailing body as a site for capturing lived gendered experiences. Much of what we know about early modern gender has developed out of a close scrutiny of embodied experiences, such as touch, violence, aging, and sex.[22] This book shows that gender, as it was performed and experienced, was also evident in physical breakdown. Infirmity compelled men and women to write about their bodies and to express a host of gendered concerns about comportment, relationships, and occupational responsibility. Laura Gowing and Mary Fissell have uncovered the complex influences of early modern culture on experiences and conceptions of the body. These valuable studies demonstrate how women's bodies provided sites for negotiating relationships and for thinking through anxieties about social, religious, and political shifts.[23] Illness offers a novel approach to exploring this relationship between culture and embodiment, a lens that brings into focus how prevailing norms and beliefs were lived on the body and reflected in varied impressions of illness. I situate patients' accounts not in prescriptive literature on gender but in the texture of early modern English life. This approach requires entering the homes of early modern men and women, in order to show how individuals constructed narratives of illness within the context of their other ways of writing and thinking.

The female authors in this book offer glimpses of how the sick body provided a rich site for self-expression, a rare venue in which women could vent their grievances and express their desires within an otherwise limiting patriarchal society. Seventeenth-century women were taught to be modest, meek, and submissive. Men, in turn, were expected to govern both their households and their wives' behavior. The model early modern man was the breadwinner in his family and exhibited strength, economic independence, and self-discipline. Overlapping feminine and masculine virtues, such as piety and chastity, were understood in ways that perpetuated these gender ideals. For example, it was commonly believed that women not only should aspire toward a pious life but were naturally suited to one. Richard Allestree, the author of popular conduct books from the period, wrote that women "have som[e]what more of a predisposition towards it in their native temper." In a seeming contradiction to this view, popular and prescriptive literature also depicted women as naturally lustful and sexual purity as tightly bound to feminine virtue. The ideal man was chaste too, but adultery did not damage a man's reputation in the same way it did for women. A man's sexual misdeeds were commonly blamed on the woman involved and were most troubling for their negative effects on her character, "robbing her of her innocency."[24]

Medical texts naturalized these ideologies in the body. One medical author argued that women were intellectually inferior to men, in part because women lacked sufficient restraint and reason. According to this author, women were servants to their passions: "That Females are more wanton and petulant then Males, wee thinke hapneth because of the impotencie of their minds; for the imaginations of lustfull women are like the imaginations of bruite beastes which have no repugnancie or contradiction of reason to restraine them." This alleged impulsiveness and intellectual incapacity was rooted in humoral physiology. Women were believed to be naturally colder and moister than men, a composition that accounted for their fleshy bodies, reproductive capabilities, and seemingly never-ending emission of fluids through processes like lactation and menstruation. But such delicate, porous bodies also made women naturally vulnerable to passion and to the powers of the imagination—"a pliableness to conviction," as Allestree put it. Reason, rather than emotion, was presumed to rule the bodies of early modern men. Medical theory of the time viewed men's warm, dry bodies as firmer, stronger, and more efficient than those of their female counterparts.[25]

These characterizations of men and women had a powerful grip on early modern mentalities but were far from reflecting reality. Many women were outspoken and sharp-witted rather than silent and meek, and manipulated established norms to suit their needs. Single women and widows who were freed from the governance of husbands or fathers were able to exercise authority and independence rather than submission and obedience. Some of these women owned property and headed their own businesses. And while married women were subordinate to their husbands, they wielded considerable authority over younger, single women, whose bodies and behaviors they policed.[26] Chapter 4 explores how suffering on the sickbed gave some women a valuable opportunity to assert agency by voicing disappointments with loved ones. These women viewed the neglect of friends and family as physically harmful to health, and they expressed disapproval in ways that highlighted their own honorable comportment.

Likewise, not all men met the patriarchal ideal of the self-sufficient householder. The final chapter of this book looks at stories of sickness by paupers who were incapable of expressing manhood in terms of economic autonomy. These men instead established their masculinity in other ways— by their thrift, prudence, and industry. Notions of ideal manhood varied not only by economic status but also by age. Alexandra Shepard has shown how old age could challenge manly markers of autonomy and self-mastery, while younger men might invert normative notions of masculinity by engaging in rituals of disorder, such as rioting, drinking, and gambling.[27] The London bachelor Dudley Ryder was concerned not so much about financial autonomy as about controlling his own unruly body. He self-consciously stood back when speaking to women, out of fear they might smell his bad breath. He continually consumed cream of tartar and spa water to try to remedy the problem. The men in this book cover a range of ages and social ranks, while the majority of the women were married or widowed members of the gentry or aristocracy who documented their lives for spiritual purposes. As a result, these women presented themselves in fairly similar terms, while notions of masculinity could be more varied.[28]

In illuminating gendered beliefs and behaviors, narratives of illness reveal how individuals understood and created a sense of self. As such, this book joins a body of literature that has investigated early modern constructions of identity in self-writing. A Hertfordshire gentlewoman writing in the early 1700s neatly summarized this process of finding and expressing herself through the act of writing: "I instruct my self by what I write and understand my self better by exercising the Notion I haue formed than I coud by priuate thoughts and internal Reflexion."[29] Illness captured such self-constructions because it elicited intense anxiety and reflection among seventeenth-century men and women. Sickness was a common feature of early modern life, one that nearly everyone faced. Yet ill health loomed large in the minds of men and women not only because so many continually battled against it but also because of associations between illness and sin. Health signified moral as well as physical fitness. A healthy body required a moderate lifestyle, wholesome habits, and self-discipline. But more important, a healthy body was believed to correspond to a healthy soul. Sickness, on the other hand, could be interpreted as a divine punishment for sin, a test of piety, or a marker along the path toward heaven. Illness brought men and women face-to-face with their own mortality, sparking a host of fears and anxieties about virtue, salvation, and proper social etiquette, as well as relationships with relatives, neighbors, friends, religious authorities, and parish administrators. As a result, ailing men and women were particularly attentive to how they presented themselves on the sickbed, as well as on the page. Responding to bodily disorders with patience rather than resistance manifested submission to God's will. Suffering "well" demonstrated a patient's respectability and also the final outcome of that patient's spiritual journey. The ailing body offers intimate glimpses of how men and women saw themselves and hoped to be seen by others.

This book draws on a range of sources to recover the words and views of seventeenth-century sufferers, including diaries, letters, account books, medical literature, healers' case notes, petitions, and devotional literature. Some of these texts, such as cases written by healers, offer indirect access to patients. Most enlightening are the stories of sickness compiled by patients themselves in more than fifty caches of correspondence and more than forty diaries. From this collection of voices, the narratives of fifty-two individuals—thirty men and twenty-two women—lie at the center of the analysis.[30] These are all of the individuals I could find from the period and region who kept firsthand accounts that include detailed discussions of health. They lived throughout England, in places ranging from urban centers like London and Manchester to country estates and villages. Some compiled their narratives while young; others wrote later in life. Sarah Cowper began documenting her days at the age of fifty-six, preserving the plights of her increasingly frail body. These men and women also embraced varying political affiliations. Brilliana Harley wrote hundreds of letters to her husband and her son that offer detailed accounts of the family's support of the Parliamentarians during the civil war. Others remained loyal to the Crown. While the narratives here are vast in number and vivid in content, they are also skewed. Firsthand accounts represent a literate minority, and certain biases emerge as a result. For example, there is a marked lack of references to witchcraft, which was a popular belief and prevalent fear in the period.

I have been referring to firsthand accounts as *diaries*, a term that can be misleading. The self-writing in this book includes a range of genres that varied in aims and conventions. The term *ego-literature* refers to the broad umbrella of self-writing that encompasses diaries, as well as spiritual journals, account books, memoirs, autobiographies, and so on.[31] Few sources fit neatly into these categories. Some authors wrote what appear to be daily diaries but focused entirely on spiritual matters. Others compiled personal experiences alongside excerpts from books, sermons, poems, or recipes—a genre of writing known as the commonplace book. A wigmaker named Edmund Harrold recorded devotional lessons and tabulated financial records together, creating a hybrid form of writing. And Alice Thornton composed her life narrative retrospectively in three different notebooks, but it was nineteenth-century editors who combined and reorganized them into a single chronological narrative. The resulting text, while valuable, provides a problematic amalgamation of Thornton's original writings.[32]

Even authors who seemed to document their lives day to day might rely on complicated recording techniques. A Catholic landowner jotted down on scraps of paper information that he later copied into his "Great Diurnal," sometimes editing it or adding new information along the way. Samuel Pepys, whose intimate, detailed entries seem closest to our modern conception of a diary, would at times compile several days' or even weeks' worth of entries in a single sitting.[33] The resulting writing does not offer immediate representations of daily life. Rather, we are faced with the challenge of navigating the unidentifiable gap between lived experience and the documentation of that experience. This book shows how gender mediated that gap, informing the ways seventeenth-century men and women perceived themselves and articulated their lives on the page.

The term *diary* is further misleading because it connotes a particular type of private, introspective writing. However, most early modern authors compiled their life stories for public or semipublic consumption.[34] Thornton circulated her narrative among friends and family, for example. Some authors were explicit about their readers, even naming them in their prose. Others kept spiritual journals for their own eyes only or wrote directly to God. Still, writing for a particular audience did not necessarily produce stilted, impersonal accounts. Sarah Cowper left behind copious pages of introspective writing, knowing that her husband would likely read every word after her death. Such readerships demonstrate the important ways that genre, authorial motivation, and audience could shape ego-literature.

Personal correspondence was no more private than journals and diaries. Authors addressed particular correspondents, but letters were rarely only two-way forms of communication. Many letters in early modern England were read and written collaboratively. Authors dictated letters to others, asked friends to revise their words, and even composed letters from drafts and notes. Illness certainly provided a common occasion for using an amanuensis. "I was so ill that I was faine to make use of another," one correspondent wrote in 1659. Likewise, requests to "pray burne this" reflect the widely held presumption that letters were semipublic documents. Both intended and unintended readers influenced the ways authors presented themselves in correspondence, compelling them to both create an inner sense of self and assert an outer presentation to others—processes that could be shaped by gendered anxieties, relationships, and occupational identities.[35]

Because particular conventions structured early modern letters, these sources offer a clear view of the dynamic relationship between written form and content. There were specific rules, addresses, and rhetorical styles for letters of varying functions, as well as for authors of diverging status, gender, and age. For example, a postscript in correspondence to a superior was considered offensive, having "the Appearance of your having almost forgot them"; however, a postscript in a love letter demonstrated the author's reluctance to say good-bye.[36] These conventions influenced correspondents' articulations of health. Many authors began or ended letters with a line or two about their bodily state or with expressions of gratitude to correspondents for inquiring after their well-being. Letter writers also commonly cited illness as an excuse for delays in writing or justification for failing to fulfill social responsibilities. While the conventions of correspondence could certainly limit authors' prose, they also enabled letters to do certain cultural work. As the historian Steven Stowe suggests, some life events only developed their fullest meaning when expressed in letters.[37]

We share a physical body with seventeenth-century men and women, yet our experiences and explanations of illness today are remarkably different. Despite its materiality, the body is a product of its cultural and historical moment. Prevailing medical frameworks, belief systems, economic conditions, and gender norms dictate the ways we interpret and even physically feel our bodies. We can better view how something as seemingly absolute as the body can be perceived so differently over time by examining a period wholly unlike ours—an era when clogged humors were believed to cause sickness and the joy of seeing a loved one walk through the door was thought to cure it. *Ill Composed* bridges this history of illness with the history of gender. It shows how ordinary patients saw and felt their bodies in the 1600s, and how those views and sensations offer a new perspective on what it meant to be a man or a woman. In early modern England, gender was propagated not only in prescriptive texts, and religion was not confined to doctrinal belief. Both religion and gender were lived on the body, shaping the ways individuals viewed health and illness and also navigated their communities, engaged in work, interacted with loved ones, and, perhaps most important for historians, documented their lives.

The phrase *ill composed* in the title of this book refers to both the physical state of sickness and the act of writing about it. Only through patients' words—the ways individuals composed suffering on the page—can we access past perceptions of the body. The experimenter Robert Hooke endured a "laziness and stiffness" in his limbs in 1677, a formulation of pain that, to us, sounds rather contradictory. James Clegg noted that his wife suffered from a "painful phlegm on her shoulder," and a man named William Handerwick characterized an ache in his head as "a sensation like an approaching swoon."[38] What did these complaints possibly feel like? Was a phlegmy shoulder tight and cramped? Was a swoonlike pain warm and fleeting? We can never know what it felt like to inhabit a seventeenth-century body but are left to decipher patients' constructions of internal, at times inexpressible, physical sensations.

1. Curing and Caring for the Early Modern Body

Before he became a widely published medical author, William Salmon made his start as an assistant to a mountebank. Mountebanks were itinerant healers who lacked formal medical education and who marketed remedies based on their alleged empirical success rather than underlying medical theories. From this inauspicious beginning, Salmon gained popularity and began promoting his own particular brand of medicine, which combined traditional treatments made of plants and herbs with those composed of salts and minerals. In one of his many publications, Salmon recounted meeting a thirty-three-year-old man who had been suffering from dropsy for more than eight months. *Dropsy* was the name for an accumulation of fluid in the body's cavities that caused massive swelling. This patient was afflicted mostly in his stomach. The failed treatments of previous healers over the course of many months had worsened his condition. Even Salmon's newfangled remedies were of little use in this case. After meeting the man and listening to his story, Salmon concluded that "nothing but Death could put a period to his Grief."[1]

In relating this episode in a compendium of cases, Salmon struggled with language. The man's stomach was "so big that the relation of it would be accounted Romantick." Salmon believed that if he provided an accurate appraisal of the man's girth, readers would suspect him of exaggerating. Even the patient himself refused to believe Salmon's assessment. Rather than accepting a prognosis of death and walking away, the patient insisted that Salmon treat him. He "little regarded my words," the healer wrote, "nor was dismayed, but desired me to undertake him, and do my best." Salmon ended up prescribing his "volatile laudanum" pills, made of opium, camphor, snake root, cloves, saffron, and other ingredients that were meant to ease pain and induce rest. He explained that he prescribed the pills to please the patient and to make his final days more comfortable. Yet to Salmon's surprise, the pills achieved these aims and more. The patient reported improved health, and he continued to assert his authority by demanding even more pills at a larger dosage. When he had consumed these too, he demanded still more and took it upon himself to increase the dose again without consulting Salmon. In the end, the man "was made perfectly well," contrary to Salmon's expectations.[2]

This "dropsical" patient ignored his practitioner again and again, insisting on treatment, altering his dosage, and demanding more pills when his supply ran low. These were not the only ways that patients exercised power in the seventeenth century. Patients could assert authority by providing or denying key information about their cases, such as a significant life event or an account of internal sensations. Patients also possessed the upper hand as shoppers in a crowded market of healers. Another of Salmon's patients had the luxury of taking her time, listening to "the opinions of many men," before settling on her healer of choice.[3] This power of the purse compelled some practitioners to alter their treatments to suit patients' demands for popular or gentler remedies. Suffering from a violent fever, Joseph Lister was frustrated with his physician's insistence on prescribing "easy cordial things." The fever developed following a frightening episode as Lister rode home one evening from the town of Hartlepool. A merchant he was meeting ran late, and it was dark by the time Lister mounted his horse to head home. In his haste and the dimming light, he decided to wade his horse across a small inlet of water. By the time he was fifteen yards from shore, he realized he had drastically miscalculated the depth. Streams of water ran over his saddle, and his boots and pockets quickly filled. He eventually made it safely to shore but was so sick when he awoke the next morning that he was unable to get out of bed. He lost his appetite and developed a high fever. After weeks of lying "in great extremity," he grew dissatisfied with his doctor's prescriptions. Cordials were sweet beverages made of syrup or liquor taken to stimulate and revive the body. Lister wanted something stronger. The physician disagreed, and so Lister paid his bill and sought out another healer twelve miles down the road.[4] Lister's resolve exposes the stubbornness, and perhaps even ignorance, of his physician. But the perseverance of Salmon's dropsical patient highlights Salmon's expertise. The determination of the patient, after all, conveyed the extremity of the case and therefore the wondrous effects of the laudanum pills. Salmon's remedy brought a dying man back to life.

How did gender shape the dynamics between these patients and their doctors? Would a female patient have contradicted her practitioner and demanded treatment, as did Salmon's dropsical patient? Gender surely influenced the negotiations at the center of Salmon's case, but it left few traces. This is not to say we know nothing about the intersections of gender and health care in this period. Historians have recovered how anxieties about masculinity were embedded in physicians' concerns about their own professional status, and how some female patients were limited more than men when negotiating disputes with male physicians. Conversely, Kevin Siena has shown how female venereal patients were not as restricted as we might think, as their preference for female healers structured the contours of the medical market.[5] Yet few historians have explored the impact of gender on patient-healer interactions.[6] After all, writing by early modern healers offers limited access to the nuances of patients' verbal expressions. In rare cases, practitioners did appropriate patients' words. Characterizing one man's ailing legs, the surgeon William Beckett wrote, "(To use his own Expression) it was hardly possible to keep Life in them."[7] Such instances are exceptional, however, and the voices of patients are mediated through the pens of practitioners. While seventeenth-century medical writing provides abundant information about diagnoses, symptoms, and cures, it offers few insights into the social practices of treatment. As a result, we know little about the gender dynamics of the seventeenth-century sickroom—how patients' and healers' gendered concerns, roles, and bodily perceptions informed their communications with one another.

This chapter opens with an overview of health and healing in early modern England from the patient's view. After examining patients' explanations of disease causation and approaches to treatment, it moves from the patient's perspective to that of healers in an exploration of medical encounters. Using more than forty medical texts, the discussion eases open the door to the sickroom to recover the exchanges between patients and practitioners and the extent to which gender shaped those interactions. I suggest two ways we might begin to recover this information. First, a close study of healers' intentions and writing practices reveals how patients' words could be critical to defining treatment yet concealed and distorted by healers' own concerns about authority. Take the case of a lawyer's son who hired Hugh Ryder to treat painful fistulas in his leg. The man knew his case was serious and that the only possible cure was amputation. But after inspecting the leg and speaking with the patient, Ryder decided that nothing could be done. The young man was indignant. He refused to accept Ryder's interpretation and instead asserted his own contradictory assessment. As Ryder explained it, "He knew he should be well, if I would cut off his Thigh; and that if I would lend him a Knife, he would cut it off himself." The patient volunteered to perform his own operation to prove the point and to demonstrate his desperation. But rather than present this case as an overt display of patient power, Ryder interpreted the patient's aggressive response as proof of Ryder's own superior surgical ability. The patient's demands displayed an "undaunted confidence in me," Ryder wrote. He operated and the man survived.[8]

Hugh Ryder, like William Salmon, published this case to promote and valorize his work. Many practitioners with similar aims wrote within an established genre of medical writing known as observations.[9] Observations were constructed with hindsight, allowing practitioners to digest information and package it into a particular genre. As a result, authors' concerns about reputation and authority could unintentionally obscure the voices of sufferers. Healers, however, did more than just listen to patients talk. They poked and prodded. They smelled. They evaluated grimaces, trembling limbs, and clenched fists. Patients' bodily behaviors could communicate important information, thereby offering a second path to recovering patient-healer interactions and the potential influences of gender. Behavioral exchanges exist in the negative spaces of healers' writings, in the background to aspects of the encounter that practitioners were eager to highlight.

The Humoral Body from the Patient's Perspective

According to traditional medical theory in early modern England, the body was composed of four fluids, or humors: phlegm, blood, black bile, and yellow bile. Each humor, in turn, was associated with a combination of the qualities hot or cold and wet or dry. The unique balance and fluctuation of these humors determined health, as well as individual constitutions. For example, those with an abundance of blood had "sanguine," or passionate, dispositions. Sanguine people were thought to be naturally warm and wet, since these were the two qualities that characterized the humor blood. Too much phlegm, on the other hand, led to listlessness and was defined by the qualities wet and cold. "Melancholic" and "choleric" defined people with depressive or disagreeable temperaments resulting from too much black or yellow bile, respectively. Originating in antiquity, humoral theory dictated ordinary understandings of health, illness, and the body into the 1700s, and treatments derived from it were employed into the nineteenth century. We even use humoral terms, such as *melancholic* and *sanguine*, to define temperaments today. Humoralism had incredible longevity because, as an explanatory system, it was logical and adaptable. Men and women could look to the humors to explain a range of bodily phenomena. Sweat, for example, was an excess of humors secreted through the pores of the skin. The wrinkles and frailty of the elderly developed from the natural cooling and drying effects of aging. Infants, on the other hand, were moister and warmer than adults, as evidenced by their near-constant gurgling and spewing. There was also a humoral logic to fertility. Women's bodies were considered to be naturally cooler and wetter than men's bodies and, as a result, burned off excess fluids less efficiently. For new mothers, their extra blood nourished the fetus and transformed into breast milk for the newborn. Women who were neither pregnant nor breastfeeding excreted this excess fluid by menstruating each month.[10] While a significant number of learned medical texts from the period record the details of this humoral framework, the first half of this chapter approaches humoral explanations of health and the body from the perspective of ordinary sufferers.

Within the humoral framework, regular intake and outgo defined health. A healthy body was in constant flux, easily taking in and expelling fluids, whereas illness resulted from clogged or corrupt fluids. Such humoral flows were susceptible to environmental, physical, and even social influences. A change in wind patterns, an altered diet, or the sight of a jarring incident could wreak profound physical alterations. Most medical remedies, discussed in further detail below, aimed at redressing imbalanced humors and therefore vacillations in the body's equilibrium of hot, cold, wet, and dry qualities. While patients' firsthand accounts suggest that imbalance was central to everyday explanations of ill health, this concept alone does not capture the complexity of ways the humors were thought to operate within the body. Some defined their conditions as *corruptions*, a medical term for putrefied matter and a morally loaded word that defined the impurity of the soul. At the root of these patients' complaints was morbid matter, often itself a particular type of humor. Patients described possessing an "ague humor," cold humors, gouty humors, sharp or pungent humors, and, in the case of Samuel Jeake, "a violent Cholerick humour, breaking out in pimples on my Nose, & Face." Jeake's pimples served as visual evidence of putrid matter propelling outward.[11] Patients also linked physical disorders to dangerous concentrations of humors that settled in discrete parts of the body. Jeake used this reasoning to connect soreness in his right eye to consuming a piece of duck in 1674. The duck, perhaps because of its richness, caused "many glutinous humours" to collect in that one part of his face. Specific ailments, themselves the results of humoral shifts, operated in similar ways. One woman was laid up for three weeks from "a Feauer wch fell into her left Eye," while her husband was confined to the house with a "Uiolent cold wch fell into my Face, but is pretty well gone off."[12] Patients viewed diseases not as discrete entities that operated the same way in all bodies but as continually shifting clusters of symptoms. Colds and fevers roamed about the body, transmuting into entirely new disorders in response to lifestyle choices, individual constitutions, and the environment.

But what caused these humoral shifts in the first place? For devout patients, the ultimate source of illness was divine. Patients commonly used the phrase "it pleased God to visit me with" when introducing a particular disorder, to convey the notion that all afflictions were valuable messages from heaven. God sent illness for the same reasons he sent any affliction: to test a believer's faith or provide a reminder of mortality. A preacher in Leeds listed these two explanations for why God might be "pleased to visit a person or people with sickness," and he also noted that illness provoked self-examination, taught humility, and reminded sufferers of the significance of prayer. This preacher delivered his sermon in 1712, a year when Leeds witnessed a raging epidemic known as "the Dunkirk distemper." The rampant fever was said to affect thousands. The preacher's words offered an important means of coping with hardship by reminding parishioners that such crushing trials imparted key spiritual lessons.[13]

Belief in divine will did not necessarily preclude the active pursuit of natural remedies. Even if God was the ultimate source of illness, he still worked through natural means. Six external factors, known as "the nonnaturals," influenced the balance, movement, and evacuation of the body's humors. The six nonnaturals were aspects of daily life, or regimen, that patients regulated to preserve health: air, diet, exercise, sleep, emotions, and the retention and expulsion of matter. Not surprisingly, the nonnaturals were also central to patients' explanations of how they got sick. Examining patients' words rather than the writing of learned medical writers reveals a common belief that the nonnaturals caused ill health by means of blockages and temperature shifts. Extreme or sudden changes in temperature altered the congestion or movement of humors, resulting in illness.

These processes are perhaps clearest in patients' accounts of how air affected health. Exposure to cold air or wind could cause headaches, fevers, numbness, and pain. Patients referred to these ailments as colds, a group of disorders wholly unlike the upper respiratory infections known as colds today. Early modern colds resulted from a sudden shift in temperature that clogged the pores and prevented the dispersal and removal of internal wastes. Samuel Pepys, who caught colds almost continually, attributed them to cool weather, dressing inadequately, drinking cool beverages, and performing mundane tasks with bare legs, such as cutting his hair or paring his corns. The ensuing cold had a physical presence in his body. An influx of cold from a drafty window, a cool beer, or even a haircut physically entered the body and afflicted a particular part. A cold could settle in an ear or be caught in one's "pole."[14] There was even a particular type of skin swelling, "pernio," that developed when cold air "shutteth up the Pores so as the Humour cannot transpire, whereupon it corrupts, and raises little Wheals or Blisters." Cold obstructed the pores and prevented the expulsion of humors, resulting in blisters and bumps on the surface of the skin. Pepys offers glimpses of what these obstructions might have felt like. Blocked pores from cold led to a "burn within," made his blood tingle and itch, and caused his "anus to be knit together."[15]

Extreme heat was also perilous to health because it created fluxes of blood that overheated the body. A rise in temperature could breed harmful humors and inflame the blood, drying up the body's strength. Resulting sweats reversed these processes by excreting the excess, noxious vapors. "I think the great Frost bound up my Rhumes," Sarah Cowper wrote in 1716, "and now the thaw brings a defluxion from my Head which causes me to cough night and day." Rheum was fluid secreted by the eyes, nose, or mouth. A flux was rheum that flowed from the head. Presumably the warm weather caused humors to shift into Cowper's brain; the brain's natural coolness made the vapors condense and drip back down into her body. Air could cause ill health in two additional ways: by its malignant quality and lack of familiarity. A common early modern remedy was to escape the impure air of crowded, filthy cities for the countryside, while those who fell ill abroad were advised to return to the familiar, healthful air of their native countries.[16]

Just as individuals were acclimated to their native air, particular constitutions were suited to specific diets. Hence, a father lectured his daughter on the merits of dry biscuits. Cold food, like a blast of cold air, could lead to debility by obstructing the body and preventing the expulsion of poisonous wastes. Using an analogy of adding cold liquid to a pot of boiling water, the author of a 1641 book on the merits of warm beer explained that cold beverages clogged the body by preventing the stomach from refining humors into food, thereby impairing digestion and health. Since beginning to drink beer "hot as bloud," the author had lived in perfect health.[17] Oppositely, some men and women moderated their intake of warm beverages and food, such as wine and spices, finding that the ensuing sweats disordered them. Jane Shakerley's son drank sherry with friends, which "made him hote and uneasy so tosing thrue ye cloes of him so came by a great cold the next day." The alcohol caused excessive heat and sweat, which opened his body and invited in cold air. Some attributed ill health to this same process when they overheated themselves with exercise, the third nonnatural, and then drank a cold beverage or were exposed to a draft of air. One man who heated his body "by hard Labour" drank too liberally from a river. His warm body was overly receptive to the cool water, which "seized uery uiolently in his throat." According to the surgeon's apprentice who recorded this case, the man's actions proved fatal. He died within days.[18]

The few patients I have found who linked ill health to the fourth nonnatural, sleep, also tended to note temperature extremes: intense heat or cold inhibited proper rest. Others associated inadequate rest to particular circumstances. Lydia Dugard offered this explanation to her cousin and lover, Samuel Dugard, upon hearing of his ailing health while he was studying at Oxford in 1671: "I'm afraid you have taken cold by so much siting up, and have done you[r] self harm as well that way as by your greife." Their cousin Harry had recently died, and, as Dugard suggests, moderating the emotions was another key dimension of maintaining a balanced lifestyle. The emotions caused ill health by triggering a series of internal changes involving the blood and heart. Emotions such as sadness, fear, and surprise sparked a contraction of the heart, which trapped blood inside it and deprived the rest of the body of heat. This reaction could cause illness and, in extreme cases, death. Emotions such as love or anger provoked a reverse set of processes: the heart expanded and dispersed heat outward to the body's extremities.[19]

Finally, sufferers linked bodily disorders to an inability to expel accumulated wastes. Several patients viewed the internal buildup of putrefied matter as the result of overeating. One man was said to have died from indulging a sudden craving for lamb. Others noted how specific kinds of food, such as milk or "curdy drinkes," clogged the stomach. Writing from Norfolk in the 1620s, Katherine Paston warned her son, a student at the University of Cambridge, to abstain from such beverages, since they are "apte to brede surffits by reson thay doe not readily disgest but many times doe corrupt in the stomake." The color, consistency, and temperature of evacuated matter could signify a surfeit, as well as a host of other health conditions. What was the hue of this morning's urine? Was the blood pooling at the bottom of the barber-surgeon's basin thick and bubbly or thin and watery? When Catherine Cary stopped menstruating, her husband surmised that the blood was trapped within her body, a judgment he made based on the smell of her breath. In an age without X-rays or MRIs, such observations offered critical insights into otherwise invisible internal processes.[20]

The vacillations of the humors corresponded to individual constitutions and lifestyle choices, as well as grander, earthly rhythms. Warm, wet blood was typically on the rise in springtime, whereas levels of cool, dry black bile increased in autumn. To counteract these seasonal shifts, some individuals routinely purged or bled themselves. One man linked an eighteen-day fever to his failure to follow such seasonal preventative measures, and also to eating a large amount of fruit in Italy. It was not foreign air or even gluttony that was so destructive to his health but the fact that the fruit was "not wholesome by reason of great rain that fell just as it was ripening." This man viewed health as intimately entwined with the environment. His body responded sensitively to seasonal shifts, but also to the air, rain, and soil. He visited a physician and began exercising, with the hope that increased activity would burn off the harmful matter in his body.[21]

A part-time healer, James Clegg believed in the six nonnatural causes of illness, as well as the four humors. And as a Presbyterian minister, he trusted that ill health ultimately reflected God's will. Yet he recorded an episode in 1730 that points to a wholly different set of meanings associated with the outbreak of illness. The story originated with the wife of John Armstrong and focused on the moment when their child fell ill with smallpox. The child contracted the disease one night when the family heard a noise "as if someone had walkd sharply over the chamber and gone under the bed." Armstrong

searched for the source of the sound and found nothing, but the child's behavior confirmed the existence of a ghost. His wife explained how the child
slept between her and her husband in the bed, "but would needs be removd
to the side next the wall but presently cryd out, the Boggard has touchd me,
and would lie betwixt them again." She heard the same noise again a week
later, when her sister's child fell ill from the same disease, "the most violent
and deadly infection I had ever seen." Smallpox afflicted the two children at
the precise moments when Armstrong heard eerie, ghostlike sounds. The
story demonstrates how a "most violent and deadly" infection could strike
quite suddenly and how fleeting sounds could signify drastic physical alterations. It also reveals supernatural interpretations of disease causation
alongside natural and spiritual explanations.[22]

Some individuals could harness these supernatural forces to inflict physical harm. Wisewomen and cunning men used occult forces to cure illness,
while witches could generate physical disorders by uttering threatening words
and conjuring evil spirits. Witchcraft accusations were dwindling in England
by the late 1600s, especially among the middling- and upper-status patients
in this book. Yet healers' casebooks suggest that belief in magic and witchcraft endured.[23] A seventeen-year-old maid to Queen Catherine of Braganza
only suspected a "poor unlearn'd woman" of witchcraft when she could come
up with no other suitable explanation for the healer's ability to cure a "rage-
ing paine" in her eyes, teeth, and neck. Suspecting that the origins of the girl's
suffering were tiny worms swimming in her blood, the healer used a quill to
painstakingly remove hundreds of worms from the chambermaid's gums. The
girl, Elizabeth Livingston, was incredulous, even when the healer brandished
a basin of wriggling creatures as proof. Livingston and "the gidy multitude"
at court insisted that the healer was a witch or cheat. Perhaps she used the
quill to insert the worms into Livingston's gums? Or she slipped lutestrings
into the basin to resemble worms? After the healer left, Livingston opened
up a worm to be certain of the matter. Sure enough, blood spurted out, and
she resigned herself to her foul condition.[24]

Witchcraft and magic were waning in this period, yet there remained a
persistent faith in sympathy, the means by which objects could alter bodies at
a distance. Sympathetic reactions were not magic per se, though they were
thought to work by means of invisible vital spirits, or what one author called
"Effluviums of the Air." The healer John Archer looked to sympathy to explain the curious burning stomach pains and convulsive fits of the wife of a

soap boiler in 1660. Archer first prescribed the woman his standard treatments, but when these proved ineffective he asked the patient's maid where she emptied her mistress's chamber pot. The maid pointed to a heap of ashes just outside the door, the remnants of the fire used to boil soap. Here was the solution to the puzzling case. By using the patient's urine to extinguish the ashes, the maid unknowingly created a sympathetic bond between the woman's excrement and belly. As the woman's urine hissed and sizzled on the fire, a similar burn churned inside her stomach. Archer's explanation of the cause of illness led him to a cure: urinating into a basin of clean, pure water soothed the patient's stomach. Sympathetic cures typically worked by transferring maladies to distant objects. Perhaps the most well-known sympathetic cure of the period was Kenelm Digby's "powder of sympathy," which purportedly healed wounds when sufferers applied it to the weapon that had caused the injury. Individuals could also dissolve the powder in a bowl with cloths bloody from the wound, which created a sympathetic connection between cloth and injury. As the bloodstains on the cloth faded, the flesh healed.[25]

Aside from sympathetic, magical, and religious approaches to healing, patients had access to a wide array of natural remedies. Most of these treatments were designed to provoke an expulsion that would rebalance, redirect, or release the body's humors. Artificial wounds opened the body and encouraged the secretion of putrid matter, for instance. Patients inserted ribbons or small objects such as dried peas into these sores to ensure they remained open. Men and women also had blood let, made use of enemas, and consumed potions and pills to induce vomit and stools. These concoctions were made from plants known to work as emetics and laxatives, such as jalap, rhubarb, and tobacco. Sudorifics provoked sweat in order to expel harmful matter out through the pores of the skin. Some feared that these harsh evacuative treatments did more harm than good, which led, in part, to movements spearheaded by Paracelsus in the sixteenth century and Johannes Baptista von Helmont in the mid-seventeenth century promoting chemical therapies composed of salts, metals, and minerals. Followers of these movements reconceived the body and disease based on the chemical properties of salt, sulfur, mercury, and water and marketed their remedies as "new, Safe and Powerful." This opposition did not, however, erode traditional medicine. Patients and healers simply folded popular chemical remedies into existing practices.[26]

Isaac Archer used a pasty dressing made from bayberries to treat numbness in his leg in 1683. Such topical treatments, known as plasters, poultices, and cataplasms, could serve varying purposes. Some, made of soothing ingredients like milk and honey, mitigated pain. Others contained abrasive ingredients that raised blisters in order to remove blockages. One seventeenth-century recipe for a poultice included chopped chickweed, mallows, parsley, and elderflower boiled in milk. White bread and oatmeal thickened the mixture, and fresh lard ensured that the dressing bound to the afflicted part. Archer first noticed his numbing sensation a full year before he tried the berry plaster. He described his complaint to his father-in-law, who seemed to be the medical expert in the family. Both his father-in-law and wife worried that the disorder would shift upward into his head, which could prove fatal. Archer also complained of a cold, stomachaches, and sweats: "I could not stand, or goe, or lie but in paine." These problems disappeared for a while but returned with force a year later, and he applied the plaster at his father-in-law's urging. The remedy caused an immediate reaction. It "dispersed the humour all over my legg, as if it had bin asleepe," Archer wrote. Yet this reaction only exacerbated his condition, causing him to lose the use of his leg altogether. He went to a druggist for a new plaster, which cured his limp in just one day, and he slowly began to regain feeling.[27]

Sensations like pins and needles or, more commonly, the discernible emission of matter generated by purges and bleedings demonstrated that remedies were producing their intended effects. There could be a blurry line, however, between a remedy "working" and its provoking new problems altogether. Archer's initial plaster seemed to deepen his disorder rather than alleviate it. When Dorothy St. John applied a topical unguent to a swelling on her lip, the affliction simply relocated to her eyes. Poultices and ointments could also be incredibly painful, sometimes causing faints, fevers, and loss of sleep.[28] Vomits and laxatives, likewise, could open the body too strongly and weaken patients rather than strengthen them. After spending four months at Tunbridge spa, Anne Dormer began to recover her health, but only after long enduring the ill effects of her treatment (fig. 1). Patients visited spas to drink or bathe in the waters in order to treat a host of complaints, including colds, melancholy, and aches and pains. Dormer was recovering not from a particular disease but from a general "languishing indisposition of body." The waters were deemed an effective remedy because of their varying temperatures and mineral content, which could work as a laxative. Dormer's room was directly next to one of the wells, which allowed her to fetch a glass of healing water in just three minutes. Months of imbibing spa water began to

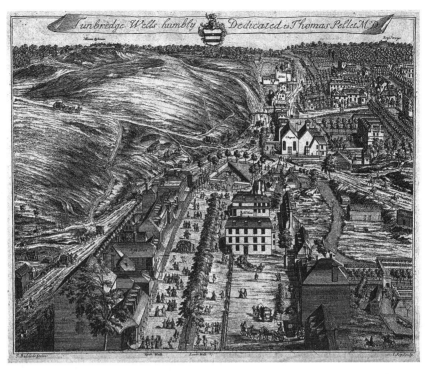

1. A bird's-eye view of Tunbridge Wells, by Jan Kip, after J. Badslade. By permission of the Wellcome Library, London.

take a toll, however. She was so indisposed by her "belly full of water" that she had to dictate some of her letters to a scribe. In one 1691 letter to her sister, Dormer explained how the waters "purg'd me so much, that I look like a Gridiron. And were it not for the scarr in my forheaed it were impossible for you to know me." A gridiron was a grill used for cooking, but a similar device was a torture implement. Dormer compared her face to a gridiron to convey her altered, emaciated state after months of consuming purgative waters. But perhaps the comparison was also meant to liken her time at Tunbridge to physical torture.[29]

Dudley Ryder was a young bachelor living in London, at a remove from his family home in Hackney. Over the course of several months in 1716, he put considerable effort into finding a cure for his shoulder pain after taking a bad fall. First he rubbed the bruised area with warming spirits, including an oily topical mixture called "Cucantellus's balsam." By the next day, the pain had spread to his neck. The anguish prevented him from leaving the house.

He tried drinking ale to provoke sweats, but this too only worsened matters. The pain deepened and extended down his thighs.[30] Many patients in this period, like Ryder, did not immediately seek help from practitioners upon falling ill but instead looked to their own gardens, cabinets, and recipe books. There were numerous medical compendiums published in the period that taught readers how to make and administer remedies at home. One popular guide, Hannah Woolley's *The Accomplish'd Ladies Delight*, lists directions for making medicaments, as well as preserving and candying fruit, concocting conserves and jellies, cooking pies, and producing cosmetic oils and waters to thicken the hair or smooth the skin. The title page portrays women carrying out some of these tasks. The middle picture shows a woman applying cosmetics as she gazes into a bedroom mirror, while the other images depict women cooking, baking, and brewing in a kitchen and producing syrups and salves in a stillroom. The following inscription is scrawled on the inside of a 1684 copy: "[S?]aney Sherrock / Her Book 1721/2." Individuals at the time commonly bequeathed books or exchanged them as gifts. Some copies boast a list of names that trace a book's transmission through numerous households over the years. The 1684 copy bears a second name too: George, followed by "His book" and "Given him to by . . ." (fig. 2). The practices Woolley's manual delineates, despite the book's title and imagery, were not considered the sole purview of women.[31]

Perhaps Ryder consulted a text like Woolley's to make his balsam, or maybe he borrowed a recipe from a relative or friend. Not everyone in early modern England was able to read, however, let alone purchase books. Nor could everyone afford to concoct their own salves, diet drinks, or plasters. Chemical ingredients, such as vitriol and mercury, could be pricey, as could imported ingredients such as nutmeg and cloves. And making cordials and distilled waters was complex, time-consuming work that required specialized equipment. A tax collector living in Somerset lacked sophisticated equipment but possessed the knowledge and wherewithal to prepare a sweating remedy for himself in his physician's workshop when the doctor was too drunk to do it.[32]

Ryder resolved to act as his own physician, or "at least to come as little into their hands as possible," after visiting his cousin Watkins's apothecary shop. Apothecaries were purveyors of remedies and medical ingredients, but many also provided advice and prescribed cures (fig. 3). A patient entered the shop to complain about one of Watkins's prescriptions, which had allegedly

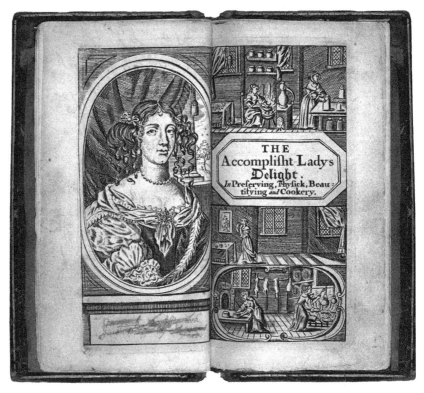

2. The so-called "accomplish'd lady" is shown here carrying out various household tasks. The name George is scrawled under the author's portrait. Title page and frontis from Hannah Woolley, *The Accomplish'd Ladies Delight in Preserving, Physick, Beautifying and Cookery* (London: Printed for Benjamin Harris, 1684). By permission of the Folger Shakespeare Library.

worsened the patient's condition. Ryder did not doubt it, noting that his cousin tended to "overload his patients with medicines" to line his own pockets. So too did physicians. As if to prove the point, the next to enter the shop was a physician who told Watkins that, despite his patient's improvement, he would still prescribe "some little thing," to the advantage of both healers. These men were acting dangerously and irresponsibly, Ryder thought, by plying their patients with "useless medicines." Yet when he was desperate for relief from his arm pain in 1716, he had Watkins apply a blister to the affected area, and he also tried one of Watkins's purges, taking it in the morning with large quantities of tea.[33]

After Ryder tried Watkins's remedy, as well as a purge prescribed by a physician, his father expressed concern about the harsh effects of his son's

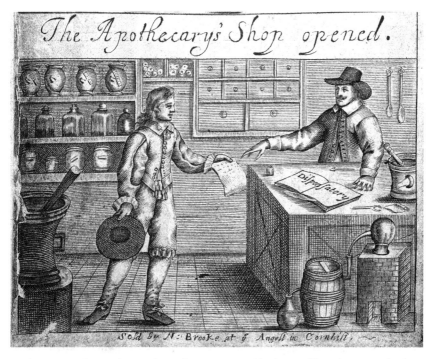

3. The interior of an apothecary shop, where patients and healers could purchase ingredients for making medicines and solicit health advice. Frontis from Michel Morel, *The Expert Doctor's Dispensatory* (London: N. Brooke, 1657). By permission of the Wellcome Library, London.

treatments. And for good reason. According to Ryder, Watkins's prescription "put me into a great faintness and lowness of spirits that I was almost ready to faint away." His father recommended a concoction made of mustard seeds bruised and steeped in wine. Ryder put hope in this cure, since "in the things the Doctor had ordered me mustard seed is one of the ingredients." He was living alone in London as a law student at the Middle Temple. When he was not studying or laid up in bed waiting for his purgative medicines to wear off, he spent his free time playing cards, frequenting coffeehouses, and attending dinners and concerts with male relatives. It was this nearly all-male social world that he turned to for medical advice. In addition to consulting his cousin and his father, Ryder visited his brother's house to be cupped four months after his initial accident. Cupping involved placing heated glasses on the skin to create a suction that drew noxious matter outward. Another cousin suggested wrapping the arm in flannel to induce sweats, as well as chewing rhubarb, "the only purge that the doctors themselves took." Physicians supposedly gnawed on the root while walking down the street, to keep their bowels regular.[34]

Ryder also looked beyond his ambit in London. He visited the same spa where Dormer turned into a gridiron, but rather than drink the waters, he immersed his body in the cold baths. He hoped the cool temperature and healing minerals would ease his pain, strengthen his body, and "purge it of ill humours." Months later, still suffering from pain, Ryder visited Bath to drink the waters. He consulted a physician about whether the spa water was suitable for his constitution. The physician "perfectly agreed" that it was, but warned that Ryder would have to consume the water for at least three to four weeks. Ryder even paid twenty-two shillings for a "quack medicine" from an empiric, a healer who derived knowledge from experience and firsthand observations rather than learned theory. Some empirics traveled from town to town, staging shows in public spaces to sell their wares (fig. 4). A cousin of Ryder's recommended the empiric, a man named Fowles who was known for treating rheumatic disorders. After first attempting to meet Fowles at his house in Derham Yard in the Strand, Ryder finally tracked down the healer at a coffeehouse in Whitehall. He described Fowles as a plain, rough man who had "nothing of the appearance of a cheat." His secret remedy allegedly purified and purged the blood, just what Ryder needed to ease his pain. Ryder was hopeful upon hearing Fowles's pitch but grew suspicious when the healer continued to promote his cure-all for disorders as varied as venereal disease and kidney stones. Fowles even offered to share testimonials from former patients who could vouch for his remedy's success. Both of these moves— touting a medicine as a panacea and listing the names and addresses of satisfied clientele—were hallmarks of the charlatan. But Ryder was desperate. Fowles brought his concoction to Ryder's home a week later, and Ryder took it with wine off and on for the next few weeks. His arm eventually improved, but he attributed his recovery to continued visits to the spa rather than to Fowles's secret formula.[35]

Ryder paid for advice from physicians and empirics as he simultaneously sought help from neighbors and relatives. A mix of home remedies and hired help constituted his care. His reliance on this array of healers reflects the shared understanding of medicine, health, and the body among individuals of varying backgrounds, training, and education levels in this period. A professional elite did not monopolize medical knowledge in seventeenth-century England. In some instances, lay healers and learned physicians doled out the

4. An empiric peddles his cure-alls from an elevated platform. Title
page from Salvator Winter, *A Pretious Treasury; or, A New Dispensatory*
(London: T. Harper for R. Harper, 1649). By permission of the
Wellcome Library, London.

very same prescriptions and cures. The eminent apothecary and naturalist
James Petiver, for instance, asked a female patient for her recipe for a wound
drink. Lay healers point to similar overlaps between domestic and commercial healing practices. Elizabeth Freke grew herbs in her garden for
making medicines and sought health advice from friends and family. Yet, as
the historian Elaine Leong has shown, this was not some quaint domestic
practice. Freke stockpiled a vast store of medicines in her home, which required purchasing exotic ingredients, performing complex techniques, and
consulting learned healers and published texts.[36]

"Sent for a Surgeon": The Medical Encounter

Alongside gentlewomen like Elizabeth Freke and cousins or neighbors who
might not have identified as healers at all, apothecaries sold their drugs, midwives delivered babies, physicians and surgeons prescribed remedies and
performed operations, and empirics peddled their cure-alls. Sarah de Heusde,
who had a medical practice in London, treated complaints that targeted particularly intimate parts of women's bodies, including hemorrhoids, uterine
disorders, venereal disease, and reproductive ailments. She claimed to have
trained under her husband and her father, both physicians. Another Londoner,

Mary Lucas, specialized in cupping.[37] A substantial number of women also worked in caregiving roles without possessing licenses, training, or even professional identities. Women worked as caregivers in hospitals, and parishes paid older women to nurse the sick and to serve as searchers who examined the ill and tabulated causes of death.[38] Men too worked in the healing trades without formal accreditation or in combination with other occupations. Ned Waters made a living as both a barber and a tailor. He cut hair and mended stockings, gowns, and caps. One client, Giles Moore, paid Waters for a blister and pills before having his head shaved, suggesting that Waters also made money purveying medicines. Edmund Harrold too was a barber, though his work entailed making and selling wigs in addition to cutting hair, shaving beards, and performing minor surgical services. The surgery was probably not very lucrative, or perhaps Harrold was not very successful at it, as his diary is full of tabulations concerning the production and sale of wigs but only mentions two patients. Both were breastfeeding women who hired him to cup their breasts in order to draw out breast milk: "Got a book given me for sucking [in] 1713 of Mrs Wismans breast, the greatest cure I did." A part-time secondhand book dealer, Harrold accepted barter in exchange for his services.[39]

Patients rarely recorded the particulars of their interactions with healers. Writing by practitioners, then, provides the most illuminating insights into medical encounters. Healers' notes and memoranda can offer just glimmers of their exchanges with patients—brief scribbles record the potency of a remedy or a reminder of an unpaid bill. John Westover kept his medical records in a notebook with columns that listed dates, patients' names, and the amount of money owed or paid. These records are interspersed with notes about the management of his farm and other tabulations, creating an amalgamation of account book and casebook. Despite its terseness, the resulting document offers some valuable information about Westover's practice. For example, he tended to ask for a portion of his fee up front and the remainder when patients were cured. Like Harrold, he also accepted barter, such as geese or eels, instead of money.[40]

As Westover eked out a living on his farm, Edmund King treated some of the wealthiest men and women in London. He recorded the following case in March 1691: "Ranalough Lady Dowager march 31 91. After a great & running at nose grew hot restless short breath uery feuerish—had a long fitt & sweat sunck her extreamly. I durst uenture a nother fitt . . . she thought this too hot. But dranke sage possit drink wch did well then she tooke it 3 times a day. at 6. in the morn at 2 & 6 at night it agreed well & her fitts abated. . . . April 5th much mended, & abated the Cordiall, to morning & euening only." This patient was Katherine Jones, Viscountess Ranelagh, the sister and confidant of Mary Rich, Countess of Warwick. Ranelagh was a leading intellectual of her age and was involved in numerous projects concerning politics, law reform, and religion. Her home in Pall Mall became a hub of scientific activity in the 1670s when her brother, the natural philosopher Robert Boyle, moved in and began carrying out experiments there. Ranelagh passed away nine months after the above episode, perhaps from the very same fever, sweats, and convulsions that King recorded. He prescribed a medicinal drink, but she found it too hot. She instead took a sage posset, a mixture of warm milk, wine, sugar, and sage. King's notes share with Westover's account book a practical utility. King might have recorded cases like Ranelagh's for some future publication, but his writing also served a more immediate means of managing information. He could look back through the notebook and ascertain how previous patients had responded to particular remedies like that sage posset. Ranelagh's fits improved after taking the drink three times a day, and after two weeks King lowered the dose to just twice a day. While valuable, this case focuses on the information King considered significant for his work. Ranelagh's words and body were at the heart of this episode, as evidenced by her demand for a cooler drink, but the aims and practices that structured the case render her barely visible.[41]

Patients' voices begin to surface in observations. A formal genre of medical writing modeled partly on the ancient Hippocratic treatise *Epidemics,* observations developed from a late Renaissance return to making empirical examinations at the bedside as opposed to documenting the progress of illness without regard to individuals' unique constitutions and circumstances. Compared to earlier genres of medical writing, observations contained substantial information about patients, including symptoms, temperaments, occupations, and lifestyle choices. By the late seventeenth century, authors no longer compiled observations solely to record rare and miraculous cases but also to classify all types of diseases from head to toe. Several published texts containing observations and circulating in England in the 1600s were translations of books by foreign authors, such as Paul Barbette's *Chirurgical and Anatomical Works* (1672), Théophile Bonet's *A Guide to the Practical Physician* (1684), and Lazare Rivière's *The Practice of Physick* (1655). The prevalence of these translations reflects the origins of the genre among physicians and surgeons from continental Europe. Low-status practitioners such as surgeons, empirics, and itinerant healers were key contributors to the genre because they tended to lack licenses or university affiliations. Instead of these more traditional forms of accreditation, healers used observations to legitimize their work. Likewise, those who propagated alternative treatments, such as chemical remedies, were unable to rely on ancient authorities to support their claims and so turned to observations to validate their practice.[42]

One such author was John Colbatch, who developed and marketed a controversial powder for treating wounds. He began his career as an apprentice to an apothecary in Worcester. Colbatch possessed no medical degrees but was able to work his way up the medical ranks, moving to London and eventually obtaining a license from the city's governing medical body, the Royal College of Physicians.[43] He published numerous books, many of which contain observations promoting his vulnerary powder and the medicinal virtues of acids and alkalis rather than traditional remedies made from plants. Like William Salmon, Colbatch used the medium of print to validate and promote his practice. He promised to provide the names of individual patients to inquiring readers, as well as the names of apothecaries "upon whose Files they may see the Prescriptions." Such concerns about reputation and custom colored Colbatch's observations. He seemed to publish severe cases that highlighted his ability to work extraordinary cures. Colbatch described one fifteen-year-old patient who suffered from "the most dreadful Fit of the Gout I ever saw" and endured "the most intolerable Pain and misery that it was possible for a Poor Creature to be in." The boy was in so much pain that he could barely move nor "suffer the Cloaths to touch him." Under Colbatch's care, the teenager was healed in a month. Colbatch tracked his various medical prescriptions, including oil of cloves, balsamic syrup, and "elixir sulphurus," alongside the fluctuations and movements of pain from deep in the boy's joints into his lower back. Tracing this progression of aches certainly depended on the patient's input. Yet far from providing unmediated access to his interactions with the boy, Colbatch focused strictly on his own remedies and the patient's improvement—a highly directed endorsement of his practice. We only seem to hear Colbatch's patients speak when they advance the healer's cause. One soldier removed his hat and affectionately thanked Colbatch for work well done: "Sir, when I came into your Company I was in most intolerable Pain and Misery, from which I was not to expect deliverance, but by the loss of my Arm; but am now as much at ease as ever I was in my whole Life." The soldier uttered these words just fifteen minutes after receiving Colbatch's cure for a wound in his hand.[44]

Practitioners seldom recorded patients' spoken words in this way. In the rare instances that we do hear patients speak, their voices seem to be used in the service of validating wondrous cures. Another example comes from a physician living and working in Gloucestershire in the late 1720s. Thomas Dover first saw his patient, a lawyer named John Goodeere, as he lay in bed with a fever. Goodeere's eyes were sunken, jaw fallen, and tongue hardened, and his face, according to Dover, was "as black as an Indian, with round Drops upon it as big as Pease." Dover asked an apothecary to bleed Goodeere, and on Dover's insistence the apothecary removed nearly fifty ounces of blood. As he bled, Goodeere also consumed a cool mixture of Rhenish wine, water, and lemon juice. A pint of the brew revived him. He moved his eyes, closed his jaw, and after a few more glasses even regained the ability to speak. Dover asked Goodeere if he could drink. "The Ocean," the patient responded. Dover then asked Goodeere how he felt. "In a strange confused Condition," Goodeere replied. An hour later, the patient flung off his bed linens, put on his slippers and nightgown, and walked to the far side of the room, where he plunked down in an armchair and invited Dover to share a flask of claret. "I told him," Dover wrote, "I would drink a Flask of Claret; but that he must stick to his Cool Tankard." The words and behaviors of the patient the next morning further confirmed his seemingly miraculous recovery. When Dover arrived at the house, Goodeere was in the stable among the horses, wearing nothing but his nightgown and slippers. "I asked him, How he did," and Goodeere replied, "Never better in all his Life."[45]

Not everyone was so lucky. In July 1706, a woman visited John Sintelaer at his home in High Holbourn, London, after consulting forty other practitioners. Sintelaer was known for treating venereal infections swiftly and discreetly, despite the fact that the standard remedies were painful, lengthy, and conspicuous. Pills, fumigations, and ointments made from mercury, guaiacum bark, and cinnabar caused excessive sweats, copious salivation, and rotting gums. Sintelaer instead prescribed therapeutics traditionally used for nonvenereal complaints: purging potions, a modified diet, and a secret drug that he dubbed his "Anti-venereal Decoction." The patient who sought him out that summer day in 1706 was five months pregnant and had "putrid corroding Ulcers" covering her head, throat, shoulders, and back. Sintelaer mentioned those forty competitors, no doubt, to highlight his superiority. Forty rivals failed where he succeeded.[46]

Other medical authors made a similar move by highlighting their competitors' unsuccessful cures and botched treatments. Hugh Ryder explained how an apprentice to a coachmaker accepted help from neighbors when a pole impaled him in the stomach. The neighbors treated the contusion using topical remedies made from turnips, but the man requested the surgeon's advice upon "finding the case to exceed their Capacity." These, of course, are the surgeon's words rather than those of the apprentice. Further demonstrating the neighbors' incompetence, Ryder noticed a horrible stench when he entered the patient's room. He removed the damp turnip compress to find that the man's excrement had seeped out the hole in his belly. Ryder filled the opening with wads of cotton drenched in a mixture of herbs and chemicals, and the man survived.[47]

If medical writers were dismissive of their competitors' work, they were even more disdainful of patients' attempts to treat themselves. Some practitioners justified their unsuccessful cases by referencing patients' bungled self-treatments or by noting how a sufferer "neglected the Rules prescribed him." One man treated a painful swelling on his leg using an ointment made of linseed oil. This topical remedy had disastrous effects, according to the healer who documented the case. Rather than opening the body, allowing it to release noxious humors, the linseed "disturbed Nature in her expulsion . . . the peccant Humor being afterwards very much impacted." The ointment clogged up the man's pores and prevented the release of virulent matter. Recording such hazardous practices allowed healers to justify complications in their own practice and to further extol their superior knowledge.[48]

Medical encounters, however, are not so easily reducible to moral tales of practitioners' virtues. Healers' concerns about displaying competence can obscure our view of sufferers, but patients' words emerge when they were crucial to determining a diagnosis, a treatment, or the progression of illness. One healer linked a woman's convulsive fits to "terror and affrightment," a causal explanation that the patient most probably provided herself. The fits contracted her entire body and caused intolerable pain. A sudden fear triggered the initial fit, but subsequent attacks followed even the faintest twinges of apprehension, brought on by walking over a bridge, peering over a high railing, or spying an insect. She even had fits in her sleep. After she suffered through these convulsive spells for weeks, the woman's entire disposition began to shift. Her face grew pale, her voice grew hoarse, and she developed a cough. As her healer put it, "she became as it were a Changling." He remarked how "the whole habit of her Body was altered . . . her mind in some sort alienated." The healer guessed that the emotional disturbances created obstructions, which he tried to release with purgative medicines. When the patient later complained of a pain in her head, the practitioner recommended shaving her hair and applying a topical ointment that created blisters to draw out the congested matter. The patient's input was crucial to the unfolding of the case, determining her diagnosis, her treatment, and her healer's interpretations of symptoms. By listening to the patient's words and observing her pale face, cough, and altered disposition, the healer developed an explanation of the problem and how to treat it. This process was informed by the assumptions and observations both patient and healer brought to the encounter.[49]

A case of dropsy that an anonymous practitioner recorded in 1726 centered around that ever illusive, invisible symptom, pain. A patient known only as "Mr Rob" diagnosed his own pain as a stiffness in his joints. His practitioner, in response, let blood. But four days later the pain moved into Rob's chest, accompanied by "a burning Heat in his shoulders." The healer noted an inflammation that corroborated Rob's report, and he applied emollients. The pain continued shifting, settling next in the patient's thigh. Rob treated himself with an infusion of chemical ingredients and "Stonehorse Dung." A few days later, the pain returned to his shoulders and struck down his chest, hindering his breathing. As the man's pain continued to morph, from a "Stupor & Numness" in his rectum and belly to a "smale suppression" in his bladder, the healer's prescriptions followed suit, running through a series of pastes, powders, and pills. Patients' words enabled healers to trace the nature and movement of such torments, as well as more subtle sensations that could signify important physical transformations—a twitch in the eyebrow or a "little Tugge in my face." The patient's narrative provided access to otherwise invisible internal trajectories.[50]

As a medium of exchange between patients and practitioners, words could enable but also inhibit the productive communication of corporeal sensations. "I must begg if you can understand any thing of my condition by this bad description," Margaret Ashburnham wrote to the eminent physician Hans Sloane in 1719. Ashburnham suffered from pain in her limbs, "with sick fitts" that were especially fierce in the morning, though she was careful to add, "I am neuer free from pain & sickness." She explained how another physician suspected "a melancholy wind that flys all ouer me." Gas swirled inside her body, dampening her spirits and deteriorating her health. She believed the disorder moved because her stomach and limbs often ached when her head was altogether free from pain. Apologetically, Ashburnham admitted that she had stopped taking Sloane's prescriptions, a diet drink and a medicinal paste known as an electuary, since she found them to be "binding." The treatments closed rather than opened her body, a determination she might have made by assessing the frequency and consistency of her stools. The letter ends with a postscript listing additional symptoms—cold shivering fits and "wind rowling in my stomack"—as though Ashburnham still struggled to express the precise nature of her ailment.[51]

Sarah Cowper found the words to express her illness, but hearing another person utter them elucidated the nature of her disorder. She was talking to a physician about snuff, pulverized tobacco that users inhaled, in 1709. The doctor admitted to loving the stuff, but just a few minutes after taking it he felt what he called "a uery ugly Feeling" in his nerves. Cowper was surprised to hear the physician use these words. He "hitt upon the phrase which I use to express my disease, and describe it more sensibly to me, than I knew how to ha[ve] done to him." Cowper long endured a "Rhumatick Humour" that raged in her hip, thigh, and eyes. She had been taking snuff for years to ward off pain in her joints and a discharge, or rheum, in her eyes and throat. In 1703 she was taking it twice a day to induce sneezing and to clear the rheum from her eyes and head. She eventually stopped carrying snuff, to avoid developing a habit, and instead asked others occasionally "for a pinch." Cowper had always attributed her "ugly feeling" to her rheumatic disorder, but after her talk with the physician she was convinced that snuff itself was the culprit.[52]

When words failed, bodily behaviors could provide a valuable means of communication. No one could explain why the daughter of a Yorkshire farmer suffered from violent convulsive fits. Demonstrating a fit, rather than attempting to describe it through speech, proved to be the most effective way to convey the problem. When a physician came to visit, the seventeen-year-old girl's mother brought out a glass of water from the kitchen. As the girl began to drink, she started shaking uncontrollably and fell to the ground. Regaining the ability to speak fifteen minutes later, she described feeling "intolerable Pain in her Breast." But she also struggled to articulate her sensations. As her physician recalled, she felt a "Weight upon her Spirits, or Anxiety which she could not express," and when asked about her pain she could only point to the upper part of her sternum.[53]

A master at Eton similarly evaluated a pupil in 1686 by not just listening to the boy's words but also making careful observations of his mannerisms. A cough, headache, and back pain confined the boy to bed for four days. The master, Lacroze, reported to the boy's mother that the most worrisome symptom was pain in his side: "He cryed so much that it seemed to be uery uiolent." As the tender patient lay in bed, irritable from his aches and pains, he shook intensely. This behavior signaled "as much fear as pain in his case." Lacroze was able to interpret the boy's behavior as a reaction to fear as opposed to pain. The boy had heard that cramping was a symptom of pleurisy, a dangerous, often fatal disease that caused inflammation in the lungs. As Lacroze soon discovered, the boy believed he had the condition, "and he was afraid it would kill him." Lacroze, on the other hand, suspected that the cramp originated from gas, a diagnosis that was such a relief to the boy that he fell asleep and awoke free from pain. Rather than assessing his pupil's articulations of pain, Lacroze observed the boy's fearful cries and trembling body.[54]

Patients like the farmer's daughter and Lacroze's pupil expressed their suffering in words but also in their contortions, trembles, howls, and whimpers. Patients afflicted with painful twitches and debilitating cramps were able to convey the nature and location of their disorders through their physical bodies. In agony, one man did not speak but instead made "many apish motions & c[on]torsions of his face & stamping w[th] his feet." Clenched fists and stomping feet could be more illuminating than words. One of William Salmon's patients suffered from head pain that "cruelly raged by Fits to the roots of his eyes." His eyes turned red and "lookt as if they would start out of his head," and hot, sharp tears streamed down his face. So vexed by the pain, the man "ran up and down like one mad, yet without any Feaver, Thirst or Inflamation." Believing the cause of the disorder to be overheated blood, Salmon made light scratches on the back of the man's head and used cupping to draw out blood from the artificial cuts. He also opened a vein in the man's forehead to alleviate the pain. Practitioners even looked to patients' behaviors while administering treatments. The surgeon Richard Wiseman peered into the faces of his patients as he let blood from them, choosing to stop when he discerned a change in their composure.[55]

Prevailing notions of femininity and masculinity could shape patients' physical expressions, as well as healers' interpretations of them. Stomping, thrashing, and raving were deemed unusual and unexpected behaviors for gentlewomen, for instance. William Petty confirmed the extremity of one female patient's pain by noting her seemingly exceptional, unfeminine strength. She had a fever, and her arms trembled and twitched "so strongly as she shooke the bed wherein shee lay and could scarce bee held by a mans strength." The patient's inability to meet expectations of gendered behavior, especially for an upper-status woman like herself, demonstrated the severity of her case. When treating external wounds or tumors, practitioners noted whether pain was intolerable, as patients "could not endure my hand to touch the place." Surgeons performed invasive and often excruciating procedures using hot irons and knives "as Age and Strength would allow" or for as long or as deep "as the Patient could well endure."[56] Assumptions about normative behavior informed these interpretations. When one man survived an excruciating amputation of his penis, his surgeon remarked how he "bore the Agonies of the Operation with such a manly Courage, as surprised all the Spectators; for he was only heard to utter a few Complaints." Stoic endurance, as demonstrated by making little noise or few complaints, demonstrated manliness. Yet the surgeon's comment also exposes his expectations of what a man should be able to endure. Men and women, children and adults, and even patients hailing from different countries were presumed to possess varying levels of tolerance for pain.[57]

Patients persuaded surgeons to undertake brutal, often unadvised interventions by expressing the severity of their suffering without appearing incapable of withstanding the pain. They came "to be cured or dye." A young apothecary's pain was "inexpressible," but he successfully communicated its severity by holding out his hand and bidding his healer to "tear it, cutt it off, or burn it."[58] There was a common belief that women were too timid or frightened to endure such procedures. Some practitioners were incredulous when female patients demanded painful treatments or attested they would be able to withstand the agony of a surgical operation. When a gentlewoman asked Richard Wiseman to treat a pain in her forefinger, he proposed making an incision to the bone, "not imagining so fearfull a creature would have permitted it." This patient, like William Petty's, was of a high social rank. Her status, as well as gender, shaped Wiseman's assumptions about her timid disposition and inability to withstand pain. She contradicted Wiseman's expectations by assenting to the procedure. Another surgeon held the opposite belief. He read that women could bear more severe pain than men, but he only believed it after removing a tumor from a woman's breast without using anesthesia. He and his colleague cut the skin, thrust in their hands, and cut out the tumor, filling the cavity with myrrh and aloe to prevent decay. The patient's endurance of this harrowing procedure altered the course of treatment. The surgical team wanted to seal up the wound and allow the patient to begin recuperating, but a distinguished surgeon who arrived late on the scene insisted that they reopen the breast to cut out more of the cancer, "since she could endure the knife."[59]

The body also spoke in other ways. Healers used candles to inspect the color and texture of afflicted areas. They smelled their patients' secretions and in some instances even relied on taste. Broken bones might reveal themselves by making a snapping, crackling, or clicking sound. And surgeons palpated patients' bodies to locate and evaluate internal congested matter. A "timpanite sounde" made by tapping, for instance, signified a tumor filled with air. Pressing enabled surgeons to locate internal swellings and to gauge their movement and consistency. After pushing down on a lump, healers noted whether the skin retained its natural color or was "yielding to Impression." When one of Thomas Willis's patients described feeling a throbbing in her ribs "as it were the leaping of some live animal," he put his hand on her side to see if he could detect the motion. He could.[60] Practitioners griped about patients who refused to bare their bodies for these examinations, pointing to another way gender shaped clinical interactions. Such cases nearly always involved female patients, male healers, and disorders of particularly intimate parts of the body. A woman with a tumor on her groin larger than a "rowl of White-bread" sent for help, but when the healer arrived she refused to let him even see the affected area. He prescribed a topical remedy, which she had her "women" apply, presumably her maids, relatives, and friends. Finally, when the abscess broke, the surgeon returned and the patient permitted him to dress the ulcer. But when he proposed a new treatment and suggested the patient seek additional help from specialists in London, she again demurred. According to Richard Wiseman, who recorded the case, this patient's unwillingness to expose her body and follow her healers' directives led to her demise. Not surprisingly, some female practitioners amassed their clientele by specializing in treating disorders that afflicted particularly intimate parts of the body.[61]

Perhaps some female patients were cautious because they heard tales of lecherous men who falsely posed as healers in order to access women's bodies. In 1661, Samuel Pepys's friend Peter Llewellyn pulled off just such a ruse at the Golden Fleece tavern near Guildhall in London. He and a man named Blurton tricked a young woman into thinking that Blurton was a physician. Llewellyn called him "Doctor," and Blurton convinced the woman to divulge her health complaint, "some ordinary infirmity belonging to women." The pretend doctor arranged to visit the woman's house with a remedy for her troubles and under the pretense of administering said remedy "hath the sight of her thing below, and did handle it—and he swears the next time that he will do more." Exposing the body could be a risky endeavor, laying oneself bare not only to harsh and painful procedures but also to sexual danger.[62]

Of course, other factors could define the nature of these clinical interactions. Practitioners diagnosed disorders in the laboring poor in accordance with beliefs about the ways particular diets and lifestyles altered bodies. And practitioners tailored their treatments for patients of varying social ranks based on concerns about cost and profit. Healers typically treated the poor for free, which meant they did not need to impress poorer clients to win their custom. One practitioner explained how, instead of treating smallpox with his favored remedy of juleps and watered-down beer mixed with orange juice, he prescribed poor patients only watery beer mixed with vinegar. He swapped out the pricier ingredients for cheaper ones "to save charges." Patients too selected treatments based on financial concerns. The maid of the eminent French physician Lazare Rivière could not afford the pricey remedies her employer prescribed for a fever. She instead chose to have blood let and cupping glasses applied, and she drank a decoction made of sorrel roots and spirit of sulfur. While status could determine the kinds of medicines physicians prescribed and patients purchased, a patient's day-to-day lifestyle and work habits could further influence treatment outcomes. A "Labouring man" had difficulty recovering from a tumor in his leg because he had to return to work. His surgeon noted that he "Exercis'd his legg uery much in part causing those symptoms & the supperation not being compleated by reason of his Impatience." What this physician called impatience the patient probably viewed as necessity. Economic need kept him from complying with his healer's direction to rest, thereby delaying his recovery.[63]

Conclusion

As opposed to presenting a play-by-play of the discussions and negotiations that transpired in the sickroom, observations provide complex and highly mediated accounts of medical practice. But patient autonomy was a key factor in many medical encounters—so much so that practitioners could not help but reveal traces of patients' words, demands, and denials in their writings. Some practitioners recorded patients' expressions and actions to validate their successful cures or to defend their failures. For others, patients' voices provided valuable access to otherwise invisible processes, such as emotional disturbances, roving pain, or previous events or accidents. A close look at healers' writing recovers the interactions between patients and their healers as the two parties determined diagnoses and negotiated treatments. Yet for all their value, observations offer only rare and often obscured access to patients. The nuances of how men and women perceived illness onset, pain, and recovery are barely visible in healers' writing. When patients' words do emerge, we must be careful about the ways practitioners' ambitions and writing practices could distort or mask their voices.

Yet we can read meaning in the silences in observations, in the moments healers chose not to record, and in the physical interactions that existed in the background of cases. Practitioners evaluated pain, engaged in physical diagnosis, and administered treatments based on sufferers' verbal and physical expressions. Assumptions about economic status or expectations of gendered behavior could inform these communications and performances. Some practitioners relied on physical observation more than others. Many of the examples here derive from writings by surgeons whose focus on external ailments, such as wounds, swellings, and fractures, required the use of touch and physical evaluation more frequently than did the treatment of internal disorders. In addition, many of the medical practitioners whose cases survive were recording observations to legitimize and promote their work. Observations provided a way to validate and defend their practice, and, as a result, concerns about reputation, custom, and professional identity are particularly strident in these texts. The following chapters turn from medical encounters to the thoughts and experiences of patients. Looking beyond the words of healers to those of ordinary sufferers uncovers vibrant imaginations, intimate conversations, and world views that seem at once incompatible and resonant with our own.

2. Learning How to Be Ill

At the age of sixteen, Elizabeth Livingston ate a significant amount of fruit just as she was recovering from a dangerous illness. This indulgence, she believed, impaired her recovery: "My great foly in pleaseing my tast for some short moment's has brought me many day's of trouble." The hazards of fruit were well known in the seventeenth century. Some, like Livingston, grew sick from overeating fruit. Others choked on fruit or fell ill after consuming rotten fruit. Early modern healers, as well as ordinary men and women, considered fruit a common source of physical disorder because its wet, cold properties could offset the body's humoral balance. By highlighting this link between fruit and ill health, sufferers like Livingston focused on the moral significance of their irresistible desires and the physical consequences of their choices. Livingston documented the episode in 1665 in order to meditate on its spiritual significance. She recorded similar episodes from her youth too: staying up late, sleeping in late, and forcing her servants to miss public prayers. In this instance, she emphasized the "transitory pleasure" of fruit, a well-known biblical symbol of sin and temptation. Her unrestrained appetite demonstrated intemperance and also disobedience toward her aunt and her physician, who both had warned her against the dangers of fruit. By viewing her illness as the consequence of her indulgence, Livingston imbued what might be seen as a wholly physical disorder, surfeit, with spiritual and moral significance.[1]

This story certainly reminds us of Eve's sin, but it also evokes a story from Saint Augustine's fourth-century conversion narrative, the *Confessions*.

Augustine was the same age as Livingston, just sixteen, when he and some friends stole pears from an orchard despite having an abundance of their own superior pears. As Augustine recalls, they stole the pears not to enjoy them but only for the thrill of taking them. He related the episode to teach the importance of acknowledging and repenting for even the slightest transgressions. His sin was not just unchecked desire but finding pleasure "in doing what was not allowed."[2] Livingston's temptation, disregard of authority, and subsequent illness echoed the very lessons Augustine sought to impart to readers. A woodturner living and working in London in the 1600s also seemed to look to Augustine to articulate the relationship between morality, illness, and fruit. When Nehemiah Wallington nearly choked on a pear, he viewed the incident as a divine portent. God was punishing him "for breaking [a] promise or vows which I haue made." He also expected to fall ill from the pear, "as some tims I am." Illness was a dimension of this divine trial and a physical affliction that Wallington associated with pears, presumably based on prior experiences. While some patients surely viewed the bodily effects of fruit in strictly humoral terms, believers like Livingston and Wallington looked to Augustine to explain the moral and physical ramifications of the temptations of fruit.[3]

Within the devout religious climate of early modern England, texts such as the *Confessions* provided important conceptual frameworks for making sense of ill health. Yet the above examples also show how devotional texts provided tangible scripts that readers appropriated to interpret lived experiences. Augustine taught believers like Wallington and Livingston how to make sense of their ailing bodies. This is what I mean by the title of this chapter, "Learning How to Be Ill." Illness entails a series of physiological developments as well as culturally determined interactions, behaviors, and expressions. Firsthand accounts offer evidence of the stories and scripts that taught early modern patients how to behave on the sickbed, as well as how to evaluate the nature and severity of illness. For instance, patients might adopt tropes or imagery from texts like the *Confessions* in their own writing. Or they might recount the experiences of friends and then draw on those experiences to analyze their own bodies. We can trace connections between these stories and subsequent accounts of illness, even when patients did not explicitly make the link and the mechanisms by which they adapted such scripts remain invisible. This chapter recovers three types of stories that patients seemed to rely upon most to make sense of bodily processes: stories of sickness about others, patients' own past experiences, and stories in devotional literature and practices. Men and women diagnosed disorders, gauged suffering, and predicted trajectories of recovery by observing their own bodies, as well as the experiences of friends, family members, and strangers who suffered from the same or similar disorders. They also learned how to respond to illness by listening to sermons, reading devotional texts, and observing the corporeal dimensions of their day-to-day spiritual exercises. Such stories did not merely model ideals for patients to emulate, though some of them surely served this purpose. Rather, these stories offered individuals a vocabulary for interpreting their ailing bodies. They helped patients understand the nature and severity of their ailments, and they taught patients how to express their suffering. All three types of stories reflect a culture in which the close study of natural processes was an important approach to viewing and experiencing the natural and supernatural worlds.

Yet patients made their observations in gendered ways. Considerably more women than men defined their illnesses by observing the experiences of other people. More than half of the women in this book continually made such comparisons, whereas I have found only a handful of discrete instances in which men did the same.[4] Rather, men tended to look to their own prior bodily experiences and interpretations. It is important to note that these patterns do not reflect hard-and-fast divisions. Some women certainly did look to their own past experiences to evaluate disorders. One woman referred to her lying-in period, the span of time women were sequestered to bed after giving birth, to communicate the extremity of her illness years later: "I am still weake, and, I thinke, allmost as weake as affter lyeing in of any of my chillderen." And in a series of letters to her physician, Hephzibah Parker compared her symptoms and sensations to those of previous days.[5] What is striking, however, is the scarcity of such self-assessments in women's writing. Any one individual could draw on a range of models to make sense of illness, yet the emphases varied between men and women. To better understand these patterns, the following discussion looks to the day-to-day lives of early modern men and women, including writing practices, occupational roles, and approaches to collecting and sharing medical knowledge. The study of gendered lived experiences in seventeenth-century England—the doing, watching, and listening that filled men's and women's days—reveals how the language of illness was grounded in the social particulars of daily life.

"Others Mortalety Might Put Me in Mind of Mine": Observing Others

Seventeenth-century diaries are full of anecdotes about other people's illnesses. Foremost, these stories served as spiritual reminders of death and divine mercy. When the Countess of Warwick Mary Rich first learned about her mother-in-law's illness in January 1667, her immediate response was to pray and meditate on death (see fig. 5). The doctors reported that the patient, Lady Manchester, might not survive the night. Rich rode from her estate in Essex to London to visit Lady Manchester the following day, spending the entire journey reflecting on death and her mother-in-law's readiness to face God's judgment. A genre of devotional literature known as *ars moriendi* taught pious men and women like Rich to make such observations as a spiritual exercise in preparation for death. The illnesses of friends and relatives, such as Lady Manchester, served as reminders of mortality, models of piety, and incidences of God's grace. Recording Lady Manchester's affliction enabled Rich to consider her own spiritual, mental, and physical readiness to meet God's judgment. As Rich eloquently put it, "Others mortalety might put me in mind of mine." After spending a week in London, Rich learned that Lady Manchester had lost her ability to speak. The news compelled Rich to consider how "my uoyce might be taken from me, and therfore it was good for me to make use of it whilst I had it to cry for mersy." Recording her mother-in-law's experience helped Rich to contemplate her own response to a potentially similar fate.[6]

Any illness could be one's last, and comporting oneself with humility and submission rather than fear and despair at the moment of death was a key indicator of salvation. The suffering of friends and family members could serve as models of this ideal suffering. Believers recorded how others endured bodily pain with calm and patience or how they peacefully quoted Scripture in spite of intense physical anguish. Individuals were explicit about documenting such examples in order to imitate them. While Rich did not provide details of Lady Manchester's final moments, she recounted the pious whispers of a friend who lay on her deathbed in 1670. This friend provided a valuable model for Rich, who prayed that she too "might upon my death bed be able to say as she did." Rich did not mention the particulars of her friend's utterances, though her words presumably included biblical passages, prayers, and expressions of gratitude that displayed piety and patience. In a spiritual diary covering the years 1721 and 1722, Ann Dawson similarly described how

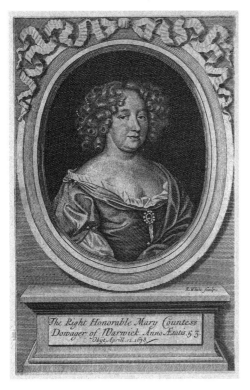

5. Portrait of Mary Rich, Countess of Warwick. Line engraving by Robert White, published in 1678, after an unknown artist's portrait. © National Portrait Gallery, London.

her sister endured a painful ailment in her neck "with a great Deal of patience oh that the same temper of mind was in me." By documenting the edifying experiences of others, believers learned how to suffer piously.[7]

Katherine Austen recorded the illness of a cousin's wife to generate feelings of gratitude toward God for her own preservation from death and also to evaluate her own relative health following a harrowing illness. The suffering of a cousin provided both a means of spiritual reflection and a tool of self-perception. Austen recorded the episode, as well as verses, meditations, prayers, and dreams, seven years after her husband's death in 1658. She described how "a uiolent cold in my head took away my hearing, my speech, my eye sight and uappours flew up almost continually as deffed [deafened] me in y^t manner I had scarce the benefit of my understanding." Shifts in body temperature resulting from colds could create emanations, or vapors, that drifted upward into the brain from the stomach. For Austen, these vapors interfered with her hearing, sight, and speech. She went on to explain how "troublesome business" accompanied the cold, though she was unable to dis-

cern whether the business matters intensified her illness or whether the illness made the "business so tedious to be endured." This "business" likely
referred to a lengthy legal battle over her family's property. The daughter of
a successful London cloth merchant, Austen married when she was just seventeen. By the age of thirty, she was a widow solely responsible for raising
three children and for resolving the unfinished business transactions of her
deceased husband and father-in-law. Austen never remarried, and she spent
a hefty portion of her twenty-five-year widowhood fighting to retain her husband's Middlesex property for their children. Though she could not clearly
discern how her financial situation affected her condition, comparing herself
to her cousin enabled Austen to make sense of her symptoms: "The original
of her illness, onely a cold in her head, caused the same effectes as fell to me
in my head." This comparison also facilitated a spiritual meditation on her
own preservation: "The Lord was pleased to let my glass run longer and giue
a final stop to this sweet good woman." Comparing herself to her cousin
helped Austen to evaluate the relative severity of her own ailment and to find
meaning in her recovery. She wrote these words during the year of a major
plague outbreak in London. Her recovery was probably even more pronounced given the death toll of the epidemic; most people who fell ill that
year did not live to write about it. She wisely fled the disease-ridden city
for Essex.[8]

A countess perhaps known best for her intellectual pursuits in philosophy suffered from lifelong debilitating headaches as a result of a fever she contracted at the age of twelve. The headaches confined Anne Conway to her
home, but not to her chamber. She frequently went on walks in the garden
and spent her days reading, writing, and contemplating complex philosophical questions. Her loved ones, particularly her longtime correspondent and
intellectual companion Henry More, marveled at the discrepancy between her
sharp intellect and frail body. "I could wish your body was in as good a plight
as your mind," he wrote to Conway in 1653. In the same letter, More shared
his suspicion that Conway's tireless study was to blame for her head pain: "You
must absteine not onely from reading but from thinking too intensely," he
commanded. She did not heed this advice but remained ever determined to
find a cure. Conway sampled a range of remedies and used her social position to consult preeminent medical men of the age, including William Harvey,
Thomas Willis, and Valentine Greatrakes, the seventh son of a seventh son,
who magically cured patients by stroking them with his hands. But even

these esteemed healers failed to relieve Conway's relentless pain. In 1657 her husband encountered a woman who had successfully recovered from the same ailment, and Conway expressed disappointment that he had not thought to ask the patient or her healer what particular remedies did the trick. She planned to "goe to towne" to visit the woman herself, though she remained pessimistic about her potential recovery, since she was "much worse then any hath been of the same distemper." Observing others enabled patients to evaluate the severity of their own ailments, as well as the potential efficacy of treatments.[9]

Elizabeth Freke diagnosed herself in 1697, in part by looking to the experiences of the maids and relatives around her. She had suffered from a string of physical trials before coming down with a violent fever while visiting her sister in London. "I fell downe quite sick att my deer sister Austins of a malignant feaver (of which my deer Lady Gettings dyed)," she recalled. She diagnosed herself with the same fever as that of her niece, Grace Gethin, the daughter of her sister Frances Norton. Freke explained how the fever kept her in bed for two months, "under the hand of doctters, apothicarys, and surgions. Affter two month this feaver fell into my left side and settled in my foott and ankle as black as cole; wher ill I lay of itt nott able to stir in my bed for neer three month more." According to the humoral framework of disease, fluxes and flows caused fevers to wander around the body and settle in discrete parts. In Freke's case, the fever resided in her ankle, as evidenced by its discoloration and eventual emission of fluid: "Itt broke when noe surjoin would meddle with itt." Perhaps Freke diagnosed herself with the same fever that her niece had because of its extremity. Gethin died just a month later, and Freke viewed their cases as part of a larger epidemic: the fever "rained much in London," Freke explained, and "aboundance dyed of itt." It is possible that the fever's location also caused Freke to make the comparison to her niece, although the fact that her maid allegedly fell ill of the same disorder, though "hers settled in her back," indicates that other symptoms led her to link the cases.[10]

Nine years after she recovered from this episode, Freke's husband, Percy, fell fatally ill from dropsy. Freke again compared her deteriorating health to that of a dying family member. Percy's illness began with shortness of breath, but just a few months later his leg and stomach swelled up, broke out in sores, and, according to Freke's calculation, excreted nine gallons of fluid. As a result of his condition, Percy had to sleep upright in a chair for months. The couple sought help from surgeons and physicians—they spent £1,150 on six healers throughout the six-month ordeal—but Freke herself also exerted a considerable amount of time and effort toward caring for Percy. She sat up with him at night and held his head "behind his chair in a fine hancher or napkin for fearc of his being choaked." In Percy's final days, Freke began to note the physical toll of this constant attendance, which led to her own "very ill condition." She compared her symptoms to those of her husband, who was also her cousin: "My left legg swell'd and broke likewise, butt nott as my deer cosins did." While Freke noted that her swelling broke differently than Percy's, she clearly viewed her ailment in relation to his condition. She suffered from "two great holles" in her leg, which excreted fluid in a manner that was eerily similar to Percy's dropsy, and she reckoned that her swellings, like her husband's, were fatal. Numerous patients in early modern England claimed to suffer in sympathy with loved ones, a phenomenon that chapter 3 discusses. These patients contracted illnesses that mirrored those of ailing friends and family members, a likeness that resulted from the supposed physiological effects of grief and sorrow. Freke looked to the body of her dying husband to better understand her own.[11]

Freke's role as nurse and healer during her husband's illness offers a possible explanation for the broader pattern in female authors' writing outlined here. Many early modern women, like Freke, spent their days tending to the bodies of others by watching and nursing ailing loved ones, delivering the children of friends and neighbors, and preparing the dead for burial. Middling- and lower-status women who worked as maidservants performed a range of other tasks that also entailed tending to bodies: they washed linens, emptied chamber pots, cooked and served food, brushed hair, and cared for children and the sick. Some older women worked as searchers in their parishes, a position that involved counting the deceased and reporting causes of death to parish officials. And women of all ranks were known to work in capacities that involved handling bodies in explicit ways: as healers, nurses, and midwives. Of course, many women were engaged in work that had nothing to do with bodies, such as single women who worked outside the family economy or those who earned wages as bakers, brewers, innkeepers, grocers, lace makers, weavers, milliners, and the like. Some women worked in trades long presumed to be dominated by men, such as engraving and printing, while independent and widowed women might own businesses or make ends meet by renting property or lending money. Decked with a ring of keys and an account book, some elite women were tasked with overseeing the management of their estates. Anne Dormer employed more than thirty servants at her home in Oxfordshire, and, as its mistress, she would have been responsible for hiring and firing maids, settling disputes, and supervising household accounts.[12]

Whether or not women actually tended to bodies day to day, prevailing representations of early modern women's work focused on domestic labor that primarily entailed "body work": bearing and rearing children; obtaining and cooking food; buying, making, and laundering linens; and nursing and treating the sick.[13] As the Spanish humanist Juan Luis Vives avowed, "the mannes duetie is to get, and the womans to kepe." These words appeared in his popular conduct manual, *The Instruction of a Christen [Christian] Woman*, originally published in 1524 and circulating in English translation five years later. The book walks through the characteristics of an ideal woman in this period and makes the case that her day-to-day duties entailed unpaid domestic work. In addition to rearing and nursing children, Vives's model woman managed the health care of her household: "She shulde knowe medicines and salves for suche diseasis as be comen, and rayne almost dayly: and have those medicines ever prepared redy in some closette, wherwith she may helpe her husbande, her lytle children, and her house holde meyne." Popular books on cookery and medicine with titles such as *The English House-Wife* and *The Good Houswife Made a Doctor* further cultivated the notion that feeding, touching, nursing, and healing other bodies were the responsibilities of women. Like Vives's prescriptive text, these books represented ideal women as virtuous and chaste but also in possession of "a Physical kind of knowledge, how to administer any wholsom receipts or medicines."[14] Such views of women's work suggest one reason why women like Freke looked to the bodies of others to make sense of their own. Female patients' tendency to observe others reflects prevailing representations of women's daily life and labor.

The ways these women used and shared medical knowledge further shaped the types of stories they told. Early modern men and women did not access knowledge in the same ways, since most women were denied entry to guilds and universities. Yet ordinary women amassed an understanding of health and healing in their daily lives that was similar and by no means inferior to that of their male counterparts. Some English gentlewomen followed Vives's above prescription by providing medical services to servants, family members, and neighbors. Recipe books illuminate these healing activities in upper-status early modern households. Recipes were not an all-female genre of writing. Men wrote and collected them too. But this is one of the only forms of early modern medical writing that substantial numbers of women authored. There are only a handful of known medical cases written by early modern women and even fewer medical treatises. Yet women collected and composed thousands of recipes. Moreover, the skills required to produce and test recipes—distilling, preserving, cooking, and gardening—were imagined to be within the compass of women's domestic labor. Recipes were the prime mode by which literate Englishwomen preserved and exchanged medical information.[15]

This method of producing and circulating medical knowledge suggests a second way women might have learned to tell stories about others' afflictions to better assess their own: recipes taught sufferers to define their ailments in relation to other people. A receipt was valued by its efficacy, which was validated by an author's name or the words *probatum est*, affirming the remedy was tried and true. Susannah Packe noted that a recipe for treating convulsions had been "Aproued by Ma:Sa: for all her Children was very successful," while a recipe Mary Hookes compiled for sore eyes included a note verifying that the remedy "cured the Lady Bechampe after the Docters had her in cure two years."[16] Assigning authorship or naming someone who had benefited from a recipe proved its worth and provided the means by which readers evaluated their own ailments, as they compared their experiences to those of the men and women recorded in the margins of recipe books. The circulation of recipes was an equally social process. Women copied down recipes that others prescribed, exchanged them as gifts, bequeathed them in wills, and transcribed them from published medical texts. When Elizabeth Hastings learned that her sister-in-law was sick, she penned a letter almost entirely devoted to the healing properties of snail water. She included a receipt for preparing the remedy, which is now lost but may have involved distilling a pasty mixture of crushed snails, milk, mint, nutmeg, and dates. Hastings also included directions for using the water (one spoonful taken with two to three spoonfuls of spa water) and even sent a bottle in the post so that her sister-in-law could "make a tryale of it." This communal production, circulation, and validation of lay medical knowledge taught sufferers to assess their ailing bodies by looking to the words and experiences of others. Hastings listed the people she knew who also found the snail water effective. "Lady

Ramsden from whom I had it has known surprizing Cases in Wastings of the Flesh," she wrote. Also, "my Sister Anns servant Mrs Dove is one instance who I believe woud not have been now alive but for it." Elizabeth Paston likewise recommended a therapy to her sister by considering their mother's experience: "If you think y^r illness proceeded in the least Manner like my mother I must repeate my petition to you to take away a little Blood this Spring time."[17] Just as other people's words and experiences verified a recipe, those words and experiences could help determine the nature, severity, and progression of sickness.

This trend of observing others' sufferings is also a consequence of what remains extant of women's writing from that period, which is overall more spiritual than self-writing by men. Pious authors recorded the afflictions of other people as meditations, as well as reminders of mortality and divine mercy. Observing others' ailments in order to express and gauge one's own was an understandable extension of this spiritual exercise. Perhaps this connection between spirituality and observation explains why, of the four men I have found who compared their ailments to others, three were deeply pious. Yet observations of others were instruments of not only spiritual self-assessment but also self-fashioning. Ego-literature provided many women with a quasi-public space in which to construct an identity for posterity. Many authors wrote to later generations, some even referring directly to their husbands, children, and grandchildren as readers. Recording the afflictions of others enabled some female authors to present themselves in particular ways— as pious, humble sufferers, for example. Lady Gethin and Percy Freke did not just suffer from symptoms similar to those of Elizabeth Freke; they died. Elizabeth could confirm the extremity of her condition by likening her disorder to the fatal ailments of others, thereby endowing her suffering with heightened spiritual significance. "Butt outt of this and all my other afflictions," she wrote as she recovered from that violent fever in 1697, "my greatt and good God delivered mee and raised mee up againe to know more of his mercyes." Freke's return from the brink of death was a remarkable mercy from heaven that demonstrated not only the intensity of her suffering but also the magnitude of her divine preservation.[18]

Stories about other people also modeled the ideal qualities authors endeavored to uphold, as well as the behaviors and characteristics writers most loathed. In this way, stories enabled individuals to formulate a particular image or self-construction through writing. Sarah Cowper recorded more stories than any other person in this book, perhaps because she was such a pro-lific writer. Her diary spans seven hefty volumes and includes detailed com-plaints about her disobedient servants, disputes with her controlling husband, and laments about her two ever-irreverent sons. Interspersed among these accounts are excerpts from sermons, books, and stories Cowper heard or read. Many of these stories documented fantastical tales for posterity, such as that of a thirty-year-old woman who bore thirty-one children. Most, however, served to provide moral lessons or kindle gratitude to God, as the above example from Katherine Austen exemplifies. Cowper neglected to ex-plain her criteria for gauging the suffering of others, but she routinely took walks to observe strangers on the street in order to evaluate her own state of health. For example, when she suffered from "a spice of rhumatism" in 1701, she described how her cough was so painful and her body so weak that she could barely move without help. Yet she somehow managed to leave the house to find people "who by their complaint seem'd to be worse case than my self. So home I came content with my own condition, nay since compared with things more greiuous I find it to be so tolerable as I ought to be uery thankfull."[19] Dwelling on the afflictions of others appeased Cowper's rela-tive sense of suffering and helped her to feel thankful for God's mercies.

Tales of others' suffering were also therapeutic, as they enabled Cow-per to express deep-seated fears and anxieties. She was particularly concerned about whether people's appearances, words, and behaviors accurately reflected their feelings, thoughts, and beliefs. She recounted how a group of ladies vis-ited a deranged countess who talked incessantly. The ladies laughed, sang ballads, and pretended to admire the countess, who in reality was "uery ridic-ulous." On witnessing this farce, Cowper noted that it "grieue'd me to see her so weak and them so false to their peers." She found the women's false sentiments distressing, even more so because she too was suffering from an aging, decaying mind. She articulated her fears by projecting her anxieties onto women who suffered from similar afflictions. Another elderly woman was overcome with a "loue whimsy," convinced that a young man with a great estate wished to marry her. The elderly woman believed the man's family "lay snares to murder her" because they disapproved of the match, and she prayed to God to deliver her from this fear where, according to Cowper, "no fear is." Cowper explained that she recorded this story in order to acknowledge gratitude for her own freedom from such "melancholly imaginations." Like this elderly woman, she was often overcome with paranoid delusions. As a result of a dream she had thirty years before beginning her diary, she was overwhelmed every year with fears of dying on June 29, her "Bodeing Day." She also suspected her sons of colluding against her, and on several occasions she believed her servants secretly threatened to harm her. Stories about others offered Cowper a means of expressing thanks to God for her preservations, and they held up mirrors of the behaviors and qualities she most vehemently feared. Telling stories allowed Cowper to fashion her identity and come to terms with it.[20]

"As I Used to Do": Observing the Self

Samuel Jeake took the time to document his life partly as a spiritual exercise. Recording God's providences enabled believers like Jeake to contemplate their spiritual progress by reflecting on past trials. Yet despite his more radical Protestant leanings, the Sussex merchant devoted little space to religious matters in his writing, instead focusing on astrological ones. He strived to link earthly events to the movements of the heavens. Jeake believed that God ordained the influence of the stars on terrestrial events, the same way pious patients believed that God's will operated through natural processes such as humoral flows. As such, he viewed astrology as a useful tool for documenting God's providences, but also for explaining terrestrial events and phenomena. Jeake fastidiously recorded significant moments in his life, including births, journeys, business ventures, and illnesses, in an attempt to connect them to astral causes. In instances of ill health, he noted the moment he fell ill, as well as significant symptoms, side effects, and the time he began to mend. He suffered primarily from agues, or recurring fevers. Jeake's meticulous attention to his habitual fevers, as well as their prevalence, influenced his understanding of illness more generally. Although he suffered from a range of health concerns, including melancholy and "noise in the ears," he perceived most of his bodily disorders within the frame of his recurring agues. When he was unsure of what ailed him, he described his body in familiar terms: as "aguish."[21]

The repetitive and quantifiable nature of this ailment—each fit began and ended at precise times and had a distinct temperature and location in the body—complemented the precise astrological computations necessary to determine the relationship between the body and the cosmos. The recurrent agues also enabled Jeake to read his own body rather than rely on the experiences of others. He discerned the nature, severity, and progression of his fevers by looking to prior sensations and experiences. He compared each bout of ague to the previous day's episode, using phrases such as "more benevolent than the former," "a greater shaking," "more sleepy," "but gentler." In addition to timing and severity, he noted where the fever lay in his body, its temperature, and the degree and timing of related processes, such as appetite, sweat, and sleep. A series of entries from December 1670 illustrates how Jeake traced these shifting symptoms over the course of several days:

> 6 About 7h 56' p.m. the 57th fit, like the 54th but my sweating was almost gone; continuing till about 11h p.m.
>
> 7 About 7h 48' p.m. the 58th fit, like the 55th but worse & some sweat: continuing till about 10h p.m. . . . .
>
> 11 About 8h 43' p.m. the 62th fit, like the 59th but without great shaking, continued till sleep came, in which I used to sweat.

According to Jeake's calculations, the fit on December 11 was the sixty-second instance of fever he endured in a row, though he compared its effects to those of the fifty-ninth fit, from a few days earlier. (During this period, he endured 142 consecutive episodes of fever.) By tracking his sickness from day to day, he could easily recognize diversions from expected disease trajectories. One day, he noted that "instead of my Ague I had 6 stools & somewhat more indisposed then ordinary." On other occasions, he struggled to fit his bodily experiences into the frame of sickness he had come to expect. When he anticipated a fever one day in 1672, he interpreted a barely perceptible physical sensation as a fit: "The 21th fit so little that the time of it's beginning was uncertain." Five years earlier he had noted having a fit that "could hardly be perceived." Based on careful observations, Jeake expected his body to behave in particular ways in accordance with the heavens.[22]

Jeake's reliance on past sensations and experiences stemmed, at least in part, from the nature of his recurring ailment and the structure and intentions of his astrological diary. And just as he looked to prior experiences to define and gauge the severity of his agues, so Ralph Thoresby noted "more severe pain in the back of my head than I have had for several years past." Thomas Mort suspected gout in his hip "because it seized me about this time twelue monith," and Samuel Pepys continually noted whether bodily disturbances reminded him of ailments from years past or caused him to feel or behave "as I used to do." Pepys was particularly observant of his body and

environment, sometimes making connections between recent and prior illnesses by comparing the weather at each time. In 1664 he thought there were
fleas in his bed when he awoke in the night from itchy, inflamed skin. After
rising, however, he noted that the weather had suddenly shifted from hot to
cold, "which (as I was two winters ago) doth stop my pores, and so my blood
tingles and iches all day all over my body and so continued to do, all the day
long just as I was then."[23] By comparing the current weather to conditions
from years earlier, Pepys was able to attribute his affliction to clogged pores,
which prevented humors from excreting outward. His surgeon reassured him
that taking remedies to provoke sweats and open the body would cure the
disorder, as it had two years earlier. Writing by other men shows a similar
tendency to look to the past in order to better understand the present. These
authors used phrases such as "my old pain" or "my old complaint" to describe
their illnesses. Like Jeake, who associated aches in his back, sweats in his sleep,
and even "twitching pain in my right Eyebrow" with his agues, these sufferers placed various aches and pains within the frames of their particular known
and recurring bodily disorders.[24]

　　These self-assessments commonly included a specific bodily process:
outflow. A healthy body in early modern England was defined partly by easy
intake and outgo. Obstructions resulting from corrupt blood, accumulated
humors, or clogged pores were dangerous to health, whereas an open body
in constant flux was desirable. As a result of these beliefs, the quality, quantity, and consistency of emitted bodily fluids could be key determinants of disease progression and severity. In particular, many observed the quantity and
quality of their stools. In a letter to his physician, Hans Sloane, Robert Herbert
described searching his excrement for "eggs," presumably some sort of foreign matter that he and Sloane believed to be at the root of his disorder.
Herbert went on to describe a range of symptoms, including cold, blackened
gums, and "a tast in my Mouth Just the same as the begining of a Flux." Yet
he seemed to view his condition nearly entirely in terms of his bowels: "But
My Bowells are so prodigiously out of order & inclinable to be lose, tho. I
haue seldom more than two stools p r day, & tho I haue no Great pain with em
yet It feels as if My Guts came away at the same time, & my Countenance
immeadiately after a stool Grows more pale and Wan than before, & my spirits Quite sunk for some time after, & am a good Deal fallen away." He felt
obliged to record the consistency and quantity of his bowel movements and,
perhaps most important, the effects of physically relieving himself. As he ex-

plained, releasing his bowels felt like a more significant evacuation, "as if My Guts came away." Perhaps he linked these bowel-related problems to his other symptoms because relieving himself caused such drastic shifts in his mood and health: he turned pale, grew depressed, and felt "a good Deal fallen away." In a follow-up letter, Herbert's wife suggested that the disorder originated from poor digestion rather than kidney stones, a prior diagnosis.[25]

Herbert's case illustrates how quantifying output could provide key insights into internal processes, enabling patients to diagnose their ailments, trace the progression of disorders, and gauge the efficacy of remedies intended to disperse humors outward. Bodily excretions visibly demonstrated a shift in the balance of humors or the release of pent-up matter. Seeing fluid emit from the body verified that a much-needed change had occurred. When James Clegg fell ill from a fever in 1731, he focused on his excretions to trace the disorder's progression. On the morning after first falling ill, he noted that he had "low urine almost blood red but let fall an encouraging sediment." Clegg was a clergyman who had taken up medicine part-time to make ends meet. Perhaps his medical expertise gave him insight into the various indications of sediment. He also self-prescribed a number of remedies over the course of his illness, including a vomit, "powders that I give in such Fevers" to expel corruptive humors through urine and sweat, and a plaster made of herbs that he applied topically to his skin to create blistering in order to release offending matter. Clegg also chewed rhubarb to open his bowels, and he counted his stools to measure its effects: "It gave me two or 3 stools and I hope did me service." A significant number of men from the period quantified their bodily output in similar ways, in order to trace the progression of illness and the efficacy of purgative remedies. In Clegg's case, the treatments were ineffective; his fever continued for weeks.[26]

Observing the bowels to evaluate health had a humoral logic, yet contemporary women rarely seemed to make this move. Men and women alike understood that the quality and quantity of stools were important indicators of illness and that a healthy body was defined, in part, by regular outflow. Reproductive processes, such as menstruation and lactation, encouraged continual attention to outflow, presumably making women more likely than men to evaluate illness by observing their bodily excretions. And women noted the benefits of open, running sores, which signified the removal of potentially harmful or imbalanced humors. Referring to a nasty, weeping wound, one woman wrote, "If it should stope sodenley it would be much wores for my health." While women clearly understood the benefits of unobstructed outflow and sometimes noted the quality or regularity of their menstrual flows in letters to physicians, I have found only three instances in which women explicitly referred to their stools in writing. All three cases were recorded in letters to Hans Sloane, perhaps because he made it a rule to inquire about this particular bodily function.[27]

It might not seem surprising that early modern patients observed others and themselves to make sense of illness. What are surprising, however, are the broad patterns in men's and women's self-writing: more women told stories about others, while men tended to focus on their own previous bodily processes, especially the quantity and quality of their stools—a clear physiological yardstick for evaluating health. One possible explanation for these findings is the nature of the ailments themselves. Perhaps more of the men here suffered from chronic disorders and so looked to their own prior experiences, while more women contracted contagious ailments that compelled them to note the experiences of others. Jeake and Pepys suffered from long-term ailments, which certainly informed their narratives. But many men endured acute disorders, while numerous women suffered from chronic ones. Cowper continually experienced rheumatic pains, sore eyes, and cramping, for instance, while Freke suffered from successive episodes of "tissick," and Conway endured chronic headaches. To explain these patterns in men's writing, I now return to the three influences that informed women's accounts: the types of personal writing these patients produced, gendered representations of lives and work, and the compilation and use of medical knowledge.

Just as pious women contemplated the significance of their suffering in self-reflective religious musings, men too kept spiritual journals. But many men possessed motivations for keeping diaries that are less common among writing by women, such as documenting political work or military feats. Astrologers like Jeake were intent on linking the details of daily life to the cosmos, a concern that resulted in careful self-observations. We can only speculate as to why the enigmatic Pepys chose to record the details of his daily life. He fastidiously noted all the items he purchased, each book he read, and every play he attended. As discussed below, his meticulous account keeping stemmed not only from his unique personality and the daily act of private writing but also from the broader influences of his intellectual community. Although Pepys's writing was by no means spiritual, he shared with pious authors a motivation for keeping a diary: self-improvement. Methodical documentation of work and worldly pleasures seemed to provide him with a means of self-evaluation and self-discipline. For the more devout, writing also provided a way to record life events in order to interpret and learn from them. Writing in the early 1700s, Dudley Ryder offered this explanation for keeping a diary: "To review any parts of my life, have the pleasure of it if it be well spent, if otherwise know how to mend it. It will help me to know myself better and give a better judgement of my own ability and what I am best qualified for." Pepys's biographer Claire Tomalin suggests another possible motivation for Pepys's diary keeping: writing enabled him to reflect on his life and also to relive it. This conflation of author and audience was also a common precept of spiritual diary keeping, which entailed rereading prior entries in order to consider God's past mercies and punishments.[28]

Many of the men in this book kept diaries to record social and spiritual concerns in combination with business matters. Thomas Tyldesley drew a line down the right side of the pages of his notebook to create a hybrid diary–account book. Next to the details of the weather and his day-to-day social engagements, he made careful tabulations of every pence he spent. The entry from February 4, 1714, notes the company he kept but also the cost of each item he purchased that day: "P^d pro horses 4s., pro servants' meat 1s., and 1s. 8d. pro ale; and gave the maide 1s., and ye boy 6d." His accounts of ill health relied on similar quantifications. Just a few days later, Tyldesley developed a headache and a "griping paine" in his body. He began taking purgatives prescribed by a doctor and meticulously calculated the number of times the pills "worked" on his body by loosening his bowels: "Only purg^d 2 or 3 time, and once in the night." The following day, February 12, Tyldesley was "very uneassy with ye gripes, and 3 purging stooles per diem, and 2 per N—tem." The conventions and aims of account keeping could lead to such terse narratives of illness, reliant on quantification and objective signifiers like stool counts. Walter Powell perhaps was most curt of all: "January I was sick all the while"; "ffebruary, I was sick"; "March, Still sick."[29]

Edmund Harrold kept his diary to document business transactions and to review and improve his life: "I pray god it may haue this effect on me to mend what I haue in my power to mend for ye time to come." He struggled to fulfill his spiritual duties, and he faced one significant secular challenge: moderating his drinking. His drunken "rambles" commonly resulted in illness that diminished his strength, impaired his reason, and exposed a lack of self-control—significant components of masculinity in early modern

England. He noted being indisposed, or "ill disordered," from drink yet unable to stop himself: "Ill al day but kept tipling." Drinking also undermined his economic autonomy, making him physically unable to complete his work. His wife had to take in washing to make ends meet. Harrold quoted sermons, recorded spiritual lessons from devotional texts, and fretted about the spiritual and financial consequences of his excessive drinking, but much of his diary concentrates on the number of wigs he sold and books he traded: "Im' begune JC's wig I'm going to seek hair but got none JW offered me but 12^s in b[oo]ks for A[mbrose's] works again I swapt 1 wig wth Rob Parley of white heauen for 1 wig & 2 boxes long ones of wood spent it wth tarbock &c 9[d] this day & night came in almost 1 a clock swapt & unswapt wth RP to please wife neglect of pub[lic] pra[yer]: 1 time priu[ate]: 2 times ye world is uanity" (fig. 6). For Harrold, self-writing was a way to document business ventures and calculate expenditures. Quantifiable accounts of illness reflect the intentions and conventions of this type of writing. In September 1712, for example, he simply noted, "I'm much indisposed as I was this day [last?] month." Indeed, accounting seemed to shape Harrold's documentation of all kinds of life experiences. In the entry about wigs above, he counts the number of private and public prayers he skipped, and he expresses spiritual anxiety by reminding himself that all attempts at worldly gain are vanity. He even routinely calculated how often and for how long he had sexual relations with his wife: "On ye 9th at night I did wife 2 tymes couch and bed in an hour an 1/2 time." As tabulations of daily minutiae rather than realms for self-expression, diaries like Harrold's facilitated such quantifications.[30]

Such modes of writing reflect authors' occupational roles. Many of the men in this study used mathematics in their day-to-day lives—to invest their fortunes, charge rents, pay taxes, calculate weights and measures, purchase supplies, and track sales. Roger Lowe probably kept a book to record debit and credit transactions for the shop he oversaw in Ashton. He also used his numerical skills by working as an accountant in his community, sometimes accepting payment in pints of ale. Merchants such as Thoresby and Jeake required a similar mastery of arithmetic for compiling invoices, drawing up bills of sale, and tracking liabilities and assets. Jeake probably learned these skills from his father, who wrote a treatise titled *Arithmetick Surveighed and Reviewed*. As a naval administrator, Pepys needed math to calculate ships' inventory, settle accounts, measure timber, and draft sea charts. Because he was not formally trained in arithmetic, he hired a tutor to help him improve

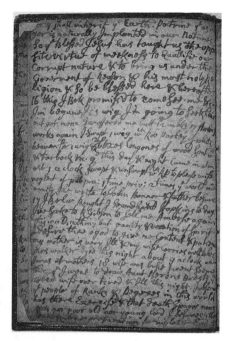

6. A page from Edmund Harrold's diary,
His Book of Remarks and Observations,
1712–16, f. 3v, MS Mun. A.2.137, Chetham's.
By permission of Chetham's Library.

the skills required for his post, and throughout July 1662 he grumbled about memorizing his multiplication tables.[31] While Pepys had to make up for lost time, merchants, carpenters, seamen, surveyors, farmers, brewers, and men of "common capacities" learned to determine interest rates and calculate the contents of casks using guides, such as John Mayne's *Arithmetick Vulgar, Decimal, and Algebraical*. A similar manual titled *Every Man His Own Gauger* instructed "the most ignorant, who can but read English, and tell twenty in figures," how to quantify the content of vessels, as well as the price of various goods according to weight.[32] These guides constituted a genre of vernacular writing that taught readers the calculations required for daily life and work. Perhaps not surprisingly, some merchants and shopkeepers evaluated their bodies the same way they approached the rest of life—by using numbers.

Women too participated in the credit economy, which required an understanding of mathematics. Some worked in the same trades as men— as laborers, shopkeepers, and helpmeets to their husbands or fathers. And gentlewomen typically kept account books in which they calculated household expenses, wages of servants, and collections of rent. Despite these realities, arithmetic was not a standard component of girls' education, nor was it typically associated with women's work. Numbers were presumed to be the preoccupation of men, even though, in practice, women also possessed and employed such knowledge.[33] Guides on accounting and bookkeeping assumed a male readership, such as John Vernon's *The Compleat Compting-House; or, The Young Lad Taken from the Writing-School, and Fully Instructed, by Way of Dialogue, in All the Mysteries of a Merchant.* In the increasingly commercial and global markets of early modern England, the labor of middling- and upper-status men was typically associated with maintaining credit relations, making calculations, and performing transactions—a world of commerce that required knowledge of numbers and the cultivation of male trust networks.[34] These views and representations of gendered work did not always map onto reality, but their prevalence in seventeenth-century England contextualizes patterns in patients' writing. Some of the men in this book quantified their bodily disorders because they documented their health in different kinds of writing than that of their female counterparts. Yet others, such as Thoresby and Pepys, did not keep hybrid diary–account books and still quantified illness in ways seldom found in writing by women. This tendency to count bodily disorders reflects the conventions of some men's personal writing but also prevailing beliefs about what it meant to be a successful artisan, merchant, or shopkeeper in early modern England. Such beliefs explicitly taught men to think and write in numbers and could implicitly inform self-presentations on the page.

Finally, several of the men in this book observed their bodies as part of a larger enterprise of exploring the operations of the natural world. Women were also deeply invested in health matters, and some carried out experiments in their homes.[35] Yet Samuel Jeake's astrological goals made him meticulously attentive to bodily signs in a way that Elizabeth Freke or Alice Thornton would never be. He made these self-observations to test and reform astrology as a set of principles for explaining life events and natural phenomena. He even codified his findings in "Astrologicall Experiments Exemplified," a treatise he presented to the London astrologer Henry Coley in 1694. While Jeake seemed to consider his ailing body in traditional humoral terms, he read books that challenged orthodox humoralism and promoted alternative, chemical frameworks for viewing the body and treating disease. He self-prescribed and administered some of these chemical remedies, including a purge composed of an "Infusion of Crocus Metallorum." He even owned a still for making these concoctions at home. Jeake's intellectual pursuits extended into areas beyond astrology and medicine as well: he read literature and theology, studied physiognomy, took up Hebrew, and recorded weather patterns and natural phenomena, such as eclipses and earthquakes.[36]

Pepys also identified with a culture of observation. Elected as a member of the Royal Society in 1665, he was immersed in an environment of experimentation intent on unlocking the secrets of the natural world. Although he was no natural philosopher, he read learned treatises, corresponded with renowned thinkers, and attended lectures and experiments at the Royal Society. He directed the same focus and curiosity toward his own body. He noted everything that went into his body and came out of it and linked weather conditions and physical sensations to those from years past. To our view, Pepys's resulting narrative documents the bodily habits of a man seemingly obsessed with illness. According to one calculation, he mentions his health 489 times in his nine-volume diary. He also took advantage of his intellectual community to develop a deeper understanding of his ordeals. He attended public anatomy lectures, including one on the kidneys, where he convinced the lecturer at the reception to show him "the manner of the disease of the stone and the cutting and all other Questions that I could think of." The empiricism that defined the intellectual community at the Royal Society perhaps encouraged Pepys to observe and assess his bodily processes. Despite the uniqueness of his and Jeake's personalities and intellectual environments, both point to how other men in this study, such as Harrold, Clegg, and Thoresby (also a fellow of the Royal Society), might have come to rely on similar empirical self-assessments to understand their bodies. This culture of observation was by no means exclusively male. Indeed, the compulsion to examine natural processes in order to better understand them underlies the inclination to monitor the ailments of others. Sarah Cowper's assertion that "want of obseruation and Experience of other folks affairs . . . made me think my self worse perplext than most people" speaks to the value of everyday observations as a means of better understanding one's ailing body and oneself.[37]

The Embodiment of Devotion

Religion offered early modern men and women a third fund of stories for making sense of suffering. Concerns about piety and morality could be deeply embedded in explanations of physical impairment, as evidenced by the appropriations of Augustine's *Confessions* that open this chapter. Believers in this period were taught to view even the most trivial events as providential signs—messages from God that imparted key spiritual lessons. Illness could be a chastisement for sin as well as a manifestation of God's grace, a means of imitating Christ, a test of faith, a reflection of moral decay, or a reminder of mortality—to name but a few possibilities. Yet religion in early modern England entailed more than just a set of doctrinal beliefs. A pious life also included day-to-day devotional activities, such as singing, praying, reading, and meditating. Devout men and women viewed these, as well as many other dimensions of religious practice, in somatic terms. Take John Bunyan's account of spiritual conversion in his popular autobiographical narrative *Grace Abounding to the Chief of Sinners:* "Then was I struck into a very great trembling, insomuch that at sometimes I could for whole days together feel my very body as well as my minde to shake and totter under the sence of the dreadful Judgement of God, that should fall on those that have sinned that most fearful and unpardonable sin. I felt also such a clogging and heat at my stomach by reason of this my terrour, that I was, especially at some times, as if my breast-bone would have split in sunder."[38] In addition to feeling his body tremble, Bunyan characterized his fear and guilt the same way a patient might describe impending illness: as a warm, clogging sensation in the stomach. Spirituality was experienced in the body, in shaking limbs and stuffed-up stomachs.

Just as Bunyan endured tightening, trembling feelings of guilt during his conversion, pious individuals were assured of properly attending to Scripture or receiving God's grace upon sensing a physical alteration, such as a stir, prick, or burn. Protestant doctrine referred to the reception of divine grace as a "quickening" of the soul, a phrase that connoted a particular bodily sensation for some women. *Quickening* also referred to the moment when a pregnant woman first felt her fetus move within the womb, marking the beginning of life. As both a medical and a religious term, *quickening* represented an acute moment of renewal and generation. Any mother surely associated the sensation of a quickened spirit with the feeling of a fetus stirring to life. Conversely, some pious authors used the term *barren* to describe the inability to pray or receive God's grace.[39] Whether quickened or barren, believers associated the physical state required for spiritual meditation and prayer with particular bodily sensations. As such, the devout were just as keen self-observers as men like Samuel Pepys and Samuel Jeake. The desired devotional disposition was a tenuous one, however. Illness could either enable or inhibit the proper meditative state required to receive God's grace. Bodily suffering was spiritually valuable because it evoked reminders of mortality and gratitude to God, but it could also be an impediment to devotion.

Mary Rich struggled at times to attain this proper devotional state. Each morning, she meditated in her garden, which she referred to as "the wilderness," perhaps borrowing from biblical accounts of prophets overcoming hardship in the wild. After two hours of meditating and preparing her soul for prayer, she retired to her closet to read Scripture and pray privately before attending family prayers. She repeated these spiritual exercises in the afternoon, in addition to reading devotional texts, fulfilling her social obligations, and completing her household chores. Rich had not always been so devout. Until her marriage to Charles Rich in 1641, Mary Boyle had lived a fairly secular life in Cork and later in London, where she spent most of her time carousing at court. She described those years as a time of "uanety, misspending my preatious time in reading romances and in seeing and reading playes, and in dressing and adorneing my uile body." When she moved into the home of her husband's parents, the political and social upheaval of the times, the piety of her father-in-law, and the religious fervor of the nonconforming preachers who visited the household all began to affect her. By 1647, Rich had experienced a full spiritual conversion.[40]

One morning in 1668 she was unable to carry out her spiritual meditations on account of a violent headache. Instead of feeling warm and open to her spiritual duties, she found herself "somthing dull and indisposed." She meditated on the suffering of Christ and "indeauered by all the awakening considerations I could to stur upe my heart and prayde to God to remoue the indisposition that was upon me." By *indisposition* Rich did not refer to her head pain; a believer accepted such a worldly affliction as an edifying sign of God's grace. Rather, she was describing her heart's inability to attain the pliable, receptive frame necessary to "poure out my soule in prayer to God." This devotional aim is a central theme throughout Rich's diary and provided the framework for her constructions of illness. Although her headache returned that afternoon and grew "uery uiolent," she was able to attend church, "though I fond still that by reason of my bodely distemper I was somthing duller then useall yet I fond the deasires of my heart went out after God." As opposed to citing the source of her ailment or recounting her symptoms, Rich defined her impairment solely in terms of its effects on her spiritual state: "somthing duller then useall." Her headache prevented her from fulfilling her spiritual duty by making her feel dull and distracted rather than sharp and ready to commune with God. The impact of her ailing body on her devotional practice shaped Rich's perceptions of ill health.[41]

At times she could successfully overcome her physical infirmity to attend to devotional duties. The process of elevating mind and soul over body in this way provoked gratitude toward God and facilitated subsequent meditations on mortality. Physical sensations, most especially bodily pain, promoted spiritual awareness by providing an opportunity to express penitence and separate oneself from worldly cares. Yet Rich and several other contemporary diarists show that, in practice, illness more often than not impeded spiritual aims. Sometimes ill health simply created scheduling problems. By remaining in bed too long, Rich squandered the allotted time in her day for spiritual duties. For the most part, however, colds, headaches, and fevers made her physically incapable of focusing her mind on religious exercises. Likewise, when a swollen face and aching teeth prevented Elias Pledger from performing his public and private prayers in 1695, he prayed for instruction: "How doe I at such a time either wholly omit my duty or performe it uery coldly & by halues." Common sources of ill health, such as social interactions and intense emotions, could also lead to physical infirmities that interfered with devotional aims. Rich often felt ill and weak following passionate arguments with her husband, which "dispirited and unfitted me for any spirituall inployment." Anxiety over domestic grievances and unsettling conversations similarly put Sarah Cowper into such disordered mental and bodily states that her soul often followed suit. At times her encounters with servants were so "sharp and so disturbing as I cou'd not attend to my accustom'd deuotion."[42]

Illness could have such profound effects on devotional exercises because praying and meditating were embodied practices. The heart had to be in a particular physical state—open, warm, broken, melted—to receive the grace of God. This pliable, repentant frame is depicted in biblical accounts of God's word inscribing the "fleshy tables of the heart" and of believers possessing a "broken and a contrite heart," like wax "melted in the midst of my bowels."[43] Pious women like Rich punctuated their spiritual meditations with moans, sighs, and groans in order to warm the heart and invite God's love to "make great worke In my breast." In 1671, Rich described achieving such a state following her daily meditation: "I was inabled to offer upe the sacrefice of a brocun and of a Contrite heart, and with many tears, grones, and sithes [sighs] to bemone my unequall walkeing with God, and in an especiall maner my heart was brocun for that dullnes that had bene upon me for some dayes." The emotional and spiritual effects of devotional reading helped to induce this receptive, supple frame. In *A Way to the Tree of Life*, John White instructed readers to discover the true sense of a passage from Scripture, apply the words directly to their own condition, and "whet them upon our hearts, till they warme, and quicken our affections." Rich noted the positive effects of devotional reading and continually reread her diary to stir and heat her heart by reflecting on past sins and divine preservations from death.[44]

Although some men in early modern England achieved a "sweet melting duty" and "wonderfull melting frame" during meditation, not all men were able to assume such vulnerability without challenging masculine ideals. Indeed, I have found that only Protestant clergymen describe devotional practice in these terms. For less pious men or for those who were not church officials, groaning, moaning, and weeping could threaten important manly markers of bodily control and self-mastery.[45] But the warm, broken frame required to receive God's grace resonated with seventeenth-century feminine virtues of docility, passivity, and humility. Moreover, there were long-lasting associations between women's flesh and piety that made this state particularly accessible to women. In the thirteenth century, female mystics commonly attributed positive spiritual significance to extreme bodily suffering and exhibited paramystical phenomena—miraculous bleeding, lactating, and fasting, or incorruptibility after death—more frequently than male saints. These women experienced and expressed piety through their bodies, often conflating the spiritual and the corporeal. They kissed God, tasted him, and entered his heart and body. Indeed, the ascetic practice of fasting so often associated with female mystics was understood to entail an ecstatic, mystical union with Christ. While Protestants like Rich did not see themselves as participating in Christ's suffering, they did describe a similar somatic connection between soul and God. The Holy Spirit penetrated and melted Rich's body, a sensual and deeply emotional experience that resulted in swoons, moans, and tears. Seventeenth-century Protestants are largely incomparable to thirteenth-century saints, yet they demonstrate the endurance of these medieval associations between women's flesh and devotion. Such continuities suggest how women in the seventeenth century might have experienced the physical dimensions of devotional practices differently than men, by being more attentive to and articulate about the connection between their spirituality and their physicality.[46]

When believers were unable to attain a warm, broken, awakened state, they characterized themselves in completely opposite terms: as cold, hard, and dull. These men and women also appropriated the vocabulary of illness, describing themselves as out of order, indisposed, frigid, senseless, languid, dead, lifeless, discomposed, out of tune, ill tempered, and frail.[47] Because illness was often the cause of such a state, authors looked to the language of the ailing body to articulate the sensations of spiritual infirmity. Furthermore, the physical sensations of ill health in this period—feeling clogged up from obstructed or imbalanced humors—directly contrasted with the open, porous frame required for spiritual duties. Believers described the origin, development, and removal of their spiritual distempers the same way they might characterize a physical ailment. The affliction lingered for a few days, growing more severe, until finally they took the necessary steps—attending church, reading Scripture—to overcome it.

Rich looked to the vocabulary of illness to articulate her devotional ability, in part because her spiritual and physical impairments were so inextricably entwined. Indeed, it is difficult to differentiate her accounts of devotional and physical infirmity because she used precisely the same terms to describe both states: ill, indisposed, given to "sithing fits." After noting an illness and her subsequent inability to pray, Rich often neglected to follow up on her physical ailment. She instead focused on her spiritual debility, as though the two disorders merged into one. For instance, after suffering from illness for nearly a week in 1675, she stopped writing about her physical suffering altogether but continued to assert that she was "sik of aspirituall lethargye." At another point she was ill and unable to perform her spiritual duties on account of exceedingly hot weather. For the next three days, she noted the progression of both disorders: "Still dull and dispirited being still much indisposed in my health." Although she presumably continued to suffer physically, the subsequent entries only mention her continued devotional deficiency: "In the mo[rning] I red, me[ditated] and prayd but my wiked heart still continued In adull and disperited temper In all my performanses." When the hot weather finally lifted, Rich only noted the removal of her spiritual infirmity, though this development implied a recovery from her physical impairment as well. Because she conceived of illness wholly in terms of its effects on her spirituality, she conflated her accounts of spiritual and physical distempers. Illness

did not just provide a vocabulary or metaphor for articulating spiritual debility; the two states were inseparable.[48]

For Rich, the body, mind, and soul were deeply entwined. There was
an imperceptible line between physical and spiritual impairment. The inability to properly meditate and pray was articulated as—and physically felt
like—being sick. As a result, spirituality provided an important frame for
Rich's assessments and descriptions of illness. Even when not attempting to
pray, she viewed physical alterations in spiritual terms. Becoming overheated
from exercise, for instance, reminded her of the warmth she felt in her heart
during meditation.[49] While her diary perhaps shows most clearly how illness
provided a vocabulary for describing devotional experience, the arrow pointed
in both directions. Devotional acts in turn shaped conceptions of illness. Rich
viewed her ailing body not according to the vicissitudes of humoral flows but
as a barometer of spirituality.

Rich's piety was central to her conceptions and constructions of illness,
and so was the genre of her writing. She probably modeled her diary on the
spiritual journal John Beadle promoted in his 1656 sermon *The Journal or Diary
of a Thankful Christian*.[50] Beadle touted diary writing as a process of spiritual
account keeping, a means of cataloguing each day's events to enforce adher-
ence to religious duties and to evaluate spiritual progress. As a result of this
prescribed mode of writing, as well as the routine nature of her days, Rich's
diary is extraordinarily formulaic. Most entries begin with an account of her
morning meditations and the frame of her heart: "In the morneing as sone as
I waked I blest God, then I reatired in to the willderness to meditate, but
finding upon my selfe auery disturbeing fitt of the spleene I was by it much
unfitted for the duty." She used this wording so often that she resorted to abbreviations by the fourth volume of her diary: "In the m as sone as I w I B G
I spent not so much time as useall at my deuotiones haueing a distemper then
upon me."[51] Rich used private writing to document the routine activities that
constituted her days. The repetitive nature of her spiritual exercises and the
dailiness of the diary enabled her to evaluate her devotions in much the same
way diary writing made it possible for men like Jeake to tabulate his agues.

Devotional texts further taught pious individuals like Rich how to respond to ill health by modeling exemplary behavior. *Ars moriendi* literature,
on the "art of dying," taught devout readers how to suffer on the deathbed in
preparation for death. Illness was a sort of practice run for the much-anticipated
moment when the soul would depart the body. Readers learned to display their

piety by quoting Scripture, to demonstrate their submission to God by accepting death patiently, and to confirm their imminent salvation by repenting their sins. As John Kettlewell explained in his 1695 *Death Made Comfortable*,
when the body falls ill, the soul is apt to fall ill along with it. The soul becomes
distressed, careless, and inattentive to religious duties. To prevent such a state,
the sufferer must "order his Carriage well under his Sickness, or to bear the
pains and weakness of his Sick bed, with Trust in God, with Resignation to
his will, with Thankfulness, and with Patience to the end."[52] We have seen
how devout women like Rich recounted stories of ailing friends as models of
this pious behavior.

Thomas Becon's popular devotional manual *The Sycke Mans Salue* outlines an exemplary response to physical suffering. Restraining fear, anger,
and uneasiness demonstrated an acceptance of God's will in the face of ill
health. Becon wrote, "I beseche thee for Christes sake, to geue me a pacient
and thankefull hart, that I neuer grudge against thy blessed will, but be obe-
dient unto it in all thinges, that whan the pains of my sicknes be most bitter:
I may lift up my hart unto thee, cal on thy blessed name, and say: O Lorde,
rebuke me not in thy indignation, nether chasten me in thy displeasure." A
true believer chose suffering over a desire to die, trusting that God would not
send an affliction that he or she would be unable to tolerate. Patience was key
to demonstrating such acceptance. Displaying patience required not necessarily a lack of sighs, groans, or complaints—what the devotional author Jeremy
Taylor called "the sad accents of a sick mans language"—but rather a lack of
despair. Fear and distress epitomized a refusal or inability to accept God's
will. Even Christ in his final moments "cried out with a loud voice, and resolved to die."[53] A patient sufferer sighed and complained without fear.
Demonstrating submission to God required expressions of humility, obedience, and repentance.

Despite deep-seated anxieties about death, Sarah Cowper exemplified
such patience and submission by resigning herself to near-constant bodily sufferings. Upon sensing pain in her shoulder in 1701, she explained how being
"ouer solicitous to haue any one Temporal Euil remou'd" was fruitless, since
"in a moment another, and perhaps a worse may succeed." A year later she
endured a series of aches and pains, particularly a cramp in her side and tenderness in her foot. After three weeks she began to mend. Her fever let up, her
spirits lifted, and she was able to perform her religious duties. She expressed gratitude to God for her improvement: "In all this time I had not

been dismay'd with the fears of Death, nor the Terror of Temptation in any kind; nor ouer eager desires of hauing my life prolong'd, but was quiet content, and as to life or Death resign'd to the will of God." Cowper presents herself here as a model sufferer. She did not complain or question her fate. She was not overwhelmed with fears of death but instead accepted her pain calmly, patiently, and, perhaps most important, "resign'd to the will of God."[54]

One woman wrote in her spiritual journal that God sent worldly trials "not as an angry judge, but as a mercifull father, not as figures of his Displeasure, but as Testimonies of his favor." According to this view, illness was an affliction from heaven but also a sign of divine grace. God chastised only his children, and all of the afflictions he sent were merciful and edifying. Demonstrating such beliefs, William Coe's account of a nineteen-day illness in 1704 ends not with dejection and despair but with the assertion that "it was good for me that I was afflicted."[55] Viewing impairment as a manifestation of godly love encouraged believers to treat illness as a valuable opportunity to acknowledge sin and exercise virtue. If there was no particular sin that had incited the illness, sufferers considered their life's sins, including past repented ones. Patients' tendencies to respond to bodily disorders with gratitude and humility reflect this view. As one woman put it, "I find my afflictions as profitable as they are unpleasing." And Rich even asked God to send "bodely torments to mind us of fleeing from eternall ones."[56] Illness was a valuable lesson from God, and devout sufferers were grateful for it as such, as well as for God's decision to spare them a worse fate.

As an opportunity to reflect on sin, illness promoted a turning toward God and away from worldly concerns. Jeremy Taylor explained, "One fit of the stone takes away from the fancies of men all relations to the world and secular interests." To demonstrate this pious turn inward, devotional literature instructed sufferers to pray fervently and continually. Prayers could not nullify past sins, but they could demonstrate virtue and communicate desire for divine pity, "piercing the clouds, and making the heavens like a pricked eye to weep over us." Religious texts on death and illness devoted a substantial number of pages to prayers in order to promote properly pious responses to debility and to discourage improper, impious ones. Compiled from Scripture, these prayers offered detailed accounts of suffering that certainly influenced patients' articulations of their ailments. A prayer in Kettlewell's *Death Made Comfortable* begins, "Lord, look upon mine Adversity and Misery, which call aloud to thee for ease. For [I am wither'd like grass, and my Bones will scarce cleave to my skin. My heart panteth, and my strength faileth me, and mine eyes are grown dim And] there is no soundness in my flesh, because of thine anger, nor rest in my bones because of my sin [Yea, my bones are burnt as an Hearth, and] I go mourning all the day long, and wearisom nights are appointed to me, and I am full of tossing to and fro unto the dawning of the day." Readers were directed to alter the bracketed expressions according to their particular ailments.[57] Pious sufferers could find the words to express their bodily afflictions by opening a book and reading from its pages.

Aside from Christ's Passion, perhaps the most influential story of suffering in this period was the Book of Job. Job lost his wealth, livestock, family, and servants, and his body was covered with ulcerous boils to the extent that his friends barely recognized him. He responded to these afflictions with patience and submission, explaining that God had only taken from him what he had once given: "The LORD gave, and the LORD hath taken away." As the archetypal pious sufferer, Job was often extolled in sermons and devotional texts as a model to imitate. In his 1679 commentary on Job's story, Simon Patrick explained that it should "incourage all pious men to indure with such wonderfull submission as he did." It is not surprising that Cowper, who owned Patrick's commentary, looked to Job for strength and guidance amid her physical and social distress. Like Job, she sought to face "all the blows of Heauen with an unwounded soul" by bearing the tedium and disappointments of life with peace and patience. Others made reference to Job to articulate the sheer severity of physical ordeals. Describing the illness of his brother, one man noted, "Job never felt what hee suffered." Job was not the only biblical model of pious suffering, but he was certainly one of the most popular.[58]

Written to instruct the living as well as eulogize the deceased, sermons also offered widely received stories of suffering. In 1657 the clergyman Isaac Ambrose published a funeral sermon for Lady Margaret Houghton, who had lived a life of contemplation, prayer, humility, and charity. The sermon served as a commemoration of her life and as a model for "perpetual instruction and imitation." Ambrose emphasized the severity of Houghton's illness, which kept her a prisoner to her bed, unable to stir a foot. Yet she exhibited ideal comportment amid her bodily torments: "She carried it as a lamb; not a word of passion or peevishnesse issued out of her lips." Rich's household chaplain and spiritual mentor, Anthony Walker, published a similar funeral sermon for Rich in 1678, accompanied by some of her meditations and diary excerpts. His intentions are abundantly clear on the text's title page, which exalts Rich for providing "the most illustrious pattern of a sincere piety, and solid goodness this age hath produced." Rich's contemporaries Sarah Cowper and Ralph Thoresby owned this work, and Thoresby confirmed the intended reception of the text when he noted that Rich was "a most virtuous, religious lady." Upon reading her summary of rules for holy living, he exclaimed, "Lord, help me to follow such excellent directions!" In life as in death, Rich served as an example for others to emulate.[59]

Some devotional texts, such as *The Sick Mans Salue*, include accounts of how precisely not to suffer. A severely ill man named Epaphroditus cursed the day he was born and bemoaned his ailing body: "That my mother had ben my graue her selfe, that the birth might not haue come out but remained styll in her. . . . My strengthe is gone, my sight faileth me, my tounge flottereth in my mouthe, my handes tremble and shake for paine, I can not hold up my head for weakenes. . . . My sences fayle me. What so euer I tast, is unplesant unto me. What other thynge am I, then a dead corps brething?" His friends condemned such complaints and pleas for the release of death. They pitied Epaphroditus, not because of his physical condition but because of his improper response to it, "whiche chaunceth unto you, not for your hurt and destruction: but for your commodity and saluatyon."[60] Rich recognized the same despair in the passionate cries of her husband, Charles, who suffered in "allmost constant paine and illnes" in the final years of his life. His recurring and excruciating episodes of gout were true tests of faith. As opposed to displaying humility and patience, however, he was continually complaining and "roaring out." Over and over, Rich described how her husband "broke out into most uiolent pationate expressions wher in he was most prouokeingly bitar." Such behavior failed to demonstrate submission to God, let alone gratitude. Rich prayed and wept for her husband's sake, fearing that his despair offended God and would keep his soul from heaven. Charles's impious suffering and lack of repentance were major blows to a woman who devoted nearly her entire adult life to converting and spiritually attending to the servants, family members, and neighbors around her. Rich blamed herself for her husband's reprobation. She believed that God had afflicted her with an ill-tempered, impious husband as punishment for her past undutiful behavior: years earlier, she had refused the match her father made for her and chose to marry Charles against her father's wishes. Moments before Charles passed away, he gave his wife a small assurance that her efforts were not entirely wasted. He briefly regained the ability to speak, and during that fleeting moment of clarity Rich implored her husband to "lift upe his heart to God for mersy." Rather than curse and swear, Charles meekly responded, "So I doe, so I doe."[61]

Conclusion

This chapter has offered three explanations for the varied ways that early modern men and women told stories about others and about themselves. Extant writing by women from the period is overall more spiritual than men's writing, thereby offering one reason for women's tendency to observe other people. Yet many women also used writing to construct an identity for posterity, a goal that could involve holding up others as foils or mirrors. Such comparisons further reflect dominant representations of women's work, as well as the most common way that early modern women collected and communicated medical information—using recipes that cited the experiences of others. Men too documented their lives in forms of writing that determined resulting accounts of illness. Their tendency to quantify their bodily disorders likewise reflects prevailing representations of men's work and the means by which several men in this book recorded and observed the natural world.

In addition to looking to others and to the self, religion offered a third source of stories for conceptualizing illness and creating meaning from it. Religion taught men and women alike how to interpret the divine significance of sickness and how to respond to it physically—how to view and feel physical sensations in spiritual terms. Providence provided a central framework for explaining the cause and meaning of natural phenomena, yet religion in early modern England entailed much more than a series of beliefs. The body provided a key site for enacting daily devotional exercises and demonstrating piety. Spirituality was embodied in trembling limbs and open, melted hearts. In monitoring their physical sensations, pious women like Mary Rich gauged their ability to perform devotional exercises, much the same way Samuel Pepys recognized similar sensations over a period of years or Samuel Jeake tracked interactions between the stars and his fevers. Religious beliefs promoted a self-focused attention to bodily processes not as a form of empirical observation to discover the secrets of the natural world but as a means of inner revelation to better understand one's spiritual progress and relationship with God. These men and women were all making observations, just in varied ways. Whether they observed their own ailments or those of others, seventeenth-century patients lived within a culture that privileged close attention to the body and its connection to other people, divine order, and the natural world.

All the approaches discussed here recognized the moral significance of suffering. When Rich conflated spiritual and physical impairment, she seemed to deflect responsibility for her spiritual failure by attributing her inability to pray to ill health. Yet illness too was deeply moralizing, and the influences of the body on the ability to pray had both physical and moral dimensions. Sarah Cowper noted, for instance, how "the fumes from the stomach of a Glutton do so ouercloud the Brain that they flag the wings of Deuotion."[62] An intemperate diet could cause ill health, which in turn could inhibit spiritual exercises. Yet in this case the word *glutton* highlights the moral implications of illness. While ill health inhibited spiritual exercises in physical ways—by clogging the body and distracting the mind—the moral ramifications of illness had a similarly powerful impact on devotional practice. Elizabeth Livingston's account of overeating fruit that opened this chapter demonstrates how physical health in early modern England was a spiritual and moral imperative.

Yet religious models of virtuous suffering did not constitute a comprehensive moral and behavioral code. Such scripts were based on the presumption that illness was a sign from heaven. While most seventeenth-century sufferers were devout and interpreted ill health as a divine message, many men and women viewed life events as signs operating within a world full of omens and correspondences. From this perspective, illnesses and accidents were still divinely ordained, but they possessed hidden meanings and affinities within the cosmos, such as symbolic connections to stars, plants, minerals, and numbers. Jeake's astrological diary reflects this world view and its compatibility with God's will. Others considered dreams, visions, and even illness itself to be portents of future events. Edmund Harrold offers a glimpse of this vision of the world in a relatively lengthy diary entry from 1712 about a mysterious crack in his wife's new pot: "What['s] y^t say's she is y^t ye pot say's Sarah Sharples ay & its a sign of death says she so as [she] was talking it gave 2 cracks more." Despite the cracks, the pot somehow remained intact. Harrold's wife "took up ye pot & Rung it & it is as sound as can be." While Harrold was unsure whether or not the episode was ominous, he jotted it down "in order to observe ye euent concerning theirs or our familyes to come."[63] This entry reflects the significance of everyday accidents as meaningful signs, as well as the social negotiations required to interpret them. Although the types of stories discussed here reflect just some of the ways seventeenth-century sufferers learned to think and write about their bodies, their significance will become more pronounced as subsequent chapters walk through various aspects of illness from the patient's point of view. Religious beliefs and practices, self-assessments, and the words and behaviors of friends and family were integral to patients' explanations of each stage of illness, from onset to recovery.

3. Emotional Causes of Illness

While some seventeenth-century sufferers told stories about the afflictions of friends and relatives to better understand their own, others modeled their ailments on the experiences of loved ones in even more explicit ways—by physically embodying their infirmities. According to early modern medical theory, witnessing the agony of an ailing friend or family member could trigger an emotional response and cause a griever to fall ill in sympathy with the aggrieved. Intense emotions, such as sorrow, surprise, or fear, could lead to illness in this way by sparking a series of internal processes involving blood and a subtle internal substance known as spirits. Alice Thornton recounted several instances of illness caused by emotions in a narrative of her life written in 1669. In one such episode, she fell ill from an emotional reaction to the sickness and subsequent death of her sister Catherine Danby. Danby was in poor health long before giving birth to her sixteenth child and remained ill for nearly a month afterward. As Thornton watched her ailing sister's increasing inability to eat or sleep following the birth, she felt such overwhelming grief that she grew sickly herself: "My greife and sorrow was soe great for her, that I had brought myselfe into a very weake condition. . . . Att which time I tooke my last leave of my dearest and only sister, never could gett to see her for my owne illnesse afftewards." Thornton was careful to note that her own illness prevented her from attending her sister's final moments. Debilitating grief justified shirking familial duties. Thornton responded similarly to the sudden death of her brother George six years later: "For the harty greifes and sorrowes I sustained, it well nigh had brought me to have died with him." In her grief, she seemed to mirror the physical trials of her loved ones. A devout Anglican, she expressed her sorrow through prayers and tears, and through her ailing body.[1]

Thornton's contemporary Ralph Thoresby also attributed ailing health to grief, but he described the process differently (see fig. 7). In 1697, following the death of his business partner Samuel Ibbetson, Thoresby endured cold sweats, dejected spirits, and an "ill state both of body and mind." Blood gushed from his nose when he glimpsed a portrait of his deceased friend—an incontrovertibly physical response. Thoresby explained, however, that his grief stemmed not from sorrow over the loss of a dear friend but rather from concern for his financial status. The two men had built a mill for processing rapeseed oil near Leeds, an investment that proved to be a spectacular failure. Thoresby's assets were tied up in Ibbetson's debt for more than £1,000, leaving Thoresby solely responsible for paying off the creditors. In addition, his brother ran off without settling a £600 debt, and his pregnant sister added a thirteenth child to the brood of children Thoresby was already supporting. He later described the effects of these financial woes in mostly physical terms: "But these afflictions, together with that of Mr. Ibbetson's, so shattered my constitution, that my spirits were sank within me, and sleep departed from my eyes; so that mostly the nights from twelve to five were spent in fruitless tossings, many faint qualms and cold clammy sweats."[2] Although Thoresby believed that his emotional response to Ibbetson's death was the ultimate source of his ill health, he viewed the process in the frame of financial anxiety rather than sorrow. Moreover, his grief did not spark an instant physical transformation, as Thornton's did. Thoresby's emotions instead triggered a series of physiological effects—"shattered" spirits, loss of sleep, cold sweats— that impaired his health. Both he and Thornton attributed their ill health to emotions, but they articulated the process differently.

As these two episodes show, early modern patients tended to attribute emotionally caused ailments to social stimuli, such as the death of a loved one or perilous credit relations. These events provoked emotional responses, which in turn sparked a series of internal mechanisms that resulted in illness. This chapter examines how men and women in seventeenth-century England articulated this relationship among the social, the emotional, and the physical in varying ways, by stressing different factors and stimuli. Thornton was just eighteen years old when she fell sick from sorrow over her sister, and she was only twenty-four when George died—ages at which the heart was

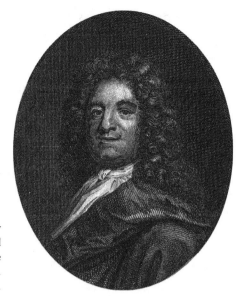

7. Portrait of Ralph Thoresby by
J. Baker, published c. 1796, based
on an engraving by George Vertue
after a painting by James Parmentier.
© National Portrait Gallery, London.

thought to be particularly vulnerable to the effects of emotions. Yet her accounts of immediate, mimetic illness reflect a common pattern in seventeenth-
century women's writing: a tendency to fall suddenly and severely ill in
response to distressing social interactions. Men like Thoresby focused more
on the physiological mechanisms underlying debilitating emotions and contextualized them within the realm of occupational concerns. Prevailing understandings of men's and women's bodies, as well as gender norms and
written conventions, are key to explaining these diverging perceptions of
emotions as a source of illness.

Patients looked to a range of factors to explain the causes of ill health,
including humoral shifts, environmental effects, and God. A careful assessment of patients' firsthand accounts reveals that emotions were a more prevalent component of sufferers' explanations of illness onset than historians have
supposed. Scholars have become increasingly interested in emotions and their
relationship to an array of early modern experiences, including conceptions
of manhood, domestic roles, clinical practice, and spiritual beliefs.[3] Much of
the scholarship on early modern illness, however, has overlooked the emotions.[4] This gap is particularly striking given that emotions were believed to
be one of six external causes of illness in the early modern period. A notable
exception is Michael MacDonald's study of the astrological physician Richard
Napier, which explores how emotional distress could lead to chronic

conditions such as madness and melancholy.[5] Examining sufferers' words rather than learned medical literature reveals the significance of the emotions to early modern understandings of disease causation. Emotions provoked serious psychological disorders, like madness and melancholy, but also everyday headaches, fevers, and colds.

Patients in early modern England did not commonly use the word *emotion*. Rather, individuals referred to grief, rage, fear, and lust as *passions*, a term loaded with negative connotations. Early modern men and women believed that the mind controlled emotional expression, which made unruly passions particularly threatening to one's rationality and morality. Surrendering to immoderate or ungoverned passions displayed a lack of self-restraint, reason, and spiritual capacity. There was a broad lexicon of early modern affect, including *feelings*, *sensibilities*, *sentiments*, and *passions*. These terms were not synonyms, but rather reflected the many characteristics and implications of emotional responses, such as sensory perceptions, moral judgments, and spiritual development.[6] The term *emotion* here encapsulates the physical, spiritual, and moral ramifications of emotive responses. Despite using this modern term, we cannot impose our present-day experiences of emotion onto the past. While emotions are, in a sense, fixed biological processes, emotive responses involve behaviors that are learned and performed.[7] Circumstances that incited fear in the 1600s may not frighten us at all. And while attributing ill health to intense emotions was common in the seventeenth century, today we might look to other explanations or references to describe our feelings, attributing different meanings to what may be similar physical sensations.

The Physiology of Emotion

According to early modern patients, emotions altered the body by means of the same processes as those of the other nonnaturals (see chapter 1). Just as a draft of air, sharp wind, or cold beverage would create a sudden shift in body temperature that could block the pores and prevent the proper dispersal and removal of corruptive humors, emotions such as fear and anxiety led to temperature changes that could "clogg the spirits." A subtle material known as the animal spirits was central to early modern explanations of the physiology of emotion. The animal spirits were one of three substances that were believed to control the internal operations of the body. Natural spirits, in the liver, were responsible for growth and nutrition; vital spirits, produced in the heart, generated the body's movement; and animal spirits, refined in the brain, imparted what Thomas Walkington called "a faculty to the nerues of sence, and real motion."[8] In other words, animal spirits provided the physical link between mind and body. The arteries and veins diffused these three spirits, propelled by natural heat, throughout the body, where they transformed into one another depending on their locations. For example, venous blood from the liver flowed to the heart, where it heated up and transformed into arterial blood, thereby refining natural spirits into vital spirits.

Upon sensing a stimulus that elicited an emotional response, the imagination communicated a message to the heart by means of the animal spirits. The imagination existed in what contemporaries called the sensible soul, along with sensory perception, common sense, and memory. Reason resided in the rational soul, the source of will and the essence of human beings. Reason could restrain the imagination in order to prevent potentially dangerous emotional responses, although the imagination had the capacity to override reason by refusing to obey its commands. As a result, one could incite illness merely by thinking about it. One woman, for instance, linked a sudden swelling on her neck to a dream that her deceased husband was tickling her under the chin. Her imagination actually created the bump beneath her skin, and, because of her "almost continual Reflection on her imaginary Husband's kind Dealing with her," the swelling grew and eventually caused death.[9] According to Richard Burton's *The Anatomy of Melancholy*, the imagination generated emotional responses by stirring the animal spirits, which signaled to the heart "what good or bad object was presented, which immediately bends it selfe to prosecute, or avoid it; and withall draweth with it other humors to help it." Emotions that caused an influx of warmth, such as joy and anger, made the heart expand and disperse heat outward. Grief and fear, on the other hand, contracted the heart, which trapped the blood and spirits and deprived the body of heat.[10]

This process could cause illness and could also exacerbate existing or dormant diseases. Sudden, severe emotion intensified a case of smallpox that Thornton contracted from her brother in 1642. Her shock upon seeing his altered appearance, perhaps compounded by fear of her own potentially similar fate, triggered a series of internal processes that worsened her condition: "Beeing strooke with feare seeing him so sadly used and all over very read,

I immediately fell very ill, and from that time grew worse till I grew so dangerously ill and inwardly sicke, that I was in much perill of my life, by theire not comeing well out but kept att my heart."[11] Fear trapped an abundance of blood in Thornton's heart, which overwhelmed the organ and extinguished the body's natural heat. Instead of manifesting externally, the smallpox remained dangerously lodged in her blood-clogged heart. Anxiety could wreak similar effects by drawing an abundance of heat and moisture from the blood, which, according to the seventeenth-century author John Harris, "tireth the Spirit and wasteth it." Diet and digestion further influenced this process, as the concoction of humors in the stomach could alter the purity of the spirits. Although mechanical frameworks of the body had begun to replace this heart-centered model by the late seventeenth century, the shift was by no means linear or simple, and the humoral model predominated in nonlearned discourse throughout the period discussed here.[12]

In *A Treatise of Melancholie*, Timothie Bright outlined how this heart-centered system accounted for an array of bodily phenomena. Tears were the "excrementitious humiditie of the brayne," a sort of liquid waste that the body expelled through the eyes. Trembling lips and sobs resulted from depleted spirits, while sighing cooled and refreshed the heart by nourishing the spirits. Medical practitioners could detect the effects of emotions in a host of physical alterations, including swellings, headaches, sweats, spots, and even excretions. By examining only the color and consistency of his urine, one physician determined that a patient suffered from an "overpowering fear."[13] To combat the effects of a flow of blood into the heart or out to the extremities, medical remedies opened up the body by purging offending humors and loosening obstructions.

Although patients rarely alluded to the intricacies of this explanatory framework, references to clogged or surprised spirits reflect a common understanding of it. Those suffering from sadness or grief tended to locate their feelings in the movements and functions of the heart. Men and women described their hearts as being physically pierced by the moans of loved ones; weakening, sinking, or lowering; possessing an "ill temper"; feeling overwhelmed; and bleeding within. Some even defined their subsequent illnesses as sickness in the heart. Such descriptions demonstrate a common understanding of both the heart's central role in generating emotional illnesses and the physical dimension and location of emotions in early modern medical discourse.[14]

"Grieued and Discomposed":
Emotionally Caused Sickness

Thornton barely mentioned the physical processes underlying the connection between her emotions and ill health. Instead she described falling immediately and severely ill in response to intense grief, fear, and surprise. We have already seen how she linked ill health to grief following the deaths of her sister and brother, and how fear and surprise exacerbated her smallpox in 1642. Similarly, when her husband William fell ill on a journey in 1665, she described how the sudden news of his condition "did soe surprize my spiritts, that I was brought into a violent passion of griefe and sorrow, with fitts of sounding, which I never knew before; and prevailed soe exceedingly that I immeadiately went sick to bed." Thornton understood the physiology of emotions, as evidenced by her reference to surprised spirits. Yet she described an instant connection between sorrow and sickness. She was so ill that everyone assumed she would die, and she was unable to tend to her ailing husband. Three years later she recounted a strikingly similar episode. Upon learning that her husband had fallen ill unexpectedly, she was so sad and frightened "that I went sicke thereupon to my sorrowfull bed."[15] She presented overwhelming grief as the sole source of these infirmities, though her narrative suggests she was also anxious about her financial situation and the livelihood of her children should her husband die. In addition, concerns about reputation compelled Thornton to narrate her life story in ways that highlighted her roles as dutiful wife, mother, and sister. Characterizing grief-induced illness as sudden and severe facilitated such self-presentations and justified an inability to care for ailing loved ones.

A significant number of women from this period recounted similar stories of illness onset. On the evening of her husband's death, Mary Rich noted how "this night with griefe I fond my selfe uery ill." When her grandmother died, Elizabeth Delaval described herself as "the person that I believe of all the world grieved most for her death. Soon after I had a very violent fit of sicknesse." The death of Ann Fanshawe's father caused her such intense grief that she was sick for six months "almost to death," and another woman, grieved over her daughter's illness, was "reduced to great Indisposition."[16] According to these accounts, grief, surprise, and fear incited illness instantly, as though these women suffered in sympathy with their ailing loved ones. In a letter to her father in October 1622, Elizabeth Trumbull described how her surgeon, a woman she referred to as "Mistris Fage," fell ill from grief when her husband and son contracted severe fevers. As Trumbull explained it, Fage was "so uflickted with it shee hath bene very il her selfe." These women rarely emphasized or even mentioned the physiological phenomena that mediated the connection between emotions and ill health, such as disturbed sleep, modified diet, or shifting humors and spirits. They described an immediate link between grief and infirmity.[17]

Similarly severe and sudden disorders resulted from grief upon separation from family members. Mothers fell "desperately sick" after leaving their children, and sisters were "grieued and discomposed" upon departing company. Elizabeth Freke endured a difficult sickness for weeks when her favorite grandson, John, left for London in 1705. The four-year-old had been staying at her Bilney estate for six months with his older brother and parents, Freke's son and daughter-in-law. Freke had grown particularly fond of John because he so closely resembled his father: "I loved him to my soule because he was the picture of my deerst son." When the family began making moves to return to London, she asked that the children stay behind. At the very least, John could remain under her care at Bilney. She characterized her son and daughter-in-law's decision not to grant this request as a cruel rebuff. Grief over the boy's departure, perhaps compounded by the sting of having been denied, left Freke gravely ill for six weeks. "I thought would have binn my last," she wrote. Most tragically, she never again saw the boy. About a month later, while staying in rented rooms on Norfolk Street in London, he, his brother, and the landlord's son found a loaded pistol that their father's servant had carelessly left in the house. John was accidentally shot and killed. Freke viewed the dreadful episode as divine punishment for her son and daughter-in-law's "undutifullness and cruellty to me."[18]

Written accounts of others' afflictions could have similarly dramatic bodily effects. Correspondents apologized for failing to report the ailments of loved ones out of fear that conveying upsetting news too suddenly might compromise readers' health. Roger North considered this outcome when he sat down to write to his sister Anne Foley in 1691. Their brother Dudley North had recently died of asthma, despite therapeutic bleedings and "extream remedys" from the best physicians. Dudley's son had passed away just three weeks earlier, and the family was already wrought with grief. North considered suppressing the news in order to allow his sister to learn about their brother's death when "comon fame had disclosed it." He hesitated to write because, as he put it, divulging the news might cause his sister to "hurt her self with Greiuing." Foley was one of three surviving sisters, so presumably he had other difficult letters to write.[19]

Patients attributed illness to words in two additional situations: in response to troubling verbal interactions and as a reaction to gossip. Like grief-induced illness, ailments provoked by speech arose from social causes, such as distressed relationships, and further illustrate women's tendency to emphasize an immediate connection between emotional disturbances and physical impairment. The power of words to cause and cure illness was not new in the seventeenth century. Charms, curses, and witchcraft accusations demonstrated enduring beliefs in the influence of words on the physical body. Patients wrote charms on pieces of paper they then burned, swallowed, or wore around their necks. These actions were thought to exact dramatic bodily alterations. According to one medical author from the period, charms "humour and feed" and "strengthen the Imagination," much the same way emotional stimuli were thought to alter the body by means of the imagination and animal spirits. The proprietor of a textile shop in Lancashire recorded the following charm for staunching blood in 1664. The charm, he noted, was used "amongst countrie persons, and not publickly knowen." He took the time to copy it down, preserving it perhaps for his own future use:

> There was a Babe in Bethlem borne
> And christiand in the water of [River] Jorden;
> The water it was both wild and wood,
> The child it was both meeke and goode—
> Stanch bloud in God's namme.[20]

This particular charm only worked when read out loud three times, a ritual that resembled the Catholic recitation of prayers to absolve sin. Charms tended to contain Christian stories and imagery, which suggests a persisting faith in the power of religious language. Even for Protestants, who did not take confession or believe in the ability of words to transform bread and wine into the body and blood of Christ, words held profound spiritual significance. The word of God is central to Christian doctrine, and Scripture substantiates the relationship between the word and the reception of divine grace in the body. According to Scripture, God's word was "written in our hearts, known and read of all men . . . written not with ink, but with the Spirit of the living God; not in tables of stone, but in fleshy tables of the heart." Piety was embodied in a soft, warm heart, which was required to receive God's spirit. Believers did not merely listen to sermons and try to live by God's word but prayed that the words "may be inwardly grafted in my Heart." The word of God indelibly marked the hearts of pious men and women.[21]

The belief that curses could cause physical harm further demonstrates the potency of spoken words in this period. Curses were rooted in medieval theology and hinged on the conviction that, if it was justified, God would ensure a curse wrought its intended effects.[22] Witchcraft also was presumed to work by means of threatening words. Accusations tended to follow menacing speech, often the result of neighborly exchanges or domestic interactions gone awry. Rewbin Bowier attributed sudden convulsive fits in 1653 to an odd conversation with one of his neighbors, for instance. He was walking past the house of John and Hellen Dishe when his dog suddenly began acting amorously toward the Dishes' hog. Hellen observed the animals and, according to Bowier, remarked that Bowier "had as good not to haue suffered this dogge to haue worried her hogge for hee should haue noe great Joy after it." Following this exchange, Bowier started experiencing painful fits several times a day. He linked this sudden and severe disorder to Dishe's threat. He also reported seeing a black cat on his bed and, later, "another thinge like a hedge-hogge." Witches were thought to have animal companions, or familiars, that embodied evil spirits. Familiars could take several forms in early modern England, including toads, rats, and rabbits. Immediately after seeing the cat and the hedgehog, Bowier felt "some thinge come up into his body . . . to his throate and then hee is almost strangled & is in great torture." He linked his convulsions to Dishe's threatening words and the choking sensation to the animal demons that did her bidding.[23]

These beliefs about the relationship between bodies and speech contextualize patients' tendencies to attribute illness to vexing words and behaviors. Relatives who displayed poor manners or friends for "want of better conuersation" could cause particularly sensitive women like Sarah Cowper to suffer from melancholy vapors, agitated blood, clogged spirits, and "grated" bowels.[24] Harmful words signified social sources of disorder—insolent servants, irreverent children, ruined relationships—and could alter the body in acute ways. Mary Rich often fell ill following passionate arguments with her husband Charles. One such instance occurred after she reproached him for his un-Christian language. As he endured a painful episode of gout, he shouted obscenities that, according to her, offended God. In response to this censure, Charles expressed "more pationate words then euer I herd," and he forbade his wife from offering any additional unsolicited "good counsel." These harsh words made a deep impact on Rich. She described awaking the following morning "with a disturbing fitt of the spleene and head ake, I fond much troble upon me, what I had mett with the day before did much discompose me." A number of women, like Rich, linked physical suffering to harsh words and troubling social interactions that provoked a broad category of emotions known as vexation.[25]

Vexing words were especially dangerous because of their ability to undermine a woman's reputation, which depended largely on sexual fidelity. Laura Gowing has shown how slander recorded in defamation litigation from the period tended to target women's sexual reputations, revealing a close connection between feminine honor and sexual honesty. Women were called whores and strumpets, while men were called names that either lacked the same sexual connotations or alluded to the sexual misbehavior of their wives: cuckolds, rogues, and knaves. Slander against men usually focused on undermining a manly status defined primarily in terms of economic self-sufficiency and self-mastery.[26] Slander afforded some women a powerful source of agency, though prescriptive literature taught that ideal women should speak calmly and sparingly, restraining emotions that could lead to dangerously passionate speech. "As their words must be few, so those few words must be reverend and meeke," one popular advice manual instructed.[27]

Given the social consequences of slander and the sensitive relationship between speech and the body, it is perhaps not surprising that some seventeenth-century women attributed their ill health to gossip. Thornton's reference to a "plague of slandorous tounges" was no mere metaphor. She first mentioned the damaging effects of slander in 1667, upon falling ill after giving birth to her ninth child. The child only survived three weeks and injured Thornton's nipple while breastfeeding, causing the breast to gangrene. The gangrene in turn led to a severe fever, headache, and toothache, all of which kept Thornton bedridden for four months. She described how the inappropriate reactions of people around her only deepened her affliction and prolonged her suffering: "The unhandsome proud carriage of those I tooke to be a comfort in my distresse, proved the greatest corisive in my sicke and weake condittion." Thornton here referred to Anne Danby, the wife of her nephew Christopher. Thornton believed that Danby possessed "a secret hatred" of her and spread nasty rumors suggesting that she only pretended to be ill and in reality "ailed nothing."[28]

The topic of slander came up a year later when Thornton once again suffered from "a very great and dangerous condittion of sickness, weakeness of body, and afflicted mind, on the account of my evill enimies' slanders." Her husband William also fell ill while traveling to Malton to help clear her name. The added grief of learning about his ailing health exacerbated Thornton's weak condition. She never fully laid out the details of the slander, but it involved her decision to marry her prepubescent daughter to a twenty-one-year-old clergyman named Thomas Comber. It also included allegations that Thornton herself planned to marry Comber upon becoming a widow. The rumors came to a head in 1668 when she, her niece Anne Danby, and their maids were in Danby's chamber. As Thornton explained it, Danby's maid, Barbara Tod, accused Thornton's maid of spreading "seuerall storeys (w:^{ch} were uery great) lies & fallshoods against my selfe." Although Thornton's maid denied the charges and defended her mistress, Tod persisted, carrying on "so unhansomly & unchristianly towards me in her [bitter?] agrauation & in false accusing ye Hon^{or} of some of ye Persons of my family." Tod claimed that the rumors originated from a woman named Mary Breaks, who sought to prevent the union between Thornton's daughter and Comber so that Breaks might marry the clergyman herself. Although Thornton neglected to provide the particulars of Tod's accusations, she recounted how the maid exclaimed that Thornton "was naught, and my parents was naught, and all that I came on was naught." Thornton represented her assailant as epitomizing typically aggressive, unfeminine speech: the maid "railed on me and scoulded at me and my poore innocent child" with "most vile expressions." Hearing his wife's emotional response, William burst into the room and threw the maid down the stairs, though Thornton refused to let him remove Danby, since she had no other place to live.[29]

This dramatic episode left Thornton bedridden for fourteen days. Hearing her name blemished felt like a "sword to my soule," and she "fell presently into a most great & sad excess of weeping & lamentable sorrow y^t it had like to haue cost me my life." When her aunt later visited, she found her niece "half dead with griefe uppon this larum that Mrs. Danby and her maide raised up." The power of the damaging words stemmed in part from the fact that someone so close to Thornton had uttered them. Danby made no attempts to warn Thornton of the slander, and she tacitly supported her maid's accusations by choosing not to defend Thornton's name. Yet Danby was a relative who had been living in Thornton's home and to whom Thornton had committed twenty years as a "continuall daily and faithfull freind."[30] The slander not only impugned Thornton's honor and challenged her sexual reputation but also exposed the betrayal and deceit of a valued, trusted friend.

Men experienced the same emotional responses as women, and some provided heart-wrenching accounts of grief, but I have found only a handful of early modern men who linked their emotions to ill health. While it is difficult to trace patterns within such a small sample, these accounts of emotionally caused ailments seem to differ from women's writing in two ways. First, these men acknowledged the physical processes that mediated their disorders. Ralph Thoresby, for example, noted how grief impaired his sleep six months after his father's death, while David Hamilton believed that grief over the death of his mother caused the "Translation of a Gouty pain, from my left foot to my Stomach." When the statesman Arthur Annesley attributed a small pain in his stomach to the "great grief and sadnesse I haue [had] for about three months past," he recognized the protracted physical processes underlying his disorder.[31] Over the span of three months, his sorrow produced an acute, localized ailment—quite unlike the instant and dramatic suffering that women recounted.

Second, these men tended to associate their emotions with economic concerns, such as shifts in property and credit relations. Indeed, several men perceived financial anxiety and its resulting bodily effects as a form of grief. Samuel Kyrk "almost broke his heart with fretting" when his business failed and he had to work overtime to compensate for the loss. So too when the bookseller Joshua Kirton lost his house and thousands of pounds' worth of books in the 1666 London fire, he allegedly died from "grief for his losses." The account by Thoresby that opens this chapter further illustrates this trend. Following the death of his business partner Samuel Ibbetson, he not only framed his ensuing illness within the context of financial anxiety but also appraised his and others' grief in economic terms. He noted how Ibbetson's son seemed to grieve less than him because the son was freed from financial obligations to his father. Thoresby's grief was more extreme because his "concerns were more intricate and dangerous."[32] Financial worries could be a significant cause of ill health for men, an understandable connection given early modern men's roles as protectors and governors of the household. Anxieties about making ends meet or securing a debt led to headaches, disturbed rest, and disordered spirits. When one man found himself unable to breathe properly, he could "attribute it to nothing but money."[33] Although women contributed to the household economy in a number of ways and also found financial security a source of deep anxiety, they rarely made this direct connection between monetary concerns and ill health. Seventeenth-century men and women relied on the same vocabulary to articulate the relationship among social stimuli, emotions, and ill health, but they perceived that relationship in gendered ways.

Explaining Gender Differences

Expectations of appropriate emotional expression partly shaped these gendered patterns. Just as men and women learned how to suffer on the sickbed, they also expressed emotions in ways that were socially dictated. Early modern women, for instance, were expected to effuse pity and sorrow in response to ailing family members. When Robert Dormer suffered from a stomach illness at his estate in Oxfordshire, he reprimanded his wife Anne for failing to express the pity and grief he had come to expect. She was in the garden at the time, unaware of her husband's condition. He wanted her to come inside and tend to him, so he sent her a message that her dog was sick. He assumed she would only respond to the distress of someone she truly loved. She saw the situation differently. Upon receiving the message about her dog, she went inside and found her husband vomiting. He felt better after three bouts of sickness, yet she "had much adoe to forbear weeping" upon witnessing his ordeal. Her pity turned to anger when her husband reproached her for displaying insufficient concern. She defended her behavior, explaining that her expressions of grief were genuine: "I did neuer weep for forms sake, being naturally too apt to it." While a family member's illness necessitated certain emotive expressions, such responses also had to be sincere. Sarah Cowper, who was acutely aware of others' behavior, noted her neighbor's display of grief with skepticism: "If weeping and wailing, and wringing of Hands be signs of Real Greif I neuer saw any more extrauagant."[34] Feigning emotion was worse than expressing none at all.

Men faced similar challenges. In 1715, Dudley Ryder was shocked to learn that his cousin Richard Ryder had died from a violent fever. He was surprised by the news not only because he did not know the fever was so serious but also because his cousin's death "did not touch me so sensibly as I should have expected." At the funeral three days later, he continued to observe his deficient grief: "I was very much displeased with myself that I could not be much affected with such a posture of affairs." He was concerned that the death of such a near relation "made so little impression," and he did what he could "to raise a little concern in me." He was similarly self-aware when his grandmother passed away a year later. This was the first death he witnessed firsthand, and he noted how it affected him less than he thought it would. But this time he took the opposite tack. He exuded an air of stoic restraint rather than pretending to grieve, and he admitted to doing so in order to live up to masculine ideals: "I did not make any great show of sorrow, but rather bore it with a kind of manly strength and firmness." Perhaps it was the particular situation that enabled him to feel confident about his lack of emotion, in contrast to the self-consciousness that overwhelmed him a year earlier. At the family's house in Hackney, everyone was suddenly called upstairs. They stood and watched Ryder's grandmother gasping for breath in her chair for seven or eight minutes before passing away. Ryder compared her dying body to a lamp that "goes out for want of oil." He saw logic and peace in her passing rather than fear and confusion, as though "nature had entirely finished her work." According to him, a lack of emotional expression in this instance displayed not callousness and detachment but rather fortitude and manliness.[35]

Others reined in their passion to demonstrate self-mastery. Upon finding his horse stolen, Roger Lowe admitted to being upset "yet bore it patiently." Similarly, when Samuel Pepys fought with his wife in front of the servants, he was vexed "to the guts" but "had the discretion to keep myself without passion."[36] Men and women expressed their emotions in ways that met cultural norms for particular situations. While a woman like Anne Dormer was expected to fulfill her wifely duty by weeping with grief, a man like Lowe displayed his manhood by moderating his anger. Such conventions are reflected in narratives of illness in which women suffered instantly and intensely in response to relational stimuli and men downplayed their emotions by focusing on physiological processes.

These gender norms were substantiated by medical conceptions of the body that deemed immoderate emotions physiologically natural for women and unnatural for men. According to early modern medical theory, women were prone to violent emotions because they were physically more malleable and mentally less rational than men. As a result, their bodies were considered to be particularly vulnerable to external influences, especially by means of vision and the imagination. This permeability is key to understanding not just the prevalence of emotionally caused illness among early modern women but also women's characterizations of these ailments as immediate and mimetic.

According to the medical theory of the time, women's wet, cool bodies were more susceptible to emotions than the dry, warm bodies of men. Women's flesh was loose, soft, and porous, thereby allowing emotions to impress upon their bodies more easily. Such spongy, open bodies required a continual emission of fluids by means of lactation and menstruation, as well as tears. According to Timothie Bright's *A Treatise of Melancholie*, women were "altogether of a moist, rare, and tender body, especially of brayne and heart, which both being of that temper, carie the rest of the parts into like disposition: this is the cause why children are more apt to weepe, then those that are of greater yeares, and women more then men, the one hauing by youth the body moist, rare & soft, and the other by sex." Women's leaky bodies offered a natural explanation for their vulnerability to emotions, thereby also confirming the presumption that they were innately inferior to men. The more desirable and allegedly perfect bodies of men were hot and dry, which made them physically compact and resistant to emotions. As Bright explained, men "hardly yeeld forth that signe of sorrow though the occasion may require it."[37] Such accounts demonstrate quite explicitly how seventeenth-century medical knowledge reinforced prevailing stereotypes and assumptions about men and women.

Women were considered more vulnerable to emotions not only because their flesh was physically looser and more porous than men's but also because they were deemed less rational. Reason could restrain the powers of the imagination and inhibit immoderate emotions, a struggle that the supposedly less rational minds of women were unlikely to win. Cowper lamented, "O how I feel the weakness of my Reason and the strength of my passions."[38] The belief that emotional outbursts could cause miscarriages further reflects prevailing assumptions about women's sensitivity to the powers of the imagination. Accordingly, some women referred to the threat of miscarriage to qualify the extremity of their grief and fear. When men stormed into Thornton's house to reclaim her husband's debt, for example, she described how "the greife I had with the fright and the rudenesse of those men had nigh gon to make me miscarrie." Pepys even found miscarriage a suitable referent for articulating the magnitude of his fear when a friend's prank woke him in the middle of the night: "It was well I was not a woman with child, for it might have made me miscarry."[39] This connection between intense emotion and miscarriage was only one of the ways the imagination was presumed to work in female bodies. Through the faculty of the imagination, pregnant women could also impress images onto the malleable flesh of their unborn babies and even create monsters. Thornton described how a quarrel with her husband and his subsequent threat to take his life with a penknife "set a marke upon my sonne." She explained how the incident "wrought so inifinitly wth greeife upon my heart" that she imagined blood on the tip of the knife. This frightful vision became imprinted on her unborn child as a mark that resembled blood in "pure & perfectly distinct round spots like as if it had been sprinkled upon his skin . . . as if it had bine cut wth a knife."[40] The powerful ways women's emotions were believed to alter their bodies internally defined a dangerous and unruly imagination as a particularly female problem.

As Thornton's account of her marked child shows, the imagination produced corporeal impressions through the medium of vision. The role of vision as a mediator between inner bodies and outer influences offers further insight into women's accounts of emotionally caused ailments. Katharine Park has studied how vision imprinted holy images, such as the cross, on the hearts of fourteenth-century female mystics. She explains how such phenomena resulted from the belief that women possessed particularly impressionable bodies, as well as from the late medieval notion that vision enabled seen objects to alter the seer—in contrast to our modern conception of active seeing subject and passive seen object.[41] This reciprocal nature of vision endured into the seventeenth century in a number of ways. Similar to women's ability to stamp seen or imagined visions onto the bodies of their unborn children, diseases such as lovesickness resulted from humoral responses to the mere sight of the beloved. When surgeons opened up the body of a man who had died from lovesickness, they found the image of his beloved's face imprinted on his heart. Demonstrating a similar concept—that an object of the imagination could somehow transform the body—the popular seventeenth-century medical writer Nicholas Culpeper explained how emotions facilitated the transmission of plague because "feare changeth the blood into the nature of the thing feared." Sympathetic medical remedies that transferred illnesses to distant objects assumed a similar correspondence between internal bodies and the external environment. One remedy for swellings on the hand entailed stroking the swollen part with the hand of a dead person. After the dead hand had been buried in the ground, the swelling would recede as the dead hand decayed. This remedy was presumed to work by transferring the affliction to the lifeless hand, a shift made possible by the likeness between the dead hand and the affected part. Such beliefs reflect a world full of sympathies and symbols, in which resemblance and the relationship between inner bodies and outer appearances held deep significance.[42]

Women's accounts of falling instantly ill in response to the words, acts, or ailments of others fit within this world view. In addition to hearing or reading distressing news, witnessing others' suffering could cause some individuals to experience similarly severe sickness. Mary Rich noted that the sight of her husband's fatal convulsions "was so uery terable to me, that after his death I fell in to uery ill fittes," and Cowper described how her "Bowels Quake to see my Dear son so Indispos'd with shaking fits." When Elizabeth Freke's husband lay dying from a running dropsy in his leg, she noted how "my left legg swell'd and broke likewise."[43] In their grief, these women embodied the illnesses of their husbands and sons. Conceptions of the seventeenth-century body outlined here—the impressionable quality of women's flesh, the powers and dangers of women's imaginations, and the mimetic relationship between viewers' bodies and viewed objects—explain how these women seemed to fall so suddenly and severely ill upon merely seeing or learning about the afflictions of others.

Conventions for expressing concern in writing could also influence the ways these women articulated the relationship between emotions and illness. Letter writers described growing sick in commiseration with their ailing correspondents: "Pray be carfoll of your heleth ore you will sowen destroy mine that has but a Litell share now." This epistolary convention echoes women's accounts of falling ill in sympathy with loved ones. Lydia Dugard's letters to her cousin and lover Samuel Dugard offer particularly rich illustrations of this trope. The cousins began writing to each other when Lydia was just fifteen years old and Samuel was a student at Oxford, and the correspondence continued until their marriage seven years later. In one letter from 1667, Lydia wrote, "If I have not had perfect health of late twas to simpathise with you for I heard you were ile. Now you are well I shall be better." She claimed to decay in health alongside her lover and to recover as his health improved.[44] Correspondents similarly referred to news of others' recoveries as cordials.

A cordial was a common remedy that revived and strengthened the body, an apt metaphor for the joy and relief that accompanied written confirmation of another's recovery. Men and women described the receipt of a letter or the sight of a loved one's handwriting—physical evidence of the author's survival—in similar terms. "I should reioyce much to see you[r] hand writing it be no great trouble to you it shall much adde to the helth of my inferme and sickly body," Elizabeth Poley wrote to her brother in 1641. The sheer volume of these kinds of statements in personal correspondence spanning the seventeenth century illustrates the popularity of this trope. As a trope, of course, such an assertion was not always meant literally. Lydia Dugard wrote, "How much am I aflicted at the bad newes of your headach it is cruel to mee now and tortures me as much as if I realy felt it."[45] She did not actually develop a headache in commiseration with her lover, but she communicated her concern by describing her emotional distress as a comparable pain. Such expressions of compassion perhaps informed more literal articulations of the sympathetic relationship between grief and illness in women's writing. When overwhelming sorrow caused women to mirror the aches and pains of loved ones, they embodied a common discourse for conveying sympathy.

Such mimetic suffering further reflects the early modern belief that actions or thoughts could be contagious. Religious and political writers, for example, used metaphors of infection to describe the potential threats of dissenting spiritual convictions.[46] Lydia Dugard articulated this concept in more literal terms. She feared adopting the poor habits and dispositions of those around her. In 1672 she made an extended visit to an aging, ailing friend of her family's, the wife of a vicar who lived six miles away in the town of Lighthorn. The elderly woman, Margaret Dodd, was fatally ill and lacked a proper nurse; Dugard felt compelled to step in and care for her. Dodd was known to be "a bad example" on account of her continual "fretting and chiding." And after a few short weeks, Dugard longed to escape from Dodd's "distemper and worss temper." But she reassured her lover that she would not "alter for the worse since my being with her." Dodd's mere presence had the potential to infect Dugard, who was particularly impressionable on account of her youth. She was just twenty-two years old at the time. Yet the much older Cowper evinced a similar notion when complaining about the harmful impact of irreverent, dissolute servants. They were a plague, an old sore "daily rubb'd upon," and a "ffreting leprosie" that stuck to the walls of the house, leaving "such infection as proues incurable at least as to the bad Effects."

Likening others' behaviors and beliefs to contagions was a clear way of expressing disdain and disapproval. The association also highlights beliefs about the sensitive relationship between individuals and the behaviors, utterances, and even thoughts of others.[47]

Men acknowledged that emotions could diminish health, but they did so in ways that were congruent with seventeenth-century masculine ideals. Shaking with fear and fainting from grief were marks of a fragile, irrational, and therefore unmanly constitution. When Dudley Ryder awoke with an intense fear that he was being robbed, he justified his emasculating emotional response by attributing it to a dream: consuming too much turkey and alcohol had caused him to have a nightmare. Of course, his fear of burglary reflected a common source of men's emotional disorders: money. Likewise, upon witnessing a fire in September 1677, Ralph Thoresby expressed his passionate fright in terms that reinforced his manhood. He was working as a merchant's apprentice in London, and just weeks earlier he had fasted in commemoration of the great fire that had raged in that city in 1666. The flames had died down by the time he arrived on the scene that day in 1677, but he caught frightening glimpses of their damage. One victim lay on the grass "sadly mangled," his head so badly burned that Thoresby could barely recognize a face. Another man passed his hand through the mouth of a charred skull. These gruesome sights "struck such a terror into my mind," Thoresby admitted, "that I fear, if left to my own poor strength, would have prejudiced me."[48] Fear did not incapacitate him, but its potential to do so enabled him to convey the intensity of the dreadful situation. By focusing on the physical processes underlying illness and by attributing emotional responses to particularly masculine concerns, men could downplay the impact of their emotional disorders and exhibit manly virtues of reason, self-governance, and strength.

Pepys offers an example of how one man understood an intense emotional response, jealousy, and its discernible effects on the body. When he came home in May 1663 and found his wife walking and talking—as opposed to practicing—with her dancing instructor, Pembleton, his "heart and head did so cast about and fret, that I could not do any business possibly." A "disease of Jealousy" consumed him over the course of the next few months. He hovered downstairs to determine whether the two were dancing, spied on Pembleton in church, and came home in the middle of the day to see if the beds were mussed. "It makes a very hell in my mind," he wrote. Although he never claimed to fall ill from his jealousy, Pepys described the various ways this emotion took a toll on his body. He awoke in the night from a "troubled" mind, experienced difficulty speaking, and described "my head akeing and my mind in trouble for my wife, being jealous." When he saw a man resembling Pembleton in a crowd, he broke into a sweat and blood rushed to his face—reactions that signified dynamic internal processes. Pepys's fear of cuckoldry reflected common masculine anxieties about authority and honor. In this period, men's reputations were severely damaged when their wives were accused of sexual infidelity, which reflected the man's loss of virility and inability to govern his wife and household. Pepys articulated these concerns by highlighting the physical effects of his jealousy. Yet he understood jealousy in terms that both defined and defended his masculinity. While he recognized that his emotions made his body behave in ways that others might label illness, he displayed self-mastery by refusing to consider himself sick.[49]

Finally, spiritual beliefs offered discourses, models, and norms concerning how and when to express emotion. Grief, fear, and anxiety were thought to represent despair and resistance to God. An ideal Christian therefore restrained such emotions and instead expressed calm, patient acceptance of worldly trials. Such a pious disposition, like reason, sat in opposition to unchecked passion. Hence, when Alice Thornton was overcome with a "flood of tears" while teaching her six-year-old son to read in 1669, she characterized her sudden outburst as overcoming both "reason and religion." She stood up to leave but "scarce gott to my bedside for falling down." It was her birthday, and her husband had recently passed away. She was lonely, grief stricken, and anxious about paying off her husband's debts and supporting the young boy. She believed that God reproved her "too great passion" but also forgave her for it. She came to this conclusion after hearing him speak to her through her son. The young boy lay next to her on the bed and guaranteed their future comfort in words that were far too sophisticated for a six-year-old.[50]

Emotional restraint was performed, and it was written on the body. Physicians who opened up corpses found evidence of the emotions in tissues and organs. The author of *The Divine Physician* explained how in cases of grief, "instead of a heart they find nothing but a dry skin like to the leaves in Autumn." One healer, on dissecting a corpse, found a sound heart and desiccated liver, which he "attributed to nothing but greif & sadness, the loss of his deare [illegible] tho it did not breake his heart because a Christian yet it dryed his Liver because a man subject to infirmities."[51] This man had remained submissive to God and focused on spiritual concerns following the loss of a loved one, an acceptance and restraint confirmed by the soundness of his heart. Yet a weak constitution allowed his grief to damage his liver. When her mother grew suddenly and dangerously sick, "ye fright of such ill tidings" caused Katherine Tylston to fall ill too. Her terse account of this episode conveys the physical as well as spiritual dimensions of her grief. The news of her mother's illness "filled me wth fears & th^n my heart was ouerwhelmed wth sorrow. . . . I labour^d for an intire resignation to his will, & he mercifully granted me mine concerning her." The young woman obviously felt deep sorrow for her mother. Yet above all, she feared that her grief demonstrated an inability to accept God's will with proper patience. She called upon God for aid, and her mother recovered "euen w^n all hope of her life was taken away f^m those ab^t her." Moreover, Tylston's journey home from her mother's house was safe and even comfortable, despite her ailing condition.[52]

Conclusion

Patients relied on an array of descriptors and metaphors to define the moment when they fell ill. They discerned the subtle shift from wellness to illness in sudden pangs or rumblings deep within the body. One woman compared the sensations that signified this moment to scampering vermin. She felt "running about in & under her breast like some liuing creature."[53] Others felt clogging, tugging, a flux, or a pricking sensation. Personal experiences, circumstances, and bodily knowledge informed the characterizations of these internal sensations and the ability to discern the fine line between health and illness.

Patients also looked to external factors to explain why and how illness occurred, including environmental, spiritual, and physical causes. This chapter has shown how, in addition to these more well-known influences, emotional responses to adverse social situations—precarious relationships, gossip, or money matters gone bad—were thought to give rise to early modern ailments. Historians have focused primarily on the first five nonnaturals when discussing disease causation in this period, reflecting a tendency to rely on learned medical writing rather than the words and views of sufferers themselves. Approaching explanations of illness onset from the patient's perspective reveals that emotions were a significant source of ill health in the seventeenth century and that gender deeply informed perceptions of the link between emotions and illness. Because early modern women were thought to be particularly prone to passion, they attributed illness to their emotions significantly more frequently than men. Yet gender also shaped patients' narratives in more subtle ways. The few accounts by men that I have found tended to place the social sources of harmful emotions within the framework of occupational concerns and to acknowledge the physical processes underlying subsequent illnesses. This concern for economic independence and focus on the acute, physical processes underlying ill health enabled men to uphold key masculine virtues. The women here emphasized the deleterious effects of interpersonal relationships and described instant physical reactions to social disturbances. They certainly understood the bodily processes that mediated the connection between emotions and sickness. Some referred to shifting and clogged spirits. Others noted how emotions disturbed rest or inhibited a proper diet. Although a loved one's recovery was "the best phisick," grieving women sometimes sought medical advice for sorrow-induced ailments or treated emotional pain with natural remedies, including spa waters and bloodletting.[54] Yet numerous women recounted how grief, fear, and vexation triggered immediate physical reactions. Perhaps most intriguingly, some women's responses to the afflictions of loved ones seemed to transpose ailments from others' bodies to their own. By linking instant ill health to their abounding sympathy and love, these female patients appropriated tropes for conveying sympathy and reflected prevailing beliefs about women's impressionable bodies and ungovernable passions. Claims such as "greefe stops my mouth" justified the neglect of social responsibilities like visiting or writing letters while presenting grievers as pitiable, loving, and sorely afflicted.[55] Just as the social was integral to patients' perceptions of how and why they fell ill, so too was it central to views of suffering and recovery. As the following chapter illustrates, social interactions could cause illness and could also cure.

4. Suffering on the Sickbed

Sarah Cowper first noticed a pain in her foot and a cramping sensation in her breast on March 1, 1702. The next day she consulted a physician and had twelve ounces of blood let out to release the corruptions in her body and ease the pain. But by March 3, her complaints had definitively worsened. She developed an inflammation in her leg known as St. Anthony's fire, as well as a cough and shortness of breath. She continued to track her ailments day by day, including the coming and going of an intermittent fever and pain that shifted from one side of her chest to the other. She was also careful to note the changing behavior of those around her, particularly her husband: "Sir W shows some regard since the Doctour (who is of his acquaintance) tells him I am considerably out of order." According to Cowper, her husband William rarely responded appropriately to her health complaints. He only expressed concern in this instance because a physician and friend convinced him that the illness was serious.[1]

In early April, Cowper "fell into a Relapse." She had not written in her diary since mid-March, presumably because she was too weak. Her next entry described her feeling wasted away from lack of proper nourishment, "hauing eat no fflesh in 21 daies." She believed her fever had collected in one of her eyes, causing what she feared to be blindness. Once again, she was attentive to how the words and behaviors of others shifted in concert with her evolving infirmities. On April 2, she wrote the following entry: "I ought in the next place to mention the Benefits and kindness I receiue from Relations Mrs Coop: hath not been wanting in any manner of help in her power to afford mee; and Sir W hath shewn care and desire of Recouery; indeed spareing for Nothing to that End, which behauiour shall euer have its due weight with, and Effect upon, mee." Cowper was grateful for the support of "Mrs Coop," presumably Margaret Cooper, Lady Shaftesbury. And while she did not specify whether the behavior of her husband, Sir W, had a particular physical, emotional, or mental effect on her, she clearly viewed his compassion as significant.[2]

Sarah Holled and William Cowper had married in 1664, just months after her mother passed away and three years following the death of her father, a London merchant. William was a lawyer who had inherited a baronetcy from his grandfather, and he became a member of Parliament in 1679. The marriage was a step up the social ladder for Sarah, and the successful political careers of her two surviving sons—the elder of whom became lord keeper of the great seal and eventually an earl—only elevated her further. But while the union seemed advantageous on paper, the reality of married life was far from idyllic. The couple seemed to disagree on nearly every matter, including money, politics, and the management of the servants. They even argued about what time to eat dinner. Cowper looked to her private writing to express her grievances and vent deep reserves of resentment. She mostly mentioned William to remark on his faults or comment on his rudeness, which made his commendable behavior in 1702 all the more noteworthy.[3]

Cowper's contemporaries made similar observations of spouses, relatives, and friends during times of ill health. Patients expected their friends and family members to behave in certain ways—to visit, dote, and pray. Likewise, early modern society taught patients to behave in particular ways on the sickbed. Illness sanctioned individuals to forgo daily work, for instance, or to ignore social obligations and make what would normally be deemed unreasonable demands. Roy and Dorothy Porter have observed how this temporary hiatus from the responsibilities of daily life could empower patients by reversing standard hierarchies: "Parents waited upon the children they normally commanded, servants were treated by physicians . . . and the powerful even sometimes submitted to doctors' orders." Scholars refer to these culturally defined behaviors, particularly the dynamic between patient and healer, as "the sick role."[4] This chapter examines that role in early modern England but draws attention to a largely overlooked aspect of it: visitors. Patients assumed a sick role, but friends and family validated the patient's new social position by responding with compassion, love, and pity.

In particular, the following discussion examines how the social dynamics between patients and their visitors could determine displays of suffering on the sickbed. Some men and women performed their suffering in ways that enabled them to negotiate relationships with friends and family—performances that differed by gender. I show, first, that many of the female authors in this study described their illnesses as extraordinarily lengthy and socially isolating and, second, that they defined their disorders as the worst ever or near fatal. Men and women alike suffered from illnesses that were exceedingly long and severe. It is the tone of their accounts, as opposed to the sheer frequency of certain formulations, that is most illuminating. Heightened narratives of suffering enabled some women to manage their domestic relationships and to assert key feminine virtues, such as patience, piety, and humility. As such, suffering was not just a means of negotiating relationships but also an important site of self-production in early modern England—a stage for constructing a sense of self. Suffering on the sickbed gave these women a tool for managing their social worlds and establishing their identities within those worlds.

Pity and the Progression of Illness

Seventeenth-century men and women expected company when they were sick, and many noted whether particular acquaintances made an effort to visit. Despite having to stay home from work on account of his own compromised health, the statesman Arthur Annesley was so intent on fulfilling his duty to his sick sister that he paid her a visit in his slippers and nightgown. Individuals like Annesley viewed the sick visit as an important social responsibility, as well as a religious exercise. Visiting the ill allowed pious authors to observe the afflictions of others, which provoked self-reflection. As Mary Rich explained after visiting a sickly neighbor, God "kept me from paine by seeing hur In so much."[5] Witnessing the suffering of others encouraged believers to contemplate their own preparedness for death and to express gratitude to God for their preservations from similar trials.

There was also a physical component to this devotional activity. Believers had to attain open, warm, broken hearts in order to receive God's spirit. These characterizations of the heart were not mere metaphors for inward sensations of piety. Visiting others evoked emotions such as pity and compassion, which were thought to assist devotion by physically opening, softening, and warming the heart. When her husband was severely ill with gout, Rich compassionately prayed for his life and grieved for his sinful ways. She noted how these emotional expressions physically facilitated her ability to pray, meditate, and receive the grace of God. Like a medical remedy, her tears offered a process of outflow that aided her spiritual health. Her tearful prayers were not emotional responses to worldly afflictions but rather pious expressions of repentance for her and her husband's sins. Immoderate grief and sorrow were frowned upon for signifying an attachment to worldly things, but emotions such as repentant sorrow could be spiritually advantageous.[6] Rich experienced a similar response when she visited a sick servant in 1677. His death was fast approaching, and she hoped to impart advice about how to prepare for the moment when he would face God's judgment. Back at home, she contemplated how these visits had affected the state of her heart: "I fond my one heart much afected with seeing that mortefyeng sight and much car[ri]ed out to pray for the saluation of his soule and when I was alone I did find my Soule to follow uery hard after G[od] for repentance and reamition of sines, for him which I did beg with much feruency and with many teares, then I red and prayd In which duty I was inabled to poure out my Soule to G[od] In strong deasires, and my heart was broken for my Sines." The "mortefyeng sight" of the dying man provoked thoughts on salvation and mortality, as well as tears, prayers, and a softened, "broken" heart. Visiting and tending to the sick enabled Rich quite literally to open her heart to God.[7]

Such compassion, however, was most commonly understood to alter the bodies of those receiving it—Rich's husband and servant, in these cases. We still believe that friendship and positive thinking have physical benefits, but there was a very different framework for explaining this phenomenon in early modern England. Positive social interactions generated feelings of hope, joy, and love in the patient, which nourished the body and hastened recovery. The healthful effects of such interactions could be intense and immediate. One woman attributed her improved health to the mere sight of her sister. Thomas Wright's *The Passions of the Minde* outlines how the elements underlying this reaction were the very same ones involved in emotional causes of illness, namely blood, spirits, and the heart: "The purer spirites retire vnto the heart, and they help maruellously the digestion of blood, so that thereby the heart engendreth great abundance, and most purified spirites, which after being dispersed thorow the body, cause a good concoction to bee made in all partes."[8] If grief caused illness by closing the heart and denying nourishing spirits to the body, emotive responses to receiving a letter or seeing concern in a loved one's face reversed this process by opening and releasing the heart. The diffusion of blood and rush of animal spirits quickened the pulse and improved digestion, which could be "highly beneficial to all parts of the body, and conduceth much to the conservation of Health." Early modern patients and healers viewed the attention and validation of friends and family as comparable to natural treatments. Some even listed the effects of social visits alongside more strictly corporeal signifiers of recovery, such as the cessation of symptoms, the return of normal functioning, or the diminution of pain. Others characterized social visits and letters as medicines, comparing the positive influences of loving interactions to the healing properties of natural remedies: "I beleeue y^r presence will be her best cordiall," one correspondent advised. When Thomas Knyvett visited a sickly cousin, he likened his presence to a common purgative: "Certainly my companye hath some Occult Quallity in it to purge malancholly, as well as a Radish ro[o]te & vinegar."[9] Given the sensitive interactions between internal bodies and external environments that the previous chapter discusses, it might come as little surprise that love and joy were thought to cure illness, just as grief and fear were believed to cause it.

Attention from friends and family did not always generate positive physical effects, however. The melancholic disposition of a visitor could impede a patient's recovery rather than accelerate it, and Cowper continually complained about the negative bodily impact of the "impertinent din" of company. Like anything in excess, affection could also harm the body by creating an overabundance of heat. Undue attachment or desire could lead to dangerous conditions, such as lovesickness. Visits from loved ones were especially dangerous if the patient was particularly sensitive to social stimulation. Anne Dormer described this problem and her "caution in my coming first out of my solitude" following the death of her husband in 1689. Her father insisted she "keepe pace" with a never-ending string of visitors, despite her ailing health and desire for solitude. She feared that such extensive amounts of time in the company of others would waste her spirits and further weaken her body. Her sister had previously experienced a similar kind of forced socialization during a spell of ill health, with damaging results. Dormer believed, like others around her, that because of "the solitude which I had to[o] long endured it was but fitt now I should enjoy and not be forced too hastily out of it." Her body was habituated to isolation, thereby making sudden or excessive interactions shocks to the system.[10]

Rich too struggled to maintain physical well-being following her husband Charles's death. Their marriage had not been an easy one. Over the years he had grown more and more unkind toward her, calling her names and bursting into angry fits that caused her to endure splitting headaches and sleepless nights. Yet his death in August 1673 was a true affliction for Rich, who was expressive about her physical and emotional decline as she nursed her husband through his final weeks. She stumbled about in a "uery stoned [stunned] and astonished Condition" in the days following his death, immobilized by grief. Day after day, she described herself as grief stricken and "bodily discomposed." Family, friends, neighbors, and preachers visited and prayed with her, offering condolences and reassurance. It was not this warm companionship that assisted her recovery, however, but rather a private connection with God. Meditating on eternal life generated feelings of joy and hope that reinvigorated her deteriorating body. "I found," she wrote, "the consideration that my afflictions ware but momentary and my hapyness hereafter would be eternall did in some weake measure reauiue my weake body and made me to rejoyce in hopes of future Glory." Her infirmity was less menacing and even less physically perilous when she acknowledged that God willed it so. Faith inspired the same healing effects as good company.[11]

Visiting the sick, then, had important social, religious, and physical implications for sufferers and visitors alike. And as with any social event, particular expectations and norms defined the sick visit in this period. Patients expressed their suffering, and visitors responded accordingly, sometimes with healthful doses of sympathy. Some visitors spent entire afternoons by a sickbed, chatting with ailing friends and neighbors. Others left too soon or failed to convey adequate expressions of pity. During her above-mentioned illness in 1702, Cowper refused to receive one friend who called at eight in the evening as Cowper was preparing for bed. It was clear the visitor took offense, as the next day she passed by Cowper's room without even saying hello. Cowper considered extending an apology but concluded that her behavior was justified. She had been sick for ten weeks; it was poor form for her friend to wait so long to visit, let alone to visit at such a late hour in the day. Cowper also detected disingenuous sentiments in her visitors. Some showed "an ouerweening concern wc may Easily be seen thro,'" while others could "scarce giue your Complaints a hearing, wc is offensive." Even seemingly proper behavior could misrepresent visitors' true sentiments. Imagining that she had fallen suddenly ill, Cowper guessed that her family would call for help only out of "Decencies sake" rather than genuine worry. Such complaints stemmed not simply from her concerns about comportment but also from her doubts about the sincerity of visitors' feelings. Visitors played a key part in the sick role, and it was just as performative as the suffering of patients.[12]

While Cowper continually lamented the poor etiquette of her visitors, she also complained about having no visitors at all. In the fall of 1702, following her initial chest pain and fever, she suffered once again from a cramp, or "stitch," in her breast. This time the stitch also reached into her throat, jaw, and head, where it settled in her eye and caused sharp pains for twenty-four hours. In addition to noting the nature and location of her complaint, Cowper added a social dimension to her suffering: "In this condition I am left uery solitary." She tended to suffer in solitude because her two grown sons were busy with their own families and political careers and her husband was continually working in London. But she complained about her family's disregard even when they were present and available. Three months after she first noted her cramp in 1702, her body bore the effects of others' neglect: "Ffor in 3 months sickness, I was not watch'd with 3 nights, but suffer'd ye want of due attendance." Staying up with a sick person, or watching, was an important component of nursing in early modern England often performed by female maidservants, neighbors, or family members. In this case, Cowper placed much of the blame on her maid, who occasionally awoke in the night to help her prepare medicines but on the whole failed to stay up and watch over her mistress. Cowper linked the deterioration of her body to the insufficient care of her fellow household members.[13]

The most egregious episodes of neglect, however, were those times when Cowper's family knowingly denied her the attention and pity she expected. On December 31, 1700, she was "uery ill of a Cold but no relation came near me." When her son Spencer and his wife invited her to dinner that day, she declined on account of ill health, and "I heard no more of 'em." Her husband had been away on business that week, and by January 2 Cowper had still had no callers, despite the fact that Spencer was fully aware of her condition—"a prodigious neglect." By noting her family's whereabouts during her episodes of ill health, she looked to her social isolation to convey the extent of her suffering. Even during times of relative health, she measured the magnitude of her misery by the long spans of time passed in solitude: "It is usual with me to be about 12 hours alone, this day made it 14." Conversely, she articulated her contempt for William by tabulating the days she was forced to endure his company—fourteen thousand as of January 1702.[14]

From their perches on their sickbeds, both Cowper and her contemporary Elizabeth Freke watched family members come and go, and both women counted the number of times their sons walked past their doors without a word or even an acknowledgment of their ailing mothers. According to Freke, "My son hass gone by my chamber doore and never called on me to see how I did butt twice (and soe I very ill)."[15] She and Cowper were expressing concerns about etiquette, but they also believed that such rude behavior could be detrimental to health. Like Cowper, Freke closely observed how her family's actions contributed to her deteriorating condition. She had a particularly tough time in 1698 when her husband Percy and their grown son, Ralph, left her alone at the family estate in Norfolk "with two maids and a man . . . and nott one peny to stock itt." Before leaving, Percy had taken Freke's inheritance of £1,000 and invested it in the East India Company in his own name. In addition to her troubling financial situation and growing loneliness, Freke suffered the "unspeakable torture" of learning about her family's rough journey to Ireland. Father and son were "tost up and downe by storms and tempest" for nearly a month, and they had to seek refuge in five different harbors before landing safely in Dublin seven weeks after leaving Norfolk. Freke was so frightened by the episode that she could not bear her solitude any longer, nor could she have "any rest night or day in my mind." She left Norfolk to seek solace from her sister Judith Austen in London. While she was certainly affected by her fear, she was most distressed by her family's neglect. She described how Austen, "commiseratting my deplorable condition to be this cruly disgarded by both my son and my husband, was soe kind to come downe with me, which I shall never forgett itt." Freke further highlighted the source of her misery by contrasting her sister's support with the absence of her husband and son. Austen stayed with her in a small bedroom "in bare walls and hardly a bed for her to lye in" for four months, a comfort that was "more then Mr Frek has afforded me this 17 yeare." Freke did not mention any particular illness during this episode, but her emotionally wrought account speaks to the impact of others' affections on her well-being.[16]

Percy and Ralph Freke's trip to Ireland in 1698 was one of several such journeys they made. The family continually moved back and forth among

London, Ireland, and Norfolk as they handled various financial and property transactions. Freke defined her physical suffering in part by the distance and neglect of her peripatetic family. Her characterizations of a chronic chest and lung disorder called tissick often included the whereabouts of her son and husband, as though their absence was another symptom of the recurring infirmity. In the summer of 1702, she attributed a lengthy illness to traveling to London and Bristol to visit her sisters. Percy left again for Ireland on August 18, and by the fall his absence had exacerbated her condition: "I have kept my chamber till this end of November. In all which time neither my husband or son have binn soe kind to lett me heer a word from either of them, which has much aded to my greatt misery and sickness." For women like Freke and Cowper, the pain caused by remote or rude friends and family members was deeply embedded in understandings of physical suffering. These women could not separate one kind of affliction from the other. Yet accounts of others' neglect also afforded them an opportunity to express dissatisfaction with their families' behavior while highlighting their own lamentable conditions. Freke emphasized her distress during a bout of fever in 1697 by reminding readers that her husband had been living in Ireland for the past three years, depriving her of much-needed support. Likewise, she conveyed the extremity of her tissick in 1712 by explaining that she lay ill for nearly eight months, "expectting my last sumons and no frind neer mee." Part of her concern had to do with the importance of having witnesses at the deathbed. An ideal death in early modern England typically involved a gathering of friends and family members who listened to the sufferer's last words and observed their final moments. This ritual was meant to demonstrate piety and inspire it in others, assuring loved ones of the patient's imminent salvation. A lack of communication from friends and family during episodes of near-fatal illness prompted Freke to enumerate her grievances in terms that were not only socially acceptable but also visible on her ailing body.[17]

The ways these women articulated the temporal progression of illness further reflects concern about social isolation. Freke recorded a succession of ailments that relegated her to bed for lengthy durations. In 1697 she was "fowre or five months sick" at her sister's house in London. At another point she was confined to her chair, "now a prisoner neer eighteen monthes with a rhumatisme and my tissick," and in March 1710 she was ill again, "haveing hardly gone cross my chamber since last November." She claimed to have barely left her room in four years during the fifth time she lived in Ireland:

"In this misserable place and condition I staid allmost frightned outt of my witts for above three years and a halfe and sick all the time with the colick and vapours, and thatt I were given over for death, and hardly ever wentt downe the staires all the time I were in Ireland, viz., 4 year and a halfe."[18] She was not unique in this tendency to record exceptionally lengthy spans of time in the sickroom. Alice Thornton reported being unable to "stand nor goe" for four months in 1666, Anne Fanshawe was ill in bed for seven months in 1658, and the noblewoman Anne Clifford was rendered immobile by a four-month-long illness in 1619.[19] Were these women truly disabled for such prolonged spans of time? We must take them at their word. But more significant than whether they were telling the truth is how their assertions of exceedingly lengthy illness emphasized both debility and its social ramifications. Those who spent months, sometimes years, sequestered in the sickbed measured suffering in part by seclusion from their social worlds.

Men too experienced lengthy ailments. Walter Calverley endured a fever "which lasted 10 days" and in 1695 a case of measles "which kept me within doors for almost a fortnight." But the men I have found who noted lengthy spans of time in the sickroom tended to refer to time as an objective means of defining sickness, like taking a pulse or noting a shade of urine. Even those afflicted with chronic ailments seemed to articulate time in accordance with individual incidences of infirmity. Samuel Pepys had a watery discharge in his eye for "about five days or six," but he neglected to report the total number of days his chronic wind and stones affected him. Likewise, Arthur Annesley seemed to suffer continually from gout, but he recorded each attack as a discrete episode of illness: "Was ill of the gout only one thursday 20 and Friday 23." Six years later, in 1683, his weakness from gout continued from early May "to May 22 inclusiue . . . yet I did busines dayly and dutyes." Annesley gives the impression of near-endless infirmity, to the extent that at times he had trouble fulfilling his political work as a baron and earl. Yet, like Pepys, he articulated the duration of his suffering within the confines of discrete episodes.[20]

Annesley's 1683 entries suggest that the nature of men's and women's work could inform patients' views and articulations of time. The men in this book who labored as booksellers, merchants, tax collectors, and ministers could not afford to remain in bed for lengthy spans of time, and they tended to measure the progression and severity of their infirmities according to their ability to work. Annesley, for example, found it noteworthy that he was able to continue his business despite his debilitating gout. When Roger Lowe was incapacitated by a cramp in his back, he gauged the extremity of his pain by his ability to tend his shop. Few of the women here worked outside the home, and unpaid domestic labor rarely served as a referent for illness. Jane Shakerley briefly mentioned, however, that "uiolent paynes in my hed an teth" prevented her from combing and sorting hair, presumably to be made into wigs. She had to find a substitute to package the hair, which, as a consequence, arrived at its destination in a disorderly state.[21] The fact that so few women here referred to work when evaluating their bodily disorders suggests that economic status had some bearing on their experiences. Although Freke concocted medical remedies in her home and others certainly worked as mistresses presiding over their estates, most of the women in this study were of upper status. Few of them bore the responsibility of supporting their families financially. They lived off their titles and land, and they could lie in bed for lengthy spans of time without contributing to the household economy.

Ralph Thoresby characterized the progression of his illness in 1723 according to his ability to attend religious services rather than meet occupational obligations. He had abandoned his earlier career as a cloth trader and now devoted most of his time to antiquary interests, namely developing a museum of curiosities and completing topographical surveys of Leeds. He remained fervently religious, and his faith provided a primary means of assessing the trajectory of his health. He lay sick for two months before building up the strength to attend church, and even then he had to sit in the vestry, where the air was cool and he could easily slip out. A few days later he regressed: "Yet worse; was not able to reach church." In some sense, tracking the capacity to get to church allowed pious authors like Thoresby a way to justify their "slender devotions." But it also provided a clear means of measuring the progression of illness. Thoresby's health continued to decline, and after one particularly harrowing night he submitted an anonymous bill to his church to ask for prayers from his fellow parishioners. Five days later he reported feeling somewhat better, an improvement he qualified with the note "not able to get to church." The vicar instead visited him in his bedchamber for private prayer.[22]

Spiritual world views informed conceptions of time and suffering in ways that extended beyond discrete episodes of illness like this one. The passing of time marked a believer's advancement on the journey toward eternal life, as reflected in pious authors' tendency to take stock of their spiritual progress on their birthdays. Thoresby lamented his "misspence" of fifty-three years on his birthday in 1711: "Lord, pardon what is irrevocably lapsed, and help me to spend the short remains more usefully!"[23] Diaries provided a tool for recording this profound relationship between time and divine order—a place to record life events and earthly rhythms as divinely determined portents. Infirmities unfolded along this grand, providential time line. Mary Fissell has found that time frames of illness in early modern England could extend far beyond the limits of immediate corporeal sensations. Men and women attributed acute afflictions to incidents or sins committed years earlier.[24] Events that seem inconsequential to our modern eyes were freighted with meaning and could wreak discernible effects on the body years after the fact.

"At the Graues Brink": Expressions of Extreme Suffering

After enduring pain and fever for nearly two months in 1702, Cowper decided to stop complaining in front of her guests, since they never responded to her grievances with the compassion she expected. As she put it, "One must be at the Graues brink, uery miserable ere it moues any pitty." The false front that she presented to friends and family contrasted sharply with the reality of her suffering. Even as she traced an improvement in her health when she was able to attend church in May 1702, a full two months after first feeling a twinge in her breast, she still experienced severe eye problems. She visited a Jewish woman who was known for treating eyes, to no avail: "She told me at first look she cou'd do me no good, there was no help for a Black Cataract; your Eie is gone and you musty submit to God." A month later, Cowper could barely see out of her eye, and she was starting to lose sight in the other one as well. In addition to her sore eyes, she endured pain and stiffness in her neck that prevented her from sitting up. She found herself in a most deplorable state, yet she made a conscious effort to hide her suffering from visitors, as it "seldom finds pitty, wheras to forbear, ofttimes much applause; wc tho' litle worth, yet Complaint if neglected, offends us." Expressing her anguish failed to elicit proper pity from loved ones. Stoic endurance, on the other hand, provoked "much applause"—less prized than pity, but appreciated nonetheless. The gulf between Cowper's disingenuous self-presentation and her actual condition led to anxieties about losing all remnants of concern from relatives and friends: "Those few hours in the Day wc I allot for Company I appear so chearfull, that I expect to lose ye compassion with wc at first meeting my friends usually accost me and 'tis like they will be apt to beleiue I haue endured nothing." Over the years, she had noticed that her continual grumbling about her eyes had eventually failed to evoke compassion, as though her visitors had grown so accustomed to the complaint that they could no longer conjure up any concern. Cowper was acutely aware of the performative nature of suffering and how her behavior could influence the actions and words of visitors.[25]

While Cowper preferred the respect and admiration bestowed upon displays of endurance, others accentuated their suffering to incite pity from friends and family members. Dudley Ryder described just such an approach when he visited his aunt in the spring of 1716. He noted how she seemed to feign suffering right on cue: the moment he knocked on the door, she "began to make a most hideous noise and crying, as if she was extremely sick, but it looked so much as if it had been done with design that I had not the least sentiments of pity." Ryder saw through his aunt's performance and, as a result, was unable to summon any genuine concern for her well-being. As the visit continued, she seemed to forget she was even ill. Rather, she "talked as well and brisk as if not at all out of order."[26] Surely not all early modern patients were as calculating as Cowper or Ryder's aunt. But illness in the seventeenth century entailed a subtle performance of sorts. A set of behaviors demonstrated pain or indicated endurance to an observant, responsive audience.

Writing was another kind of performance—a textual display of suffering for posterity. Cowper reined in her complaints before visitors but resorted to hyperbolic characterizations of suffering in writing. She described her 1702 bout of cramps and pain as the most intense and difficult she had ever endured—"I neuer ail'd so much in all my life"—and at one point her fever was "worse than euer." She characterized her ensuing eye trouble in similarly extreme terms, as an "Exquisite pain." She used superlative descriptors when recounting other kinds of health conditions too. When she had felt a stiffness in her back and legs the preceding winter, she described the episode as "a sudden stroak I neuer felt in all my life." And suffering from stomach pain the next summer, she asserted that "no [other] disease or pain hath afflicted me to extremeity in all my Life." For Mary Shirley, defining an illness as the worst ever provided an immediately identifiable means of communicating debility. She was confined to bed for three weeks while visiting Rome in the early 1700s, seized with fever, "giddiness" in the head, and a "Uiolent pain" in her limbs. As she explained it, "Ye Discharge was beyond any thing I euer had experience'd & ye pain & soreness aboue any thing I euer felt before."[27] I have found fourteen instances of ailments described as the "worst ever" by women and four by men.[28] Male and female patients seemed to stress the severity of their illnesses with varying frequency, but it was their tones that diverged the most.

Rather than use such extreme language again and again, as Cowper did, Rowland Davies defined a single episode of hemorrhoids as truly the most severe he had ever experienced. He had only just arrived in England, in 1689. His family hailed from Hertfordshire, but his father had settled in Ireland, and Davies had traveled to England to escape political upheaval at home. With the help of some friends, he was appointed minister of Great Yarmouth, and it was there that he developed his debilitating condition. He linked his troubles to walking ten miles in the rain with his landlord's brother. He offered no further explanation, though the rain might have led to a cold, in turn provoking the hemorrhoids. Davies was in so much agony that he was unable to kneel in church and could barely walk, "having never in my life had so severe a fit before." Although his characterization of his disorder resembled Cowper's, this was the sole occasion when he described his health in such terms, and he supported the interpretation with his analytical measure of debility—a failure to perform everyday functions like praying and walking. As a clergyman who worked part time as a healer, he prescribed himself a soothing emollient made of honey and cerium, a chemical ingredient, which seems to have proved effective, since he only mentioned the condition once more the following day and then was silent on the matter.[29]

References to death provided another common approach to expressing the severity of suffering. Even as Cowper began to mend in 1702, she viewed her illness as fatal. She feared she might have consumption, which "tho' a slower, yet is as sure a way of Dying no doubt." When Henry More developed scurvy, spleen (melancholy), sinking spirits, and weakness in his legs in 1653, he considered his impending demise: "I suspect myself not far of[f] from an Apoplexy which is an easy death." The particular mix of symptoms led him to suspect an oncoming loss of motion and sensation known as apoplexy, and he began imagining his ensuing end. He predicted only surviving another year, possibly two. The Cambridge philosopher and theologian was mistaken: he ended up living another thirty-four years.[30] Such morbid assessments were distinct from claims that disorders literally felt like the onset of death. For instance, Francis Conway found himself "very ill although not in my former violent paynes." As he explained in a letter to his older brother, "My Condition now is weakness and often suden soundings, just as if I were dyeing." He did not define his condition as seemingly fatal in order to articulate the magnitude of his suffering; indeed, he admitted that his present disorder was less painful than previous episodes. Rather, he believed that certain bodily sensations—weakness and sudden swoons, or "soundings"—felt the way he imagined dying would feel. His doctor recommended sweating in a "hott house" in the springtime.[31]

Men and women alike viewed their disorders as dire and potentially fatal, yet several female authors provided heightened accounts of suffering as if teetering on the brink of death, while men's articulations of potentially deadly ailments tended to be more matter-of-fact: "My right eye began to faile & I fell sick shortly after and was like to dye at Christmas"; "All doubted my recovery"; "very neer death."[32] Isaac Archer almost died from a violent fever after catching cold while traveling in 1677. He believed the illness was possibly fatal, but he communicated the extremity of the situation by coolly interpreting his bodily signs. The ailment was unusual in that he claimed not to feel very ill, although he was disordered by a fever and inability to sleep. Only after he had recovered did he realize that he had survived a fever that others in his community had died from that year, "the nature of which is not to make the patient sick but to kill suddainly." A doctor was visiting unexpectedly when Archer arrived home, and he convinced Archer that the condition was possibly fatal. Indeed, he predicted that Archer would die if he did not improve in two days. Archer viewed the doctor's presence as a divine providence. Had the doctor not been there, he probably "should not have sought out for helpe til I might have bin past helpe." The physician was able to convince Archer of the severity of his illness by feeling his pulse, which Archer unhelpfully characterized as "bad." The doctor prescribed a powder that induced sweats and caused Archer to "breake out with heat," positive developments that enabled him to enjoy "sweet sleepe." Like Davies, Archer articulated the intensity of his condition and the nature of his recovery using specific signifiers—in this case, a dangerously slow pulse and improved rest.[33]

Women such as Freke, Thornton, and Cowper recounted harrowing stories of near-fatal sickness in ways that conveyed remarkably intense suffering. Freke was so frequently on her deathbed that her readers might begin to doubt her sincerity. She was "laid for dead" with a cough in 1702, and after remaining in London in 1711 "all the while allmost dead with my tisick," traveled home two days later, "did itt allmost kill me." In all, she defined eleven episodes of illness as fatal.[34] Some female patients' references to death were so frequent and fervent, they even appeared in men's writing. Archer's wife Anne gave birth to a large, lusty boy in 1672. She had already had two children, only one of whom survived infancy. Two weeks following the birth, she grew severely sick as a result of "noxious and venemous impurities" that remained in her body. The entire family grieved for her life, fearing that death was near. This interpretation seemed to reflect her own reading of the situation. Her husband explained how "she had the very agonies of death, as she thought, and was seized all over with intolerable paine, and possessed with a persuasion she should die that night." Although Archer recorded the incident, it was Anne who interpreted her pain as "the very agonies of death." Likewise, it was she who was "possessed with a persuasion" that death was imminent. Her family trusted her reading of the situation, perhaps because the disorder was rooted in reproductive processes that were otherwise mysterious to them. She took a mixture of boiled herbs, and "nature did its office" by cleansing her body of impurities.[35]

Thornton was recuperating at Scarborough spa in 1666 when she learned she had to travel to York to settle pending financial matters. On the morning she set out, she felt faint and ate nothing, and the horse ride catalyzed the purgative effects of the spa waters. When she asked to stop and rest, her travel companion, an uncle named Francis Darley, refused. She chose not to press the matter, for fear of "displeasing" him. But the decision to continue the journey only worsened her condition, and she subtly noted that if her husband had been present he would have responded to the situation quite differently. Thornton highlighted the intensity of her ensuing illness by noting her proximity to death. Her lengthy suffering, compounded by her declining spirits, "seized soe extremely upon my person with such violency and danger to my life, I could not be insensable of my daily decay and dieing condittion." She indicated the severity of her situation through the intensity of her prose. She was not simply ill but "exceeding feeble and weake" for weeks on end. She endured "continuall faintings upon the reneuall of the extreamity," and she referred to the ailment as a "terrible visitation and languishing condition." In the manuscript version of her account, she provided additional details, such as an excess of blood "perpetualy flowing," which led her to suspect a consumption.[36] She was not fabricating the seriousness of her disorder; she trusted that she was at death's door. Yet she recorded her brush with death quite differently than did Archer or More.

Thornton further verified the magnitude of her condition by citing the opinions and judgments of other people, a move that both men and women made. She wrote that "it was expected I should haue fallen into a deepe consumption," suggesting that those monitoring her health predicted that particular outcome. She had experienced a similar episode of weakness, illness, and dangerous flux of blood while giving birth to her seventh child four years earlier. Then too she had confirmed the extremity of her condition by recounting the observations of other people: "It was terrible to behold to those about me, bringing me into a most desperat condittion, without hopes of life; spiritts, soule, and strength seemed all gon from me." Rather than detail her bodily sensations, Thornton took the perspective of those who tended to her. She went on to note how her husband, children, and friends "had taken theire last fairewell." She survived this ordeal thanks to her healing abilities and what she considered an act of providence. After lying immobile and speechless for five hours, she suddenly remembered a powder that she had administered to others in similar situations. As a cousin wept over her, Thornton was able to whisper in her ear, "Goe into closet, right hand shelfe, box, pouder, syrup of cloves, give me." The powder worked. Thornton delivered the child and recovered, but the effects of the incident "lasted till Candlemass upon my body by fitts"—five full months.[37]

Narratives of lengthy, socially isolating, and severe debility enabled these women to articulate dissatisfaction with their domestic lives in ways that also depicted them as gracious recipients of divine mercy and archetypes of female suffering. In other words, bodily infirmity gave them an opportunity to demonstrate their distress and their virtue.[38] As Freke lay ill for months on end and Thornton's family crowded around what they believed to be her deathbed, these women presented themselves as patient, dutiful, pious sufferers. Bodily suffering provided an outlet for articulating their frustrations within a limiting patriarchal society, as well as a means of demonstrating feminine ideals. Two slightly different accounts of an accidental fall down a flight of stairs in 1704 reveal Freke's attempts to present her life narrative in just this way—as a series of life-threatening trials. In the earlier version she noted letting blood five or six times, while the later account puts the number of bloodlettings at sixteen.[39]

When men and women defined their illnesses as incurable, they surely meant it. Yet this tendency to interpret every illness as one's last stemmed partly from the religious context in which so many seventeenth-century individuals viewed and wrote about their lives. Most of the men and women in this book were pious and regularly contemplated death as the all-important moment when their souls would join God in heaven. A shopkeeper living in Lancashire had a morbid habit of routinely visiting cemeteries to ruminate on the impermanence and frailty of life.[40] Preparing for death was a subject of substantial thought and anxiety among the more devout, and even the most trivial accidents could serve as key lessons or reminders of mortality. This pervasive, almost compulsive focus on death offers another explanation for patients' interpretations of everyday ailments as signs of their impending demise. Feeling slightly out of sorts in 1665, Owen Stockton was provoked to contemplate "w^t grounde I had to expect to eternall life when I should dy." Perhaps he considered his death more readily than he might have otherwise because it was the Sabbath, as well as a year of a major plague epidemic in England. Death surrounded him. Yet other pious individuals, such as Sarah Savage, made similar moves in response to day-to-day disorders. Upon experiencing pain, she could "feel death working, as it were shaking at this Earthly Tabernacle." For such devout sufferers, everyday ailments were small exercises in how to die.[41]

This focus on mortality could impart valuable spiritual lessons. Near-fatal illnesses reminded believers of their potential salvation and how God might judge them. By documenting life-threatening trials, men and women were able to relive their brushes with death and to continue benefiting from the lessons of their harrowing ordeals. For individuals who were not wholly confident about the state of their souls, the specter of death was particularly rife with anxiety and doubt. When Joseph Lister fell ill from a "death-threatening distemper," his spiritual anxiety seemed more acute than any physical suffering. He was then an apprentice living and working in the Yorkshire town of Halifax. He first felt stirrings of doubt about his salvation one afternoon as he sat listening to a sermon about the "day of gracious visitation." That he might not pass this test—his own day of visitation, when God would assess his readiness for heaven—hit Lister "like a thunder-bolt." He began experiencing what he called "a troubled heart," and his ill health only deepened those doubts and revived his "soul-trouble." Anxiety about salvation heightened his physical suffering. He was severely ill, but he interpreted his disorder in wholly spiritual terms. Illness combined with thoughts of death and his past sins left him "oppressed under the burden of gilt." He did not mention humors or rheums but instead described how his fear and anxiety were "more sharp and piercing than before." Only a brush with death could incite such fearful self-reflection.[42]

As Lister's illness began to fade, so too did his fear. He linked his recovery to the will of God, who "was pleased to step in with light, and love, and clear satisfaction." Lister broke out into passionate cries, grateful for what he believed to be a divine intervention: "I could not hold, but cried out loud, 'He is come! He is come!'" Lister trusted that God's grace ultimately spared him his life. Considering this divine mercy alleviated the burden of his bodily suffering, much the way Mary Rich described feeling physical ease while ruminating on her eternal salvation. Thinking about his divine preservation from death "made the affliction on my body the more light and easy," Lister wrote.[43] Narrow escapes from death were deliverances—palpable reminders of God's grace. And tales of near-death experiences followed by recovery echoed Christ's death and resurrection, allowing ordinary believers like Lister to imbue their adversities with deeper, divine import.

Even non-life-threatening incidents imparted similar meditations by reminding individuals of their mortality. While she was walking along Grays Inn, a stone the size of an egg flew over a wall and hit Cowper on the neck. Later that afternoon she received an accidental blow in the chest, this time by a warming pan used to heat up a bed. Pious authors commonly used personal writing to record these kinds of incidents as edifying acts of God. Neither the stone nor the warming pan injured Cowper. She took the time to document both episodes not because these objects harmed her but because she escaped unscathed. She linked her preservations from danger to God's providence; indeed, she believed guardian angels were watching over her.[44] She and Lister continually pondered their fatality. They saw death in everyday accidents and in agonizing sickness. All such occurrences were divine portents to be recorded, studied, and interpreted in search of God's grace. Surviving a close encounter with death was the most definitive sign of all.

The Social World of Treatment

When Samuel Pepys felt spasms of pain in his groin in 1663, he visited a surgeon for advice. The surgeon wrote up a prescription for an enema made from ale, sugar, and butter, which Pepys took home to manufacture. But it was his wife Elizabeth who filled a syringe and injected the mixture in his backside.[45] This chapter has explored how the words, actions, and neglect of visitors could influence patients' expressions of suffering and evaluations of recovery. Loved ones further determined patients' experiences by providing treatment and care. Maids sat up and watched their mistresses through the night. Spouses administered enemas and inserted lancets into arms and feet, holding up basins to catch the blood. Friends encouraged patients to stomach foul-tasting pills and potions. Visitors also shared opinions and observations that could be crucial to patients' understandings of their ailing bodies. Loved ones might recognize a symptom from their own lives or share a recipe known to be effective for similar cases. And the interjections and opinions of friends and visitors could play important roles in negotiating diagnoses and cures with healers. Medical treatment in early modern England was just as social as suffering (fig. 8).

Remedies like Pepys's enema, which opened the body by releasing obstructions, were called *physick*. This was a term for medicine in general, but it also came to be used to define any remedy that provoked outflow—enemas, pills, or drinks that purged the body by releasing the bowels or inducing vomit. Physick could be incredibly debilitating and therefore isolating. One patient reported taking physick made from manna and cream of tartar that produced twenty-seven stools, a near-constant emission that made it all but impossible for him to leave the sickroom, let alone receive visitors.[46] When the effects of his physick faded, however, Pepys found himself "at leisure," relaxing in his chamber. He spent his mornings bent over a bedpan but whiled away the afternoons reading romances, writing songs, and chatting with friends. He took physick one night in 1663, which successfully produced "a good stool" the following morning. When he rose from bed later that day, he had three or four more. He kept to his chamber for most of the morning but began receiving visitors when he was assured the medicine had worn off. Around noon he went downstairs for a meal and spent portions of the afternoon reading Cicero. He passed similarly peaceful days with his wife when the two took physick together, sometimes for their respective infirmities and at other times as a preventative measure—not to treat a known disorder but to keep their bodies open and healthy. Taking physick provided rare opportunities for the couple to rest and commune with each other. Rather than heading off to work or the theater, Pepys spent those afternoons lying beside his wife, "with some

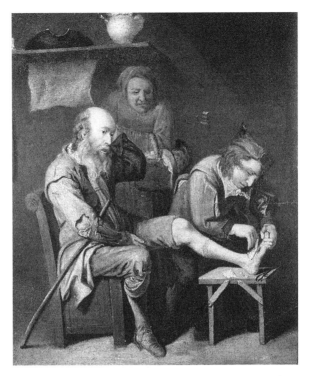

8. A surgeon tends to a patient's foot as a woman watches. Oil
painting after David Ryckaert, 1600s. By permission of the
Wellcome Library, London.

pleasure talking." She used one such opportunity to remind her husband of
the £20 he had promised her for purchasing new Easter clothes.[47]

"Taking the waters" at a spa could be similarly leisurely. Patients traveled to spa towns, many of which developed into extensive leisure resorts,
to treat a range of disorders, including consumption, dizziness, pain, convulsions, bladder stones, stomach trouble, and emotional distress. Rhoda Delves
lived just three miles from Islington spa, which afforded her the ability to
spend three hours drinking the waters each morning to treat "giddiness" in
her head. The minerals in spa waters—which one man described as tasting
"inkish"—opened and purged the body, helping to remove obstructions and
ease pain.[48] Certain ailments called for hot waters, while others required cooling springs, so sufferers chose particular spas based on their disorders, as
well as their constitutions. One physician instructed his patient to treat a kidney
ailment by visiting Knaresborough spa, known for its particularly cold
spring: "I . . . shall not advise you to goe to the Bathe, those waters are too

hott for yor kidneys & will encrease the bleeding, I shall rather advise yor Lad to goe to Knaresborough Spaw, wch are of the nature of Tumbrige waters wch I take to be better for yor Lad." There was a key social dimension to the healing capabilities of spas. Some patients' accounts of their time spent at spas include more details about social engagements than health matters. Nicholas Blundell made no mention of health when he visited Lathom Spa in 1702 but only noted that "we dansed with Young Mr Hesketh of Oughton, Mrs Entisely, Mrs Ann Bold &c." Others explicitly noted how the atmosphere of spas wrought positive bodily effects. William Burrell traveled to Tunbridge Wells "in hopes air and company at this place might help me." Another man had "aduice of at least 20 Phisitians and haue swallow'd a Cart load of Drugs" but only found relief after drinking the waters at Bath. He attributed this success not to the water itself but to the "free air" and "respite from all bussines for some time." The relaxing environment, good company, and clean air of the spa rejuvenated these men.[49]

To treat his hemorrhoids, Philip Gawdy wrote to his brother in search of a recipe: "I knowe you haue had experience of this disease, and that you haue tried uerye excellent medycynes for the ease thereof." Individuals like Gawdy requested advice from relatives and acquaintances in correspondence, the same way they sometimes sought such information from practitioners. Gawdy proceeded to provide more detail about his condition than his brother probably cared to hear: "Myne as all inwards, and they now beginn to bleede a little, I haue kepte my bedd this fyue dayes for the moste parte neither able to go, nor sytt, the outer parts of my tuell is not swelled awhitt, but it is more inwards uery whott, angrye, and beating uery paynefull."[50] Some correspondents responded to such testimonials with helpful instructions. Over the course of several years George Weckherlin shared a huge amount of health advice with his daughter, Elizabeth Trumbull. He provided exercises for curing a bad back, a diet for treating weakness, and a recipe for a salve that purportedly loosened obstructions caused by breastfeeding. He even shared an artificial nipple that she might use to draw out congested matter. As this last, sex-specific remedy illustrates, men and women exchanged treatments that did not necessarily originate in their own firsthand experiences. One woman directed her correspondent to a remedy in her own receipt book: "If you could get a stiling tracle [treacle] water it would do well, it is called in my book jandis water." Patients commonly named the person who provided a particular recipe, as a way of acknowledging gratitude as much as recording that remedy for future use. Blundell's wife concocted a purgative "by Advice of Betty Morrice," and Arthur Annesley took a purge and a cordial "all of Lady Prats praescription."[51] While recipes were exchanged as gifts and commodities, they were also an important means of expressing sympathy and displaying concern. Recipes known to benefit others were a tangible form of pity—words that communicated compassion and concern, reassurance and hope.

The family members and friends who shared recipes, administered enemas, or accompanied loved ones to spas could be present when a healer arrived, and many were quick to offer up their observations and judgments. Historians have suggested that early modern female patients were more restricted than their male counterparts when negotiating medical treatment, as the concerns and demands of relatives could limit their choices.[52] While this may have been the case in some instances, writing by medical practitioners suggests that friends and relatives mediated the treatment of male and female patients alike. Friends, neighbors, and kin were often present in the rooms of sufferers of all ages and genders, and they could be actively involved in negotiating procedures and cures on behalf of loved ones. The patient's family and friends were especially crucial when they disagreed with a healer's interpretation of the case. A surgeon at St. Thomas's Hospital in London noted how "a Person" present during one consultation objected to his proposed course of treatment. The surgical team, James Molins and his father, were preparing to amputate a man's foot the "authentick way" when the unnamed speaker demanded they instead apply to the affected area a concoction called "Aqua Regalis Stiptica." This course of treatment "was agreed on more by ye Desire of ye party himslfe & his freinds y^n by ye free consent of ye Chururg [surgeon]." As another surgeon prepared to trepan a patient, a procedure that entailed boring a hole into the skull to alleviate tension, he allowed the patient's friends to inspect and even test his various instruments. He ended up using the trepanning device that they preferred.[53]

While practitioners lamented the pushiness of patients' loved ones, the voices and views of family members could provide valuable, otherwise unobtainable information. John Douglas asked a patient whether he had taken his prescribed medicine, but it was the patient's family who responded: "Yes, yes, said they, he has not miss'd taking it once; that is nott the Cause of his Disorder, he has been talk'd to too much, and upon a very improper Subject." They explained that the patient's health had deteriorated when a "Limb of the Law" entered the sickroom and divulged that a stranger would likely inherit his estate. The patient was physically present for this conversation, but communication seemed to exist solely between the sufferer's friends and practitioners. The man was suffering from a mortified foot that had broken out into ulcerous tumors. Amputation was the most common treatment for such disorders. Douglas asked the patient whether he had ever noticed a bruise or wound on the afflicted foot. Although the patient could not recall anything noteworthy, "some Persons about him talk'd of a strait Shoe, which he had complain'd of some time before." Again, the patient's friends provided key information about the man's past, which enabled Douglas to determine the source of the disorder. In the end, thanks to the input of his friends and family, the patient recovered without having to lose a limb.[54]

John Colbatch was influenced not so much by the words and appeals of one patient's friends as by their emotive expressions. He was called to see a gentlewoman suffering from a high fever, faintness, and weakness. The patient had not slept in ten days, and her physician had given up all hope. Colbatch was called in "only to look upon her, and see her expire." But upon witnessing the sorrow of those who grieved for her, he instead chose to make a last-ditch attempt at a cure: "Seeing her Relations all in Tears, bewailing the great loss they were like to have, I told them there were still some sparks of hopes." He successfully treated the patient with juleps made of lemons and oranges, as well as a complex remedy made from acids. While pity was believed to have real effects on early modern bodies, in this particular case it was the compassion of a healer that mediated the healthful influences of a patient's social world.[55]

Conclusion

We still believe in mind over matter. Many trust that a placebo, a positive attitude, or the power of suggestion can have discernible physiological effects. The notion that "A merry heart doth good like a Medicine" is long enduring.[56] There was a complex physiological framework underlying this phenomenon in early modern England, one that involved vacillating humors, nourishing spirits, surges of blood, and the heart. By the eighteenth century, the positive effects of sociability had been reinterpreted within the frame of new medical models that came to replace humoralism. Sociable activity and polite conversation were thought to affect the tautness of the body's nerves or to transmit healthful qualities by means of invisible airborne particles. Positive social interactions still contributed to health and were even believed to prolong life, but patients and healers looked to new frameworks to explain the phenomenon.[57]

As a key determinant of recovery, social interactions could have a significant impact on patients' verbal and behavioral expressions of suffering. Some patients communicated their bodily distress in ways that enabled them to elicit certain kinds of responses from friends and family members. Others measured their anguish on the sickbed in terms of the caliber and frequency of their interactions with visitors. This chapter shows that we must view patients' words and behaviors within the context of their relationships with visiting friends, relatives, colleagues, and neighbors. It is within this social matrix that patients occupied the sick role. Suffering differed according to individual personalities and circumstances, yet broad, gendered patterns emerge in similar forms of writing by patients. Several accounts by women reflect a tendency to describe time in the sickroom as uncommonly lengthy, lonely, and painful. Illness afforded these women a rare opportunity to present themselves as patient, humble sufferers and to communicate their dissatisfactions with friends and family. One female author, Ann Fanshawe, remarked that she recorded her illness so that "you may see how near dying we were."[58] She was conscious of her readership, and this awareness shaped the record of her life. For many women, like Fanshawe, bodily suffering provided a means of constructing and asserting a sense of self. Men too endured long, terrifying disorders, but they seem to have described their experiences in more objective, less heightened tones.

Work and religion further informed these varied expressions of suffering on the sickbed. Men who labored outside the home tended to track the progression of illness in brief, quantifiable time spans and to rely on work as a key measure of that time. More pious individuals evaluated recovery according to their ability to attend church or perform devotional duties. While defining ailments as life threatening could convey the severity of suffering and the significance of social isolation, this compulsion could also reflect a tendency to view life's trials as valuable spiritual opportunities to meditate on mortality. The following chapter continues to explore the impact of these gendered, religious, and economic concerns by concentrating on patients' perceptions of one common dimension of ill health: physical pain.

5. Perceptions of Pain

Samuel Pepys woke up in pain from a cold he had caught the previous day. It was the spring of 1664. He was rising in the ranks as an administrator in the navy and had recently been appointed to the commission of the royal fishery (see fig. 9). He decided to head to his office that day despite his discomfort but soon returned home, "being in extraordinary pain." After dinner, the agony was so exquisite that he was forced to retire early. He evaluated his pain by looking to past experiences: it was "as great for an hour or two as ever I remember it was in any fit of the stone." Kidney stones plagued Pepys throughout his adult life. He continually complained about twinges in his back, tenderness while urinating, bruised testicles, and incapacitating gas. Though he did not always view these disorders as symptoms of a single chronic ailment as we might today, he lived in perpetual fear of the stone and its debilitating effects. And his anguish was so extreme that day in 1664 that he compared it to the excruciating sensation of stones. Pepys's account of this episode is particularly detailed and intimate: "I took a glister [enema], but it brought away but a little and my heighth of pain fallowed it. At last, after two hours lying thus in most extraordinary anguish, crying and roaring, I know not what whether it was my great sweating that [made] me do it, but upon getting by chance among my other tumblings, upon my knees in bed, my pain began to grow less." Sitting on his knees somehow lessened the sensation, but it was only a temporary relief. Over the course of the next few weeks he endured pain from an inability to urinate or pass gas. He had to miss work and other social obligations for several days, and he took a series of medical treatments,

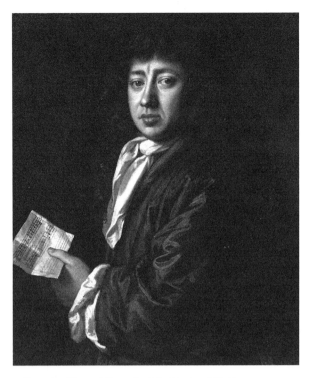

9. Portrait of Samuel Pepys by John Hayls, 1666. Pepys at age
thirty-three poses here holding sheet music by William Davenant.
© National Portrait Gallery, London.

including a concoction of buttermilk and whey, to try to alleviate the
symptoms.[1]

Pepys continually looked to prior episodes of the stone to evaluate his
various bodily pains. He made careful observations of the location, cause, severity, and timing of his aches in order to determine whether they predicted the
reemergence of his "old pain" or rather another trouble altogether. Experience
allowed him to discern that a "stopping" in his urine signaled the early stages of
stones, as did wind, or gas, on a coach ride home. When he felt twinges or
irritations without familiar symptoms, he was able to attribute them to other
causes, such as stooping or straining to lift heavy objects. Based on these careful
self-observations, he was able to diagnose his own body, and even those of others. At one point he surmised that his servant suffered from the stone "or some
other pain like it," and a surgeon later confirmed this evaluation.[2]

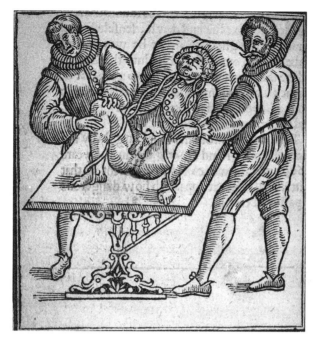

10. A man prepares to be "cut for the stone." Wilhelm Fabricius Hildamus, *Lithotomia Vesicae* (London: Printed by John Norton, 1640), pg. 88. This item is reproduced by permission of The Huntington Library, San Marino, California.

The gravity of Pepys's particular case made the stone a suitable reference for all kinds of bodily complaints. In 1658 he survived an invasive and dangerous procedure to remove a kidney stone the size of a tennis ball. The successful operation was one of the most significant events of his life. He recounted the story to anyone who would listen and even paid twenty-four shillings for a special case in which to preserve and display the extracted specimen. The magnitude of the event is perhaps most clearly reflected in his annual "feast-days" commemorating the successful intervention. In March 1661, Pepys wrote, "This is my great day, that three years ago I was cut of the stone—and blessed be God, I do yet find myself very free from pain again." On the sixth anniversary of the operation he thanked God that he was raised from "a condition of constant and dangerous and most painful sickness."[3] The surgery was noteworthy not only because it alleviated his intense suffering but also because he survived it (fig. 10).

Kidney stones dominated Pepys's thoughts and dictated his day-to-day life. They even permeated his dreams. In 1661, three years after the operation, he dreamed that one of his testicles swelled, "and in such pain that I waked with it." Years later he dreamed that he again had the stone, "and that once I looked upon my yard in making water at the steps before my door, and there I took hold of the end of a thing and pulled it out, and it was a turd." As opposed to analyzing the Freudian dimensions of this dream, I only want to highlight that Pepys exhibited deep anxiety about the stone, perhaps because a series of related ailments continued to afflict him throughout his adulthood. He nearly relived his surgery when the wound from the operation ruptured in 1700, "so as to make another issue for my urine to sally at, besides that of its natural channel." He underwent two attempts to remedy the fissure, both of which involved reopening the wound so that it could heal anew. These procedures incapacitated Pepys for four months, as his legs were bound to enable the flesh to heal.[4]

Pepys was an exceptional character, and he offers a uniquely detailed narrative of health. As chapter 2 discusses, he scrutinized his body and provided a meticulous record of interactions among his health, his diet, his exercise, and the weather, occasionally interspersed with sordid accounts, such as that of awaking "wet with my spewing" after a night of heavy drinking.[5] Despite his individuality, he reveals some common ways sufferers made sense of recurring and debilitating bodily sensations. Like Pepys, other men and women made observations to locate pain internally, to assess its shifts and pulses, and to capture resulting sensations on the page. Such assessments were important because pain was both a common symptom and source of early modern bodily disorders. Evaluating the location, movement, and quality of pain could also be integral to medical treatment. Such information enabled healers to make diagnoses and gauge the effects of remedies. Yet as Esther Cohen has noted, historians of pain have tended to focus more on the management of sensation than on modes of expression. This chapter opens by examining patients' approaches to diagnosing and describing pain as a physical, internal process.[6]

Attempts to explain the physiology of pain coexisted with religious conceptions of suffering. Patients did everything in their power to alleviate physical suffering, but they also accepted pain, and some even embraced it as an ennobling spiritual opportunity.[7] While patients drew on a range of devotional texts, images, and beliefs to articulate their bodily torments, this chapter focuses on their use of martyrdom—one of the most popular and resonant narratives of the period. Popular accounts of religious martyrs circulated orally, visually, and textually in the seventeenth century and provided a key script for voicing pain. Stories of martyrdom provided patients with a language, a set of metaphors, and also models for expressing pain as pious Christians. One book in particular, John Foxe's *Actes and Monuments*, largely informed prevailing views and beliefs about martyrdom in early modern England. It is a sensational account of the persecution of Protestants under the Catholic queen Mary Tudor in the sixteenth century, and it remained immensely popular well into the 1600s. Like martyrs at the stake, Protestant patients aspired to endure their pain with calm and composure.

Alongside religious models and medical knowledge, gender ideals and concerns determined expressions of bodily suffering. The aim here is to pull all these strands together. As opposed to analyzing pain solely within a spiritual context or exclusively focusing on medicine, which can obscure the influences of gender on patients' perceptions, this chapter pieces together how both male and female sufferers relied on a range of scripts to write about and respond to pain.[8] Severe episodes of pain enabled some patients to emphasize ideal gendered and Christian behavior simultaneously. Feminine humility and submission, as well as masculine strength and self-control, nicely complemented Christian concerns about enduring physical afflictions with patience, passivity, reflection, and hope. In practice, however, gendered and religious ideals could complicate one another. Excruciating, redemptive pain that was so significant to believers could undermine displays of feminine patience and masculine endurance. Women in anguish could not remain silent and meek but instead cried out. And both middling- and upper-status men lamented having to forgo occupational responsibilities. These men and women expressed the intensity of their suffering in ways that defied established gender norms. Indeed, it is the very defiance of normative gendered behavior that enabled these men and women to communicate the severity of their suffering most effectively. Not everyone expressed physical distress in such terms, but those who did reveal overlapping and conflicting influences on patients' perceptions of pain.

Giving Pain a Name

Catherine Cary went on a brisk walk in 1733, which caused her to break into a sweat. At the precise moment when she arrived back home, she later realized, her cold struck. The walls in the house were damp and the air was chilly, in sharp contrast to the heat she had generated on the walk. Patients in this period often linked colds to cool air that breached the body through warm, receptive skin. The air then became trapped inside the body as the pores tightened and closed. Cary determined that her cold sparked the return of a throbbing sensation in her breast. It was "as if a dart had struck into it," she later explained to her husband. She looked to a range of metaphors to communicate her pain: it felt like stabbing forks, a gnawing sensation, and a tugging. She even drew on the iconic symbol of early modern women's work, the needle, by comparing her aches to "broken-pointed needles pricking her lightly." The pain in her breast likewise felt "as if the part were stitching up with a needle & thread." She had first felt the sensation sixteen years earlier, and it returned year after year, sometimes in her hip, at other times in her hand. Now it was localized in her left breast. The feeling reappeared whenever the weather turned cool or right before a rainstorm. In this instance, the pain was more intense than ever. Within days she was unable to lift her left arm above her head. She felt the pain settle deep within her bones.[9]

Cary used an ointment made of white bread, milk, and brandy to soothe her pain. When this proved ineffective, she applied a topical remedy made of bruised herbs fried in lard, which softened the swelling forming on her breast. She drank a quart of spa waters each morning before breakfast, in the hope that the minerals would further open her body, release corruptions, and ease her suffering. Physicians wrote prescriptions for these various treatments, though Cary added or removed ingredients based on her own sense of what would work best. One recipe for a purgative, for instance, included an ingredient that induced menstruation. But by the time she took the recipe to an apothecary to purchase the ingredients, Cary was menstruating without trouble. The apothecary recommended adding twenty grains of mercury instead, and she complied. In addition to seeking help from apothecaries and physicians, she tried an ointment that some neighbors recommended, as well as a topical cream made of white lily root and butter prescribed by an older woman who specialized in treating sore breasts. More than a year later Cary's health had improved, but she was still taking medicines regularly to keep the pain at bay.[10]

Patients like Cary possessed substantial knowledge of medicine and the body, which afforded them leverage as they shopped for healers and cures. Previous chapters of this book explored the ways patients used that knowledge in procuring treatments, interacting with healers, and interpreting the cause and duration of illnesses. This knowledge is further evidenced in the sensations and internal maps of the body that individuals relied on to make sense of pain. Patients evaluated throbbing and tingling physical complaints by determining their location, severity, and movement deep within the body. Henry Ireton demonstrates an attentive reading of pain quite similar to those provided by Cary and Pepys. Ireton was a member of Parliament from Gloucestershire and the son of a famous civil war Parliamentarian. In 1709, he noticed that his urine was tinged with blood, yet he only suspected the stone upon feeling "a little paine on the left side of my Belly, Inwardly." He shared this experience in a lengthy letter outlining five fits of stone in excruciating detail. He evaluated himself by feeling around the area below his ribs, finding it firmer than the same spot on the other side. When he pressed down, he noticed that the part was hard and his pain spiked. He spent the rest of the night in "Excessiuely Uiolent" torment. The pain was so severe it made him vomit, and, unlike for Pepys, no change in position alleviated the sensation.[11]

Ireton claimed to have "no Skill In Anatomy," yet he was able to locate his pain in a remarkably specific part of his body: "I feele not any paine on the outside of my back, but all Inwardly: But if it be not in ye kidney, I fancy it must be betweene ye kidney & the upper part of ye bladder, & not in ye bladder, for I thinke my paine is not low enouf to proceede from any thing within ye bladder or below it." Like Pepys, who only suspected the stone upon feeling aches in his lower back and groin, Ireton was able to diagnose his complaint by locating specific sensations internally. He calculated the cause and progression of his disorder by evaluating its location and severity and by measuring these factors against other observations, such as the quantity of gravel, or sediment, in his urine. He noted making "6 spoonfuls of uery bloudy water, wth some Grauel in it," but then explained that it was "not enouf grauel to account for ye ceasing of so greate pain as I had then bin in." After another fit, he similarly explained, "w^t I had brought away was not a sufficient reason for my being Eas'd from so greate pain." Ireton associated a certain amount of excreted sediment with a particular level of physical distress. His diagnosis also colored his reading of otherwise imperceptible sensations. A few days after his initial discovery of blood in his urine, he felt light twinges, but "not enouf to haue bin noticed by me, were it not or w^t has preceded."[12] When Pepys's tenderness did not fit his expectations or prior experiences of the stone, he altered his diagnosis. After a particularly difficult day in 1661, for example, he awoke the following morning completely free from pain, "which makes me think that my pain yesterday was nothing but from my drinking too much the day before."[13] The sudden relief led him to consider other possible explanations for his discomfort.

Rather than relying on bodily memory and past experiences to evaluate tenderness in her joints, Sarah Cowper looked to the behaviors of other people. By the time she reached the age of seventy-one, her health had deteriorated substantially. She described herself as "Lame, Half Blind, Half Deaf, but 3 Teeth beside stumps." Added to these complaints, she suffered from hemorrhoids, a sore back, and aching legs. The palsy in her hands was so severe that she could no longer safely hold a cup of coffee. And her hearing was so impaired that she stopped attending church, since she was unable to make out the sermons. Her diary entries from that year reflect a growing preoccupation with the physical effects of old age. She increasingly recorded stories and aphorisms about aging, including the tale of a ninety-six-year-old man who suddenly grew a new set of teeth. But rather than evaluate her sore back and limbs relative to her own experiences over the years, as Pepys or Ireton might have done, she made sense of her pain by watching strangers walk beneath her window: "Perhaps it may proceed from ye extream Rainy weather, for I obserue that people of all sorts who walk the streets do Hobble and go lame more than euer."[14] Cowper definitively linked her disorder to the weather by recognizing her own distress in the postures of others.

In some instances, pain was more elusive. When patients were unable to connect their physical distress to a particular disorder or experience, they relied on familiar sensations to give pain a name. Sufferers described feeling a "drawing and sucking," a weight or oppression, a burning, pricking, or "tensive" feeling, and even scraping. Others looked to ailments or symptoms that most closely resembled their sensations: an aching knee joint was "like that of a Sprain," or a smarting rib felt like a cramp.[15] George Weckherlin suffered from "raging paine" as a result of gout. He traced the rise and fall of swellings in his joints and surges of incapacitating pangs in his legs, a recurring debility that sometimes prevented him from writing. In 1647 he communicated these sensations by comparing them to a feeling that surely anyone in the period was equipped to evaluate: his pain felt like "a colde in all my bones." Others referred to daily experiences to articulate physical discomfort, such as a harsh remedy working on the stomach "like barm on new beer." Barm was the froth that formed on fermenting liquor, an evocative comparison to the bubbling sensation of a purgative at work.[16] While comparing pain to a needle and thread, as did Cary, is one way that patients looked to gendered work to express their bodily torments, I have found surprisingly little evidence that women compared the pains of illness and accidents to the sensations of childbirth. Yet one man, Samuel Crew, found childbirth a compelling referent. He likened the anguish of releasing his bowels to the pain of giving birth: "No Woman in extream Labour could have more Pain, caused through contraction of my Fundiment."[17] The location of his pain no doubt led him to make this comparison.

Crew felt anguish throughout his entire body in 1696, from his right elbow to the insteps of his feet. Even his skin hurt. He described a contraction in his legs "as hard as any Iron Wedg" and a beating in his ears as though a "Red-hot Iron had been run into them." Such violent language provided one of the most common approaches to articulating the nature and intensity of physical suffering. Sharp, sudden sensations were compared to daggers or caused body parts to "smart as if they had been cut with a razor." Others likened their anguish to various forms of bodily harm. One man's thigh felt "as if the Bone had been grinding to pieces."[18] Such comparisons reflect their historical moment. Most people today have little contact with irons or daggers and so look to other objects—even if just as violent ones—to express their anguish. These linguistic expressions can, in turn, influence sensations. There was a certain understanding of what it felt like to have a dagger tear into your muscle or a hot iron sear your skin. Such descriptors communicated bodily torments, and they informed perceptions of them.

If the language of pain in early modern England is unlike our own, the disparity stems in part from a very different understanding of how pain operated within the body. Circulating pain was a key symptom of some disorders, such as gout and rheumatism. But roving, raging pain also had a physical existence. Pain was a symptom and also a disorder unto itself. Patients described pain as running, shooting, darting, and wandering throughout the body. These movements created dramatic alterations and could lead to new complaints altogether. One woman, for example, endured a headache for years before it suddenly fell into her pelvis, where it "fix'd on ye os pubis & uesica sphincter." This unexpected shift from headache to kidney stone occurred while she was riding in a field.[19] Pain was mutable, and the body was a flow-ing, holistic composition. As concentrations of humors dispersed, rheums fell, or spirits shifted, sufferers felt entirely new ailments emerge. Sometimes pain sparked new conditions that, to our minds, seem entirely unrelated. In one such instance, a pin from a head scarf pierced a woman's throat, which "caus'd so much anguish as cast her in a Feauor." This particular woman was grief stricken over the recent death of her mother. In her distress, she had accidentally knocked over a candle on the rail of her bed, igniting a small fire. The flames caught her clothing before she could call for help. She was in this state of sorrow, confusion, and fear when the pin impaled her neck and the ensuing pain generated fever. Other factors within the early modern framework of disease, such as the emotions or the environment, possibly contributed to her sudden fever, yet a number of other patients in the period similarly linked acute stabs of pain to subsequent fevers.[20]

Hephzibah Parker, who was living in Waddon Court, just south of Lon-don, in the early 1700s, withstood a variety of debilitating disorders. She convulsed in ways that constricted her breathing, and she felt a frightening rising sensation in her throat. Her health slowly improved after a few months, a progression that her mother determined by her daughter's ability to move around the house. But Parker walked on the sides of her feet, which strained the tendons in her ankles. Her ankles grew so tender that merely "touching of them puts her into a Conuolsion." She was living almost entirely on green tea, and her mother grew increasingly concerned. She bled her daughter and gave her purgative medicines, but these proved too potent for the patient's delicate stomach. The purge was so harsh that Parker refused to take it, de-spite her mother's urging that she consume it every day "till newe." By the peak of her illness, Parker was experiencing seven convulsive fits a day, which lasted as long as thirty minutes at a stretch. While some developed in response to pain, for instance when someone touched her sensitive ankles, others were the cause of Parker's uneasiness. She would draw in a breath, "which is very Painfull to her side," and then "it flys into her head & is uery painfull." The breath generated pain that instantly afflicted various parts of her body, as fast as the breath could carry it.[21]

Pain roamed, generating fevers and morphing into new complaints, and it also disrupted and redirected internal flows. For instance, when a physi-cian attempted to let blood from a patient to alleviate her chest pain, he was unable to complete the procedure. Upon the insertion of the lancet in the woman's arm, no blood came out. The physician explained that because "the Blood was drawn so strongly towards the Breast through the very violent pain thereof, that hardly any would spurt out of the opened Vein." Pain was an internal force that, like wind or cold, could alter the movement and evacuation of bodily substances such as blood, humors, and spirits. In this case, blood was drawn toward the source of the pain and away from the patient's limbs. The remedy was simple: the patient coughed as hard as she could to drive the blood toward her extremities. If internal matter like pain or blood could move, then patients could direct those travels by coughing, running, or jumping up and down. Such forceful movements were thought to transfer offending matter to other regions of the body. Hence, a man with a throbbing shoulder rode his horse to "moue it off." Patients also imbibed remedies more quickly or slowly in order to alter their potency, or they lay down or went on walks to guide medicines toward particular parts.[22] This relationship between external behaviors and internal processes reflects, once again, the permeable boundary between the early modern body and its world. Just as disturbing social interactions could trigger fevers and distressing news could cause colds, manipulating the external body could produce significant internal transformations.

Some seventeenth-century patients endured medical procedures that were more excruciating than their illnesses. Bloodletting, purging pills, and enemas could be extraordinarily unpleasant. And surgeons set bones, inserted probes into lesions, and cauterized wounds using hot irons—all without anesthesia. While these practices were believed to be effective, many shared Anne North's sentiment that "a great part of there trade is to tortor."[23] Some patients refused to consume remedies or to undergo operations, instead seeking out practitioners who would comply with their demands for gentler, less invasive treatments. Medical preparations made from chemicals and minerals that were purported to be less painful than traditional evacuative remedies became increasingly popular over the course of the century. Patients might also prepare for operations by drinking alcohol or imbibing tobacco, which served as a numbing agent. And some healers prescribed analgesics or altered their procedures to spare patients. But for the most part, palliatives in the seventeenth century were purges, bleedings, and ointments that differed little from other common therapies. In 1695, Magdalen Coward recorded recipes for relieving various types of pain, including sore arms and legs, stomachaches, and "a setled paine" in the hips. They called for similar strategies and ingredients as those listed for other conditions, such as colds, convulsions, and jaundice. One required deer suet and boar's grease, for instance, while another made use of pulverized saffron boiled in milk and salt.[24] Pain-killers such as henbane and laudanum were common ingredients in pills and ointments that targeted pain, but these ingredients were prohibitively expensive and could cause dangerous side effects. Opium was known to induce sleep from which some patients never awoke, as well as to slow the pulse and diminish the ability to breathe. Safe doses failed to relieve the acute pain of surgical interventions. Writing in 1712, one practitioner explained how narcotics are "of little use" for treating severe pain, "for they only stupifie, and seldom remove the Cause." For all of these reasons, opiates were rarely taken on their own and were considered a means of last resort. Moreover, observing the nature, location, and movement of pain provided a valuable means of diagnosing and tracking the progression of disorders. Numbing such sensations could be detrimental to healing, as well as to the natural process of recovery.[25]

"I Was as It Were Set upon a Rack": Martyrdom and Narratives of Pain

Patients made every attempt to diagnose and treat their bodily afflictions, yet many were also resigned to a lifetime of physical distress. The pious viewed pain, after all, as an enduring and necessary component of life. By the time Sarah Cowper awoke at seven every morning, she wrote, "my Bones ake, with weariness of my Bed." Sufferers like Cowper calmly accepted sore feet, throbbing heads, and aching joints in order to demonstrate an elevation of spiritual concerns over corporeal considerations. Protestant literature taught believers to respond to corporeal suffering as patiently as possible, and many evaluated the progression of their pain according to their ability to fulfill devotional duties. The challenge of transcending bodily suffering points to the double nature of pain as both trial and gift: pain could inhibit proper prayer, but it could also promote spiritual meditation. The word *pain* derives from *poena*, or "punishment," and as such was viewed as an affliction from God for human sin—a concept reflected in the belief that women experienced pain in childbirth as punishment for Eve's transgression. As a divine punishment, bodily torment encouraged sufferers to meditate on their sins and frailties, as well as on their potential salvation.[26]

Ralph Thoresby viewed pain as "a memento of mortality," a reminder of death's inevitability. In one such instance, he had recently attended the funeral of Mrs. Whitaker, the wife of a minister in his community. She died only two weeks after giving birth to her first child. Thoresby was affected by her death in part because he had nearly lost his wife to childbirth. But it was also the suddenness of Whitaker's demise that was so unsettling. An unexpected death denied the dying adequate time to prepare spiritually, emotionally, and physically for God's judgment. In the following weeks, Thoresby felt two sharp stabs in his head, which sparked reflections on his own inevitable demise: "Morning, as once before this week, had a memento of mortality, perhaps of sudden dissolution, in violent pain in the back parts of head." His smarting head was not only a reminder of death but also a potential sign of its imminence—a "sudden dissolution." Whitaker's death perhaps colored Thoresby's interpretation of his headaches. Yet he used the phrase in other instances too. Years later he again felt an ache in his head, which was so intense he had to stop working: "A memento of a sudden dissolution. Lord, prepare me for thy pleasure!" Pain reminded the faithful to prepare for death, and it aided in that preparation by encouraging sufferers to fix their thoughts on what Thoresby called "the great change" after life. Just the memory of past torments could continue to serve these important functions long after sensations faded.[27]

Pious patients struggled to withstand pain without displaying fear or despair. Complaints were admissible, but only if they exuded patience and hope. As Jeremy Taylor explained in *The Rule and Exercises of Holy Dying*, "He that is afraid of pain is afraid of his own nature; and if his fear be violent, it is a sign his Patience is none at all; and an impatient person is not ready dressed for Heaven."[28] Although responding to suffering with passive endurance was not always easy, accepting that God was the ultimate source of all afflictions provided much needed comfort. Reflecting on the pain of childbirth as she waited to begin labor, Elizabeth Egerton feared the forthcoming torments. Yet she also trusted that God would enable her to bear "this height of torture, without grudging at thy holy will." A clergyman described the challenge of embracing physical pain in spiritual as well as economic terms: "I desyre the dissolution of this earthly tabernacle, sighing and longing to rest from my Labors and to be at peace with the Lord. But yet in regard of the needfull dependency of my louing wife and poore chyldren on my temporary life, I must confesse that I haue mainly st⸀yuen and doe yet daily struggle against many uiolent pangs."[29] The author of this account, Richard Carpenter, described his impending death to his father-in-law following a fifteen-day sickness. He accepted his imminent demise and even longed to rest "at peace with the Lord." Yet anxiety about the welfare of his family lest he should die compelled him to fight his illness and subdue his pain. Carpenter survived the ordeal, only to pass away eight years later.

While pain was essential to being human, it was also the means of Christ's redemption. Scripture taught that Christ, through pain, atoned for human sin and granted believers the promise of salvation from the suffering of mortal life. For the devout, then, exemplary responses to pain were modeled on Christ, the most virtuous sufferer of all. As one prescriptive text on the art of dying attested, "Those shall nearest resemble the Glory of Christ himself, who suffer as he did." Christ's pain offered an important model for Catholics above all. Catholics believed that by imitating Christ, they actually participated in his suffering and developed a closer relationship to God. Bodily pain was a means of experiencing God's immanence, an act of penance that, like good works, was essential to salvation. The French philosopher Blaise Pascal eloquently described this desire to share Christ's agony: "Make me truly understand that the ills of the body are nothing more than punishment and the complete manifestation of the ills of the soul. . . . I find nothing in me that could please you. I see nothing there, Lord, apart from my pain that in some way resembles yours."[30] Because God took human form as Christ, believers were able to partake in God's corporeal suffering. Catholic martyrs' responses to pain perhaps reflect this belief most explicitly. In 1642 a Mohawk raiding party captured and brutally beat a Jesuit missionary named Isaac Jogues. He recounted his calm reception of bodily torments by likening his torture to Christ's: "God alone knows for how long a time and how many were the blows that landed on my body, but the sufferings undertaken for His love and His glory are filled with joy and honor." Jogues described the sticks and rods that his captors wielded as "weapons of the Passion" and his suffering as a sacrificial act that enabled him to participate in Christ's affliction: God "was making us share his suffering and admitting us to participation in his crosses." Ascetic practices of self-punishment took this notion of partaking in Christ's redemptive pain to its furthest extreme. Flagellants whipped themselves with knotted ropes, trusting that such torments settled a debt owed to God. By reenacting Christ's pain, they assumed some of the suffering that he had endured. Self-inflicted pain could serve several purposes, but it was most overtly a means of pursuing a union with Christ by imitating, and thus sharing, his torments. For Catholics, pain itself was a central site of piety.[31]

Few individuals had to face the kind of anguish that Jogues endured, and judicial torture was only used briefly and sporadically in England in the sixteenth century. Yet torture became a lasting model of suffering well into the 1600s. John Foxe's sensational account of the persecution of Protestant martyrs under the Catholic Mary Tudor, popularly known as the *Book of Martyrs*, was integral to developing and popularizing this discourse. Several of the men and women here read or at the very least purchased Foxe's book. Thoresby read its second and third volumes, finding it "solid, useful, notwithstanding the clamours of some bigots against it." Both Samuel Jeake and Pepys owned the book, and Mary Rich mentioned having "som storyes red to me out of the booke of Martyres."[32] Others made remarks that reveal the internalization of Foxe's imagery in early modern vernacular consciousness. Embodying the heroic suffering of the persecuted, Cowper noted that "it is a sort of Martyrdom to liue with wicked seruants," and Elizabeth Freke's grandson was "martered with the small pox." The impact of Foxe's text is further evident in literature from the period. There are traces of martyrological imagery in, for instance, Aphra Behn's novel *Oroonoko*. Like the martyrs who calmly endured torture in Foxe's book, some seeming to wash their hands in flames, the protagonist in this story passively smokes a pipe "as if nothing had touch'd him" while his executioners dismember him at the stake. Foxe's vividly illustrated book provided a fund of stories and habits of interpretation that were accessible to literate and illiterate audiences alike (fig. 11).[33]

Stories of martyrdom shaped seventeenth-century narratives of pain in two key ways. First, patients used martyrdom as a metaphor to articulate the severity of their pain. Defining bodily suffering as torture on the rack enabled them to express the extremity of their anguish in spiritually significant terms. Alice Thornton relied on just such a metaphor to describe giving birth. She spent much of her adulthood either pregnant or recovering from pregnancy. She had nine children in all, three of whom survived childhood, and she was continually suffering from ailments related to childbirth. Reflecting on the labor of her fifth pregnancy, in 1657, she wrote, "I was upon the racke in bearing my childe with such exquisitt torment as if each lime [limb] weare divided from other, for the space of two houers." Comparing her pain to torture highlighted the intensity of her suffering, as well as the spiritual

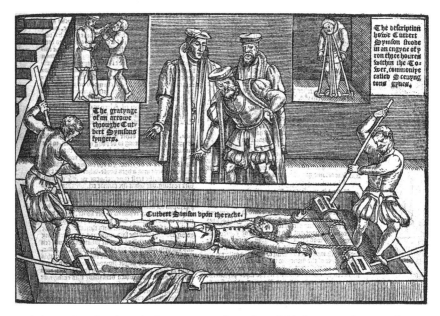

The description howe Cutbert Symnfon ftoode in an engyne of yron three houres within the Tower, commonlye called Ω ceuyng tons gyues.

The gratynge of an arrowe throughe Cutbert Symfons fyngers.

Cutbert Simfon vpon the racke.

11. A deacon from London submits to an arrow thrust through his fingers, an "engyne of yron," and the rack. John Foxe, *Actes and Monuments* (London: Iohn Day, 1563), pg. 1651. This item is reproduced by permission of The Huntington Library, San Marino, California.

significance of her deliverance from danger. Thornton's pain, like that of a martyr, was harsh and harrowing, and surviving such an ordeal demonstrated God's profound grace and mercy. Part of the metaphor's power lay in the overlapping imagery of a body split on the rack and a body torn apart in childbirth.[34] The discourse of martyrdom gave deep and positive meaning to the spiritual as well as physical experience of suffering.

Patients employed the rack imagery to articulate the sheer severity of pain even when physical sensations did not map so neatly onto Foxe's text. One woman who experienced what we would call menstrual cramps endured torments that were "so extreame y^t she is upon ye rack," while a 1699 anonymous letter describes a patient whose chief complaint was "uiolent pains cross his belly, being still more upon the rack when he went to stool." References to judicial procedures beyond the rack, such as pain that felt worse than being "broke on the wheel," further reflect the widespread use of torture as a frame for expressing bodily sufferings.[35] Oliver Heywood drew readily on the language of martyrdom to describe his bodily suffering. He lived and worked as a preacher in the town of Halifax, though he was prevented from preaching to his congregation in 1662 when he refused to conform to the

Church of England. For years afterward he traveled around the area preaching in private homes. He was heading back to Halifax from Manchester one afternoon when he suddenly felt the symptoms of a cold. He endured "excessiue paines" for five long hours. He rushed home and took two pills to open his body, but by the following day he had developed what he called "an aguish fit of cold." Despite his disorder, he preached twice that day. The work deepened the shooting pains in his head, but he found comfort in the thought that his distemper provided an "advantage" to his congregants—others could learn from his affliction. He was let blood, but this only made matters worse. Heywood suffered from intense aches all over his body for ten hours. "I was as it were set upon a rack," he wrote, "but god was mercifull to this poore worme."[36]

John Sintelaer drew on the imagery of martyrdom not to articulate the pain of illness but rather to condemn the harsh effects of mercury as a treatment for venereal disease. Early modern healers typically administered mercury directly by mouth, topically to the skin, or in fumigations that patients inhaled. The ingestion of mercury caused excessive sweats and salivation. Today we associate such responses with mercury poisoning, but within the humoral framework of the body, salivating and sweating signaled that the medicine was working. Mercury also caused a host of other harsh side effects, including fevers, severe shaking, and rotting palates. Some patients' teeth fell out from a combination of decayed gums and trembling fits. Many believed that venereal patients deserved the punishing effects of mercury—a punitive treatment for a sinful disease. But Sintelaer, who specialized in curing venereal disorders, was opposed to the severity of mercurial regimens. He communicated his critique in his 1709 *The Scourge of Venus and Mercury*, which includes an image of patients languishing as healers administer mercurial fumigations or apply topical ointments to decaying limbs and faces (fig. 12). A skeletal figure reclines in the foreground, covered in sores, as a dog sniffs at his feet. By titling this gruesome scene *The Martyrdom of Mercury*, Sintelaer likened the anguish of mercurial remedies to redemptive torture. Rather than an effective cure for syphilis, the "Mercurial Rack" was only a means of achieving atonement through physical suffering.[37]

Martyrdom offered scripts for expressing the torments of pain, as well as models of heroic endurance. This is the second way patients employed the discourse of martyrdom: in imitation of martyrs themselves. Anne Dormer relied on the language of martyrdom to articulate her tolerance of a long,

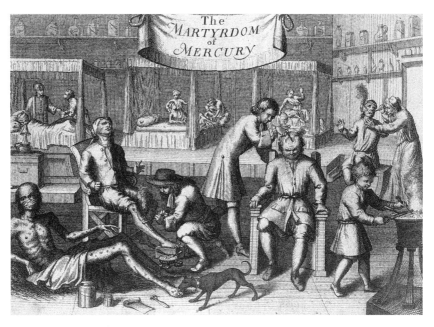

12. Corpselike patients undergo various mercurial treatments. John Sintelaer, *The Scourge of Venus and Mercury* (London: G. Harris, 1709), sig. A9r–v. By permission of the Wellcome Library, London.

uneasy marriage. Her husband Robert was a wealthy landowner who had become increasingly tyrannical toward his wife by monitoring her correspondence and refusing to let her visit neighbors and friends. A captive in her own home, Dormer submitted "most cheerfully to his absolute dominion ouer me." She divulged the details of this fraught relationship in a series of letters to her sister, Elizabeth Trumbull, who lived in France and later Constantinople, where her husband worked as ambassador. Not only did Robert display possessiveness, poor manners, and an ill temper, but his affections were insincere, "more like a jeere then a commondation" and merely a "pretence to the being a fond kinde husband." Dormer welled with disdain and resentment, yet she also revered her wedding vows and obediently strived to fulfill her role as a dutiful wife. After lying sick in bed for more than a week, she lamented, "I . . . found none of the tenderness I had showed him retourned to me." On the contrary, her husband "studdyed all the ways he could to afflict me," and when he expressed any affection at all, she reminded herself not to be fooled by his wiles: "I told him amongst many things too long to write that I had neuer found his kindness other then as a cordiall giuen to one upon the rack to preserue them to endure the torments." Like Thornton, Dormer identified with the persecuted. She was the body on the rack, passively and quietly enduring the afflictions of holy matrimony. Yet she did not look to torture to convey an acute physical sensation. Although "torments" referred to her immediate illness, she suffered most from the emotional pain of a turbulent domestic life. Nor did she draw on the rack imagery to express the severity of her suffering. Rather, for her the rack provided a metaphor for her heroic endurance. Her husband's intermitting affections were not true salves for Dormer's suffering but only false sentiments that lengthened her pain by allowing her to endure it that much longer.[38]

The ability of martyrs to respond so serenely to intense physical distress stemmed from a much older tradition of saints and ascetics who experienced pain without seeming to feel its effects. By the thirteenth century, pain was thought to originate in the soul, while the body served merely as a vehicle for its expression. Medieval saints and martyrs submitted to bodily abuses, but because their souls remained free from pain they were able to withstand the torture without flinching.[39] The sixteenth-century martyrs in Foxe's text maintained this tradition of demonstrating piety through the acceptance of pain with calm, courage, and what appeared to be insensibility. As opposed to emphasizing the brutality of their torture or the magnitude of their pain, Protestant martyrs calmly and quietly submitted to unspeakable torments. Foxe described in gruesome detail the forty-five minutes that John Hooper, a Gloucester bishop, burned at the stake: "Euen as a Lambe, paciently he abode the extremitie therof, neither mouying forwardes, backwardes, or to any side: but hauying his nether partes burne, and his bowels fallen out, he died as quietly as a childe in his bed." As his limbs burned and his insides fell out, Hooper appeared calm and composed (fig. 13). He remained impassive— almost comfortable—as he sustained unimaginable physical anguish. Just as Protestant sufferers viewed illness as an impediment to overcome in order to pray and meditate, Foxe's martyrs exhibited a remarkable ability to transcend the corporeal.[40]

Some patients in seventeenth-century England embodied this martyrological ideal on the deathbed. These men and women experienced excruciating pain yet remained unresponsive to it. Calm composure and pious speech in life's final moments were key signifiers of salvation. Attempts to die in this ideal way were epitomized by sufferers who experienced agonizing pain in the throes of death but remained insensible to the torments. These individuals

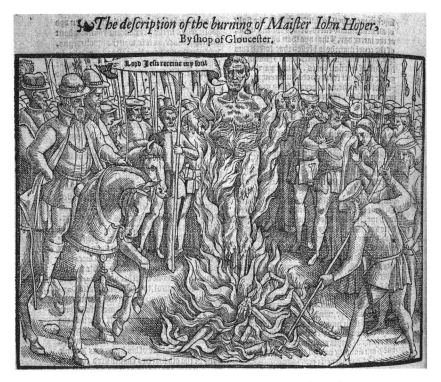

The description of the burning of Maister Iohn Hoper, Byshop of Gloucester.

Lord Iesu receiue my soul

13. John Hooper at the stake. John Foxe, *Actes and Monuments* (London: Iohn Day, 1563), pg. 1064. This item is reproduced by permission of The Huntington Library, San Marino, California.

were not ascetics or martyrs but ordinary individuals. Onlookers described how one such woman, Lady Lucy, suffered "much pain" in her final moments: "It pleased God so to continue her Pain, that those that Valued her Life aboue any Earthly Blessing, did more Grieue to see her Torment, then at the nearness of her End: but God was so Mercyfull to her, that Four or Five hours before her Death, none could perceiue she had any pain, in her Greatest Agonies; her thoughts were bent on Heaven."[41] The author does not suggest that Lucy was free from suffering. Indeed, she experienced "her Greatest Agonies." Yet onlookers saw no clenched fists, grinding teeth, or contorted facial expressions. The dying woman could withstand the pain because she concentrated so completely on the afterlife.

Isaac Archer noted his son's similar ability to calmly tolerate the torments of death even as Archer witnessed their terrifying effects. He traced the course of young Will's sickness in 1675, from fever and the voiding of worms to a relapse a few months later, when he "suddainly lost his strength, and stomach." Will's imminent death was an even greater than ordinary trial, but Archer found solace in the fact that his boy "felt nothing." Peering at his gaunt, convulsing son, Archer expressed "feare he should have come to him-selfe, and felt those paines which, with griefe, we saw." He was confident that Will's body was racked with pain, as the grieving father witnessed wasting, vomiting, spasms, and other symptoms that he incontrovertibly identified as painful. Yet he reasoned that his son was "senseles," and when a doctor confirmed that the boy experienced the pain without feeling it, Archer was grateful for God's mercy. All believed the pain actually existed even as the dying child lay unresponsive to it. Oliver Heywood recounted this same phenomenon in his father-in-law John Angier: "Altho the pangs of death were on him; yet he said, Blessed be God, I feel no pain, but your cold hand." The inability to feel pain in life's final moments reflected concerns about privileging the spiritual over the corporeal at the all-important moment of God's judgment. To die well was to die like a martyr, with pious thoughts of heaven.[42]

Some individuals were unresponsive to pain not because they had reached a deep spiritual state but rather because their ailments rendered them senseless—incapable of feeling, thinking, or speaking. Two brief examples demonstrate how this type of insensibility was associated with severe, immobilizing pain. William Salmon described a case of headache in a thirty-five-year-old woman who caught cold by swimming: "The violence of it was so great, that at sometimes it created Raving, and sometimes senselessness." The patient's "raving" and insensitivity to the world provided proof, according to Salmon, of the pain's severity. Conversely, the preacher John Bowle was able to confirm the mildness of a man's condition because it "neither tooke away the power of his memory and understandinge."[43] The pain could not have been too severe, since the man was still able to talk and function normally. The acuity of the senses served as a barometer of patients' physical suffering.

When pain caused individuals to lose the ability to speak or see, it was commonly understood that death was fast approaching. This type of death was far from ideal. The model death in early modern England entailed stoic endurance of pain and a lucid mind. Witnesses at the deathbed reassured absent friends and family that the dying experienced an awakened state in their final moments. When Grace Nettleton wrote to Sir Francis Leicester about his son's death in 1725, for example, she softened the news by affirming that his son's "head was neuer in ye least touchd but sencible to ye uery last

moment." The association between senselessness and death endured for centuries. Physicians opposed to anesthesia in the 1800s argued that the ability
to feel pain was essential to life and, conversely, dulling pain was tantamount
to death. Insensibility was also associated with death linguistically; patients
commonly used the word *dead* to describe a lack of sensation.[44]

"Like an Old Man for Tendernes": Gender and Pain

The senselessness of Archer's son on the deathbed was more pronounced
given the extremity of pain that Archer himself witnessed. And Lady Lucy's
calm acceptance of physical distress was commendable in part because onlookers could see the intensity and duration of her suffering. The fathers and
friends who compiled these accounts were not exaggerating the pain of their
loved ones. Indeed, many recorded their own and others' agonies as a means
of expressing and coping with suffering. Yet these men and women were also
conscientious about presenting themselves in certain ways for onlookers and
for posterity. Patients strove to suffer well. They did so in part by responding to pain in ways that upheld prevailing assumptions about what it meant
to be a model Christian man or woman.

Thornton's lengthy account of the death of her mother, Alice Wandesford, in 1659 made much of Wandesford's "inexpressable paines and torments," an emphasis on suffering that served to highlight her patience.
Wandesford suffered from "an exceeding great Cough, which tormented her
bodie with stitches in her breast." The cramps were so acute that she had trouble breathing and was unable to sleep or rest for weeks. Thornton found it
"wonderfull how she could subsist." Next, a hard lump developed in Wandesford's stomach, causing intense pain to rise up her throat. She had trouble
swallowing and breathing and was unable to eat for days, save for small drops
of beer administered by a syringe. Through it all, the patient exhibited
"extraordinary patience, still saing it was the Lord that sent it to her, and
none else could take it from her." Rather than complain or howl in pain, she
quietly quoted Scripture: "Why art though soe full of heavinesse, oh my soul,
and why art thou soe disquietted within me? I will still hope in my God, and
putt my trust in the God of my salvation, who is the helpe of my countenance,
and my God." Wandesford carried out her spiritual duties with zeal despite
her obvious unease. She asked the friends and relatives who collected at her
bedside to pray with her—not to prolong her life, "for she was weary of it,"

but to ask God to forgive her sins and grant her "true faith in Him to believe all His promises." Wandesford's submission and poised, pious speech provided a model of faith as well as femininity.[45]

In 1690, Dormer described the seven-week illness of her sister-in-law Elizabeth Cottrell as "most cruel." Cottrell's troublesome cough and sore chest "increased till now her oppression there is extreame and shee fetches her breath with greate difficultie and has suffred uery much." Through her pain, Cottrell possessed "invioleable patience"; in life and death she was a model Christian woman. Like Thornton's account of her mother, Dormer's description of the pain's brutality emphasized her sister-in-law's calm disposition—a depiction most overtly formulated in her reference to Cottrell as a "happy saint."[46] Similarly, when Archer's six-year-old daughter cried in the night from illness in 1679, he justified her behavior by defining the intensity of her pain, so visible in her tremors and seizures. At first the family was unaware of the child's fever. She was able to walk, eat, and drink, and her mother was ill from grief over the death of another child, drawing the family's attention elsewhere. As Archer's wife improved, however, his daughter worsened. The child was "naturally patient," yet her condition was so grave that she lay awake shrieking through the night. Archer's father-in-law rushed to the house in the middle of the night to try everything he could to save his granddaughter. As her death drew near, the child assumed the ideal Christian response: despite fits of pain "she made no noise" and was able to talk, think sensibly, and even say her catechism. When Archer asked the child if he could sit with her, she replied, " 'Yes if you please,' speaking with difficulty, but shewing her selfe dutifull, as all her life long so, to the last." Excruciating pain excused the child's cries and complaints and also heightened her display of patience and obedience.[47]

Archer, Dormer, and Thornton were each describing the pain of loved ones at the moment of death, when martyrlike composure was of utmost significance. Others characterized all kinds of bodily torments in similarly heightened terms. Cowper surmised that a daggerlike pain in her back would have killed her if it had struck her head. And in 1678, Lady Francis Clifton was in so much pain that she was "ready to give up the Ghost. . . . I can hardly gasp, or moove, or stirr my selfe the least in my bed, or from one chair to another though but a yards space without excessive torment." Her stomach and legs were swollen, and she had a high fever and "lethargie." Two weeks later her symptoms grew even more severe. Her feet and legs were as large as "mill posts," and she could "scarce breath yet or walke halfe a chamber length . . . panting worse then if I had run to London." She eventually did travel to London, to consult physicians.[48]

These accounts can be difficult to read. Detailed descriptions of distress and debility communicated patients' pain and their impressive calm in the face of unbearable anguish. Some women expressed the magnitude of their pain by admitting to an inability to conform to normative gendered behavior. Rather than remain poised and peaceful, they complained and cried out. As she was combing her hair one day in 1651, Thornton suddenly experienced a searing burn in the sinews of her neck. She described feeling "soe violently tormented with a paine . . . which caused me to cry out in extreamity." Such behavior certainly contrasted with the measured speech of her mother on the deathbed eight years later. At the sound of the cries, Thornton's mother came rushing into the room and applied rose oil to soothe her daughter's neck. Thornton later interpreted the "strainge paine" as an omen. She felt its presence just as she heard her brother George on the stairs. He was coming upstairs to say good-bye before embarking on a trip to settle his estate: "Deare sister," he remarked, upon finding Thornton paralyzed in pain, "I hope to find you better at my returne home." He left the house, mounted his horse, and began his journey. Two men walking along the Swale River reported that he descended the bank "cairfully and slowly as foot could fall." A flood of water suddenly surged when he was halfway across the river, and only his horse emerged from the rough waters. Perhaps the connection Thornton later made between George's death and the sudden stab in her neck caused her to emphasize the intensity of her pain. It lasted approximately half an hour—the time it took George to leave the house and reach the river where he met his tragic end.[49]

Dormer similarly expressed the extremity of her pain by articulating her struggle to uphold certain feminine virtues. In a letter to her sister, she wrote, "My head is all the time in the most uiolent paine which forces me somtimes to complain of it." She suspected her trouble originated from lack of sleep. She was especially sensitive to her duties as mother, sister, and wife. But rather than neglect her obligation to friends and family, she chose to exacerbate her pain by continuing to write letters and update loved ones on her life: "Tho I do with an expressible difficulty compass the doing my duty and as farr as I am able the being gratefull to all I am obliged to, and therefore do and must tugg out this poore leane shattred carcase."[50] For Dormer, fulfilling social expectations was worth intensifying her physical discomfort.

The social performance of pain was equally important for men, but the venues and meanings were different. Dudley Ryder expressed anxiety about properly responding to unexpected pain at the dinner table. He suffered from toothache when a hollow tooth was worn down so low that it exposed a nerve, causing intolerable anguish when anything touched it. He had to be particularly cautious when eating. His fear of pain, rather than pain itself, made him "angry and fretful" at dinner. He recounted how "every little thing that was done raised my anger, but I had prudence not in the least to show it." Nine months later he again faced the challenge of mastering pain at the dinner table. A wasp sting had made his hand swell up, yet he "bore it with a great deal of patience on purpose to have it taken notice of by Aunt Billio who dined with us and I laughed it off pretty well." Like Dormer, who described her sister as a happy saint, Ryder was anxious about the performative aspects of suffering. The son of a linen draper, he was of middling rank and struggled to meet the standards of London polite society. He was particularly self-conscious about his social interactions and comportment, and he deliberately moderated his behavior at the table in order to appear manly in front of his guests. He quelled his anger and endured the sting with fortitude. The swelling in his hand eventually diminished, and Ryder later had the offending tooth drawn. He noted that, despite his fear, he kept his resolve and bore the procedure without crying out or even moving—sure signs of strength and bravery.[51]

A considerable number of men from the period expressed the severity of their physical ordeals by noting an inability to meet expectations of masculine behavior, namely occupational roles and responsibilities. William Stout's uneasiness was so extreme he was unable to stir or move without help. James Clegg was indisposed and unable to preach due to stabbing pain and heaviness in his head. John Cannon had a boil on his belly that did not hinder him from work, "tho' painful enough especialy by Obstructing my rest." And Samuel Pepys displayed fortitude when he injured his finger while hammering a nail. He applied "balsam of Mrs. Turners" to the wound and "though in great pain, yet went on with my business."[52] While Cannon and Pepys exhibited resilience by working through their anguish, others measured the agony of a sore finger by its incapacitating effects. Humphrey Mildmay stayed home all day with an ache in his toe, and on several occasions the anguish of a single digit debilitated Thomas Tyldesley: "Alday in my room very bad with a swell ^d ffing^r." Sick from rheum and toothache in 1678, Archer did not compare his physical discomfort to torture but instead noted how he was "like an old man for tendernes."[53] He was vulnerable and weak, physically incapable of studying, eating solid foods, or, perhaps most important, fulfilling his occupational obligations. Pain stripped away the key components of his manhood: virility, strength, and livelihood.

These patients were aware of their readerships and of the implications of their behaviors, whether on the deathbed or at the dinner table. Highlighting the nature and extent of their pain enabled individuals to convey and cope with their conditions and also to make certain self-constructions. Both religion and gender are essential to fully understand these self-presentations. Concerns about suffering as a proper Christian and ideal man or woman could be complementary, as evidenced by Wandesford's last illness and the death of Dormer's sister-in-law. In these accounts, heightened narratives of pain enabled sufferers to display overlapping feminine and Christian virtues of patience, humility, and calm acceptance of God and of death. But some patients struggled to endure spiritually ennobling pain and also behave in socially sanctioned ways. Men could not work. Women screamed out in agony. Normative gendered behavior gave these men and women a vocabulary for expressing the intensity of their bodily afflictions. Even martyrs did not always exhibit prevailing gendered virtues. Take, for instance, the Protestant martyr Anne Askew:

> Then they did put me on the racke, because I confessed no Ladies or Gentlewomen to be of my opinion, & thereon they kept me a long time. And because I lay still I dyd not cry, my L. Chau[n]cellour & sr Joh. Baker tooke paines to racke me with their owne handes, till I was nigh dead. . . . After that I sat two long houres reasonyng with my Lord Chauncellour upon the bare flore, whereas he with many flatteryng wordes, perswaded me to leaue my opinion. But my Lord God (I thanke his euerlastyng goodness) gaue me grace to perseuer. . . . I sent him agayne word, that I would rather dye, then to breake my fayth.[54]

Askew was opinionated, disobedient, and outspoken—hardly a model of early modern femininity. The dying Lady Lucy, who was unresponsive to pain in her final moments, resembled a martyr in some ways. Yet she did not act like the assertive Askew. She instead remained quiet, patient, and submissive. Both narratives of martyrdom and deeply ingrained gender norms shaped Lucy's behavior. By acknowledging the influences of both gender and religion on patients' words and behaviors, we can begin to see each more clearly.

A final example from a rare, firsthand account by a Catholic man illustrates how concerns about both gender and piety could be embedded in patients' responses to physical suffering. Thomas Tyldesley lived in Blackpool, Lancashire, and was a member of the upper gentry. Pain accompanied nearly all of his ailments, including stomachache, cold, wind, stone, gout, and a cramping disorder that he called "the grips." In November 1712, at the age of fifty-five, he began recording the details of his developing gout, tracking its severity and location day by day. He applied warm cabbage leaves to his left hand and cleansed his stomach by taking a remedy that caused him to vomit. By the end of the month, the gout in his hand had eased, but he also noted new pain from a cramp: "My stitch eassior, and my left hand ffreeor ffrom paine." By early December the pain had returned, but this time "by could." Tyldesley tried to combat this development by removing twelve to fourteen ounces of blood from the afflicted arm. The pain persisted, however, and he continued to trace it daily until, by December 19, he was "something eassy ʳ off the gout but in paine with the gravell." His ailments evolved over time, but pain remained a constant descriptor of ill health and determinant of recovery. The movement, severity, or appearance of "new" aches and pains defined the progression of his various, transmuting disorders.[55]

Alongside these complaints and his various attempts to alleviate them, Tyldesley noted whether pain prevented him from performing certain tasks or sequestered him to his chamber. "Very ffull of pain," he noted in January 1713, "and not able to writ[e]." He listed varying gradations of debility alongside his recurring and transmuting pain: "helpless and in great paine; alday on yᵉ beed"; "all day in my chamber, very lame"; "in very much paine; not able to help myselfe"; "in much paine; not well able to move." Several of these entries include few additional remarks, as though pain itself occupied the greater part of his day.[56] Such terse daily records suggest that he found little else worth recording. These accounts also demonstrate the significance of helplessness to his articulations of physical suffering. Unlike many of the men in this book, Tyldesley did not have a shop to open or patients to treat. He was a gentleman living off his landed estate in Lancashire, and in times of health he spent his days pursuing leisurely activities such as hunting and visiting friends. Yet, as with middling-status and impoverished men, incapacity provided the primary means by which he expressed the severity of his suffering. He conveyed his physical torture by measuring its impact on the key masculine ideals of independence and self-sufficiency.

Tyldesley seemed to view the extremity of his pain in gendered terms. Yet his attention to debility might also reflect his particular beliefs about the relationship between God's grace and suffering. For Catholics like him, God's grace fluctuated in relation to human merit or charitable works. According to this belief system, enduring bodily pain was a redemptive act that atoned for sin and enabled individuals to share in Christ's suffering. Accordingly, Catholics viewed pain as penance that was integral to salvation. Lying in bed all day, immobilized by pain, was a devotional act of suffering and self-denial that brought believers closer to God. From this religious perspective, Tyldesley's inability to get out of bed, write, or even move signified the intensity of a critical religious experience. Perhaps, then, the ravages of stitches and stones provided him with a spiritually virtuous means of redeeming his compromised masculinity. He lost his ability to function independently, but the spiritual significance of his bodily torments mitigated this loss. Much of the recent literature on pain in this period has placed patients like Tyldesley solely within a medical context.[57] Analyzing his words exclusively in medical or spiritual terms, divorced from prevailing views of the male body, would provide only a partial view of his account. Individuals like Tyldesley drew on a range of scripts to construct meaningful narratives of suffering—scripts that could intersect with one another. Tyldesley's expressions of pain simultaneously reflected concerns about his imperiled masculinity and the spiritual significance of his physical anguish.

Conclusion

Even Samuel Pepys's body-focused assessments of his stones were probably shaped by implicit spiritual attitudes. He was not especially forthcoming about his personal beliefs. He was a member of the Church of England, although this affiliation may be more reflective of his political maneuverings than of any profound belief. He attended church regularly, but he spent most of his time there ogling women rather than listening to sermons. He also attended Catholic masses on several occasions to listen to the music, and he was even the godfather of a Catholic child. He described the rituals during the child's baptism as "foolish," yet he gratefully accepted the family's thank-you gift, a painting of the Passion.[58]

A brief episode in 1663 offers one of the few instances when Pepys seemed to attribute sickness to God. He complained of a pain in his chest and head, as well as impaired hearing in his right ear: "It is a cold, which God Almighty in justice did give me while I sat lewdly sporting with Mrs. Lane the other day with the broken window in my neck." Pepys had a lengthy affair with Betty Lane, who worked at a draper's stall in Westminster Hall. Given his skeptical attitude toward religion, he most probably attributed his cold that day to the drafty window rather than to God's hand. His reference to divine punishment was an expression of guilt regarding his adulterous ways. His other references to God are few and fleeting: "This day, by the blessing of God, I have lived 31 years in the world." Such instances seem to reflect common parlance as opposed to genuine belief.[59]

Another infidelity—this time with his wife's maid Deb Willet—offers perhaps the most revealing insights into Pepys's spirituality. After supper one day in 1668, Elizabeth Pepys unexpectedly walked in on her husband embracing Willet. In a mix of English slang and French, his language of preference when documenting sexual exploits, Pepys divulged the details of his undeniable guilt: "Endeed, I was with my main in her cunny." That night Elizabeth woke her husband at two in the morning to share "a great secret": she was a Roman Catholic. She no doubt made this admission to upset her husband in retaliation for his affair. Elizabeth was raised a French Protestant and never converted to Catholicism, but on at least one other occasion she vowed to die a Catholic. Such declarations were potent weapons in marital disputes that deeply rankled Pepys, compelling him to write more openly about his religious sentiments than at any other points in the diary. A few days after this incident, following yet another tryst with Willet, he articulated his feelings of guilt and remorse in religious terms: "I did this night promise to my wife never to go to bed without calling upon God upon my knees by prayer; and I begun this night, and hope I shall never forget to do the like all my life—for I do find that it is much the best for my soul and body to live pleasing to God and my poor wife—and will ease me of much care, as well as much expense."[60] Whether or not he adhered to Anglicanism because of guilt, political gain, social ease, or sincere faith, the above excerpt reflects the significant power of God and prayer in Pepys's life. There are few traces of religion in his descriptions of pain or in his diary altogether, yet religion was critical to his marital relationship, daily life, and world view—a factor that surely influenced the meanings and experience of his suffering.

Conceptions of the body's internal operations, models of suffering in discourses of martyrdom, and gendered concerns about enduring pain with stoicism and patience all informed patients' expressions and behaviors in the sickroom. The ways men and women drew on these disparate beliefs surely varied by writing forms, individual personalities, and circumstances. Yet common concerns emerge across multiple lives and writing styles: anxieties about salvation and piety, about diagnosing and articulating sensations in order to suitably alleviate them, and about conforming to ideas of proper comportment in the face of physical ordeals. Patients expressed the magnitude of their suffering in part by defying normative gendered behavior: women in pain were unable to remain meek and submissive, while afflicted men were incapable of fulfilling financial obligations or exhibiting self-sufficiency. Yet the spiritually significant, instructive meanings of physical anguish could endow such nonnormative behavior with divine import. Although some men and women struggled with language and perhaps never found the right metaphor to communicate their experiences, narratives of pain provide intimate views of how seventeenth-century individuals understood and perceived their bodies. Pain darted and snapped, tickled and popped. It foamed "like barm on new beer" and had the capacity to morph into fevers and stones. These formulations illuminate how early modern individuals imagined and expressed bodily sensations, and also what it might have felt like to endure the physical torments of seventeenth-century life.

6. Illness Narratives by the Poor

Roger Smaley was able to pinpoint the day he fell ill two years after the fact. He had been suddenly paralyzed on one side of his body, unable to stand or move without help, and he had lost the ability to speak. He recorded this episode in a 1658 petition to poor law authorities in Preston, Lancashire. He was too weak to support himself, his wife, and their four small children, so he appealed to the parish for support.[1] Smaley was likely illiterate and narrated his story orally to a scribe, who then wrote up the petition using stock legal language (fig. 14). Much of what we know about patients and illness in early modern England has overlooked the experiences of sufferers like Smaley by focusing instead on wealthier men and women who had the time, ability, and inclination to write about their lives. This chapter captures a broader view of illness experiences by examining how the very poorest members of seventeenth-century society defined disease causation, diagnosis, and the social dimensions of suffering. Like their wealthier counterparts, lower-status patients relied on informal networks of healing. They solicited advice, treatments, and assistance from friends, neighbors, and family members. But when these approaches were insufficient or unavailable they could access more formal support, such as private alms, donations from charitable trusts, and hospitals. They also drew on parish-administered relief, the focus of this chapter.

Smaley's story resembles more introspective firsthand accounts in some aspects. For example, he recounted the duration of his suffering and its impact on his ability to move and function, much like the men and women we

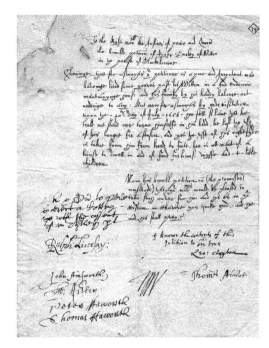

14. Petitions used fairly formulaic legal language and formatting, as shown here. Roger Smaley, petition to Quarter Sessions, 1658, QSP/158/14, Lancashire Archives, Preston. Reproduced by permission of Lancashire Archives.

have met in preceding chapters. Indeed, just as he "could not stand nor turne himselfe in his bedd," Sarah Cowper was "so indispos'd I cannot well turn in my Bed." But there are also key differences between narratives by paupers and those by upper-status individuals like Cowper, beyond the obvious fact that Smaley did not write his report himself. This chapter highlights three distinctions in particular. First, petitioners provided fairly different explanations of illness onset than did their wealthier counterparts. They underemphasized the influences of the six nonnaturals on humoral congestion and balance and instead focused on accidents and misfortunes beyond their control. They also cited different kinds of illnesses than upper-status patients did, focusing on external, physically debilitating disorders rather than internal, humoral ones. Third, paupers noted the material toll of illness—"we were forced to sell the beds from under us," for example—while wealthier individuals tended to gloss over or omit such concerns altogether.[2] The conventions and demands of the petition as a genre of legal writing surely informed these differences, as did the social circumstances that compelled paupers to submit one.

More subtly, expressions and concerns that are prevalent in ego-literature take on new meanings in the context of petitioning for relief. Much like accounts by upper-status patients, petitioners' stories of sickness employed the language of morality and pity. Yet petitioners couched this language in terms of hard work, responsibility, and need rather than piety, gender, and posterity. Even references to God seem to indicate different types of concerns in paupers' writing. Smaley attributed his paralysis in 1658 to "gods uisitation," yet he did not reflect on the spiritual implications of this providential event. Like those of so many of his fellow petitioners, Smaley's allusions to God are brief and routine. Perhaps it was even the scribe who inserted religious references in order to increase his client's chances of winning parish support. Petitioners also adapted gender norms to suit their particular circumstances. Male paupers could not uphold the ideal of the independent householder, and poor female petitioners were incapable of remaining silent and meek. These men and women instead presented themselves in seemingly contradictory terms to secure parish funds: as industrious and resilient yet also dependent and weak. Situating pauper petitions within the broader realm of health and healing illuminates the ways economic circumstances could shape the language and experience of suffering.

Historical sources that capture the lives of the poor in the seventeenth century are less detailed and less abundant than those from later centuries. Charitable health care institutions only began to proliferate in England in the eighteenth century, and it was only in the mid-1700s that more and more paupers began sending letters in search of aid to parish officials. Because the seventeenth century offers a relative paucity of narrative sources by the poor, this chapter focuses on terse, mediated petitions like Smaley's.[3] Under the legal system that governed public welfare in this period, the Old Poor Law, parish officials known as overseers administered funds to the needy. Two overseers in each parish collected a poor rate and dispersed monthly payments or in-kind allowances to individuals like Smaley. Because overseers administered relief locally, norms could vary from parish to parish. For instance, northern counties tended to provide less-generous stipends than southern ones, while begging seemed to be an acceptable last resort only in particular regions, such as Cumbria, Lancashire, and Yorkshire. To account for such variation, this chapter analyzes petitions from ten archives across England (fig. 15).[4]

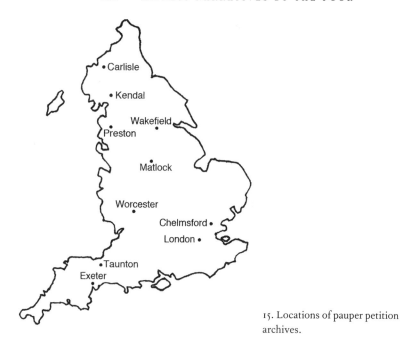

15. Locations of pauper petition archives.

Most men and women became dependent on parish relief following a sudden accident, illness, or what historians call life-cycle poverty: vulnerability resulting from life stages such as old age, widowhood, or parenthood. The petitioners examined here were writing to dispute overseers' decisions to discontinue, reduce, or refuse an allowance. Paupers made their appeals to the next tier of poor law administrators, magistrates at county criminal courts known as Quarter Sessions.[5] Individuals could petition Quarter Sessions for a range of reasons—for instance, to dismiss an apprentice or to press charges for burglary. Those petitioning to overturn overseers' decisions to cancel or lower a stipend might cite a number of justifications, including sudden blindness, old age, or the loss of employment. This chapter draws on petitions that specifically requested relief on account of ailing health. Some petitioners asked for the continuation of a stipend or an increase to a current one, while others requested discrete sums of money to pay for cures or to finance trips to procure remedies. I have omitted petitions that reference disabilities such as deafness and blindness unless such impairment also accompanied sickness or physical weakness. For the period covered in this book, I found 648 petitions that specifically cited ill health; the earliest dates from 1623 and the latest from 1730. In this sample, 342 petitioners were men and 238 were women. Sixty-seven couples submitted petitions together, and one person of unidentified gender submitted a petition. Not all petitioners in my sample, however, wrote about themselves. Fourteen of the male petitioners wrote on behalf of women, while eight women wrote on behalf of men.

Petitions offer rare insights into the lives of illiterate men and women, but the pens of legal clerks mediate these glimpses of the poor. The scribes who drafted petitions for the most part adhered to formulaic legal phrases and deferential language rather than the words paupers might have used themselves. A 1653 petition to the Essex Quarter Sessions in Chelmsford illustrates some common patterns. It opens by introducing the claimant, Mary Grave, a widow from the town of Writtle. The bulk of the text provides biographical information about the aptly named Grave, as well as a summary of her situation:

> Tha yor pet^r beinge ffouer score yeares old & extreame poore hath for the spase of 5 yeares last past receiued 12^d pe[r] weeke of the Ouerseers of the P[ar]ish towards the maintenance of her selfe and one Mary Graue her daughter who is uery lame & impotent & noe longer capable to gett any thinge towards a liuing with which small allowance together with the Charitye of well disposed people they haue with the blessinge of God kept themselues aliue. But so it is that about a weeke of it hence yor petitioner beinge uery weake & feeble receiued a fall wherewith its conseiued shee hath uery much bruised her Body or Dislocated her Bones or both, & at this instant lyes languishinge in that miserable torture hauinge noe meanes at all whereby to seeke out remedye or in the (interim) to support her Droopinge Spiritte.

Petitioners commonly noted the cause and duration of their incapacitation. In this instance, a fall resulted in bruises and possibly dislocated bones. Accounts of illness are brief. They can provide colorful but also limited information, such as the petitioner's "languishinge in that miserable torture." Petitions might also include references to the debilities and dependency of claimants' family members, in this case Grave's daughter, who was too sickly to provide for her ailing mother. The remainder of the petition outlines the amount and nature of relief requested: "P[ro]uide her a Chirurgeon thereby (if it may bee) to remoue the greiuous paynes shee now Graones under and to giue some Competent allowance for the Releife of her selfe & poore lame daughter."[6] The petitioner asked for a supplement to her monthly twelve-pence allowance to cover the cost of treating her injury. The outcome of her case is not recorded.

Petitioners rarely composed these documents themselves. As a result, it can be difficult to parse sufferers' words from clerks' interpretations. I have found a few petitions written in the first person, though in several cases this seems like a rhetorical strategy rather than evidence of literacy. One petition to the Middlesex Sessions of the Peace describes a seventy-seven-year-old petitioner "greatly afflicted wth distempers of body as y[e] stone and wind Collick." About halfway through the text, the writing shifts to the petitioner's perspective: "I hope y[e] honourable Bench will take my Condicon in Consideration for my want is uery great." Whoever wrote this petition probably changed pronouns to evoke readers' pity. Nineteenth-century pauper letters reveal similar shifts in perspective. A widowed wife, for example, might take on the voice of her deceased husband.[7] Such language reminds us that scribes composed these documents from petitioners' narrated accounts, and perhaps in some cases they even directly recorded paupers' words as they were spoken.

A parish clerk from Lancashire had his own petition drawn up and submitted to Quarter Sessions in 1636. The petitioner, John Lapphinch, sought protection from a man named Thomas Dalton. Dalton had allegedly barged into Lapphinch's home, stolen his personal possessions, and threatened his life, all on account of an unsettled debt of three pence: "Dalton . . . came furiously like a mad-man (as hee is indeed in his raging-fitts) into your Pet:[rs] house, uiolently and in a ryotous-manner took & caryed away out of the house of your Pet:[r] your Pet:[rs] goods, swearing most fearefull, that y[f] any one should assay to hinder or w[th]stand him so doing, hee would either kill or bee kild." Petitioners' goals of securing support could shape their accounts of suffering. Dalton was not just rude and greedy but also irrational and "rebellious"—a word that carried particular weight in the tumultuous political climate of 1636. He was overcome by "raging-fitts" and acted "uiolently and in a ryotous-manner." He swore, stole, and threatened murder. The petition depicts Lapphinch in completely opposite terms. Pained and crippled by gout, he was physically incapable of chasing Dalton. Indeed, the ailing petitioner "cannot so much as put his owne meat & drink into his owne mouth, but is fedd by others." This characterization of Lapphinch as frail, immobile, and reliant on charity was compounded by his peaceful response to Dalton's violent intrusion. He "most kindly in a uery louing-manner entreated the said Dalton to bee quiet and not to take away his goods." In contrast to the violent madman barging into his home, Lapphinch remained quiet, calm, and reasonable, speaking in a "louing" way and promising to pay any debts.[8]

Paupers like Lapphinch submitted petitions with particular objectives in mind, and they commonly employed deferential, supplicating language to win the favor of poor law authorities. Petitioners referred to the "accustomed goodnes & Christian compassion" of their readers and attested "that your poore Petitioner is euer bound to praie for your healthes and longe liues for by your Louinge and nourishfull fauours . . . you haue beene supporters & p[ro]longers of mine."[9] While such language might seem contrived or even deceitful to us, it was integral to petitioners' constructions of illness, and therefore we can learn something from it regardless of its veracity. Like firsthand accounts recorded in diaries and letters, petitions reflect not the collective experiences of a particular social group but rather the fractured, mediated articulations of those experiences. The expectations, motivations, and circumstances that informed paupers' narratives, then, do not inhibit our access to some more accurate reality but were instead integral to petitioners' versions of that reality. We may never know whether Lapphinch actually acted lovingly toward Dalton in 1636, but we can learn something from the fact that he said he did.

Like Lapphinch, claimants asking for relief on account of illness presented themselves in terms that attested to their moral worth—as honest, respectful, creditworthy, and "in good repute & creditt." Diarists too made this move by describing their ailments in ways that deflected blame. After all, maintaining health in the early modern period was a deeply moralistic endeavor. It was the patient's responsibility to monitor daily lifestyle choices in order to maintain health, in part by moderating the six nonnaturals. Attributing causation to an external factor—whether an airborne contagion or a loved one's behavior—enabled the patient to shift some responsibility for illness. Paupers show a similar concern about the moral implications of ill health, but they articulate it differently. Petitioners had to prove they deserved support, and key aspects of such characterizations were a lengthy amount of time spent in residence in the parish and a record of contributing to poor relief. John Clove of Southwark was "78 yeares old & upwardes & so long as he was able did releiue others and pay . . . for 30 yeares togeather towards the releife of the poore there."[10] After charitably supporting his neighbors for more than thirty years, he looked to his fellow parishioners to reciprocate.

Petitioners like Clove emphasized their long-standing contributions to the community and the brevity of their reliance on parish support. The category of "pauper" in early modern England was an administrative label that reflected dependency. It was a state that individuals could pass through at various points in their lives rather than a fixed economic status, as we view it today.[11] By establishing the brevity of their dependence in the past, petitioners demonstrated that they were responsible, industrious members of the parish. Men and women alike conveyed these attributes by emphasizing their strength, self-sufficiency, and resilience, describing themselves as "Labouring night & day" or "uery diligent and industrious." Others characterized themselves as thrifty or "uery Carefull" with money. Rather than frivoling away their income, claimants explained, they exhausted their wealth on necessary expenses, such as medical care. Petitioners further proved their industry by stressing their former ability to sustain themselves without burdening the parish. A crippled man from North Curry, Somerset, was unable to subsist after his father died, and so took it upon himself to build a room on the end of his mother's cottage where he could make money by mending shoes. Others characterized themselves in similar terms by describing how they continued to work in spite of painful, debilitating injuries. One Lancashire farmer lost the use of one of his hands, yet he continued to work "without burdening others about him." For these men and women, parish aid was truly a last resort.[12]

Petitioners altered these expressions of toil and industry to meet the social realities of early modern life. Men tended to emphasize strength and productivity more often than female petitioners did, most certainly as a result of the physicality of their work as smelters, smiths, miners, and the like. But, unlike those of higher ranks, these men were unable to assert their manhood in terms of independence and self-sufficiency. Indeed, they were asking for help because they were incapable of financially supporting their families. These petitioners instead looked to other characterizations of manhood, defining themselves as conscientious and hardworking. In his petition for a charitable gift from a hospital in Somerset, William Smart described himself as an "honest man" who had been "euer laborious and industrious in his calling." This characterization of reliability, productivity, and able-bodiedness certainly stood in stark contrast to the tender, submissive man pleading for help. While emphasizing the rigor and duration of their work enabled men like Smart to establish their masculinity in terms that fit their social station, such characterizations also allowed petitioners to demonstrate the extremity of their current conditions. Smart manifested his need in part by highlighting his loss of physical ability: he had grown old, frail, and "disabled for labour." Thomas Boradale was blind for eight years and unable to work on account of disabled limbs. He and his family would have starved "but for ye industry of his wife who now onely for want of imploymt & onely by her aged & bodily infirmity can no longer contribute to ye mentanance of yor petitionr." This gender role reversal conveyed the petitioner's condition and established his wife's worth as a surrogate breadwinner. Both Smart and Boradale received relief.[13]

While some female petitioners referred to their physical labor, others contextualized their strength and industry within the realm of child rearing. The eighty-year-old Marian Sibson of Cumbria was "an ould infirme Crazy body." Yet she also "hath all along liued honestly & truly amongst her Neighbors . . . and hath brought upp a great Charge of Children by her industry & hard labour." Elizabeth Bone had ten children and was "uery well knowne in the sayd Towne to bee a paynfull woman for the breeding upp of them." She was finally cured after lying immobile for five weeks in 1663 but lacked the funds to pay her surgeon. While some men also referred to their large families, to show how diligently they worked to provide for them, it was the work required to rear children—not just support them materially—that attested to these female petitioners' moral worth. A "uery hard laboring woman in her caling" was also careful to note that she raised "her Charge in sum desent manner." The work of raising children into responsible adults made these women fit recipients of parish funds and underlined their distance from bastard bearers.[14]

Others established their moral standing by underscoring their capacity for self-improvement. Impotent, lame, and destitute, George Clarke petitioned the Cumbria Quarter Sessions in May 1690 when his parish stopped paying his weekly stipend of twelve pence. Rather than detail his former industry, Clarke established his moral status by explaining that he needed the stipend to finance an education "for his future Livlyhood." This tack, like those outlined above, defined the petitioner as a respectable member of the community, in part by attesting to his future independence from public assistance. This approach proved successful; the justices instructed Clarke's parish to begin paying him ten pence each week.[15]

The principles that structured the poor law could inform these articulations of morality. The law characterized individuals who were dependent on the parish in three ways. First, the laboring poor could be unemployed but physically capable. Overseers commonly assigned these individuals work or apprenticeships. The second group, idle vagrants, wandering beggars, and victims of "incorrigible diseases," were associated with vice and therefore were punished and forced to work. The third group, the impotent, included nearly all of the petitioners discussed here. These individuals were physically incapable of supporting themselves, often as a result of illness, accidents, or life-cycle poverty. Scholars have pointed to the arbitrary nature of these categories and have shown that early modern individuals did not think in simple binaries of deserving versus undeserving.[16] Nonetheless, concerns about morality were bound up in the intentions of the law. Dependency of any sort was shameful in this period. Just like wealthier patients, paupers attempted to compensate for the moral implications of falling ill and asking for help. It was the scripts with which they chose to do so that varied. Unlike so many diarists and letter writers, paupers did not express morality in terms of personal salvation or lifestyle choices, but instead situated it within the context of work and community.

Such concerns about morality and industry are further evident in petitioners' explanations of illness onset. In my sample, 278 petitioners noted a cause of illness, and for the most part they cited factors beyond their control: 166 attributed their ailments to old age, and 62 mentioned God's will. The high number of references to old age is certainly due to the fact that, of the 143 petitioners who included their exact age, all were over fifty except four, who were under fifteen.[17] Accidents were the third most common source of ill health; 14 percent attributed their conditions to mishaps such as falling off a horse, tumbling out of bed, or receiving a crippling blow from an object or animal. Of course, poor and rich alike endured the perils of early modern life. A shower of glass and tiles blew into Sarah Cowper's home during a storm in 1702. She somehow escaped unscathed. Elizabeth Freke slipped and fell down her stairs on more than one occasion, and she witnessed the collapse of her kitchen chimney in 1711: "I were like againe to bee burnt to death and to be knock'd att hed by the fall." What is unique among petitioners, relative to the wealthier patients in this book, is the frequency with which their illnesses resulted from accidents, as well as the ways they contextualized their mishaps to mitigate responsibility and highlight integrity. For instance, Margaret Wood tripped and fell over a stone in the dark, which left her "weake &

sickly and decrepit in her lyms." She was careful to note that the accident occurred on her way to church.[18]

More commonly, petitioners faced misfortunes associated with their
occupations. Falling rocks injured coal miners working in the pits. Farmers
suffered from the particular hazards of their jobs; one man lost his sight when
a branch struck his eye. Others attributed illness not to specific incidents but
more broadly to their diligent "hard Labour and Industry."[19] Such sources of
illness characterized petitioners in morally virtuous terms, establishing both
their industry and their inability to subsist without help. Upper-status patients
were less likely to incur occupational injuries, since they either did not work or
toiled in less hazardous trades—as apothecaries and merchants rather than as
blacksmiths and miners. The middling-status men who did link poor health to
work tended to cite internal, less visibly debilitating disorders. They developed headaches, colds, and fevers from sustained, strained, or anxious thought.
On several occasions, for instance, Samuel Pepys attributed headaches and
physical disorder to overworking. Elias Pledger even visited the baths at Islington to treat melancholy that developed in part from his unsuccessful business as an apothecary: "Want of trade much discomposes me & makes me
frequently distrust yᵉ prouidence of god." Perhaps his religious doubts contributed as much as his anxiety about work to his melancholic state.[20]

The ministry was one middling-status occupation that seemed to elicit
complaints about the physical demands of the job. One minister compared
preaching to a kind of physical labor that he might never have experienced
firsthand: it felt "as if I had been at plough all day." Another, James Clegg,
continually noted the physical effects of his work. He lived in Derbyshire, a
farming and milling area in the north of England, and to supplement his income as a preacher he moved to a farm in 1713 and began working part time
as a physician. The obligations of these multiple occupations took a toll on
his health. He traveled throughout the area to treat patients and devoted significant time at home to concocting remedies and ordering medicaments from
London. He also refused to deliver the same sermon twice, so he stayed up
late on Saturdays to prepare for the following morning. Clegg continually
complained about fatigue and often developed hoarseness and overheating
from the act of preaching.[21]

Some paupers linked their ailments to occupational hazards in seemingly
tangential ways. Susannah Rose submitted a petition to the justices of the

bench in Worcester in 1688 in search of a monthly stipend for her brother George Gilbert. A former servant to a blacksmith, Gilbert was no longer able to work, on account of recurrent fevers. As the petition explained, "By accident his hammer fell Upon his foot and bruised on of his Toes, the which did soe much disable him, that he hath not binn able to doe any worke for a liuely hood, and after a longe tyme of suffer[ing] feuers, he was perswaded it was gon to the kings euell, Then went to London & was tuched by his majestie, And Affter, was fforced to goe to A Sirjant at Rushocke under cure aboue halfe a yeare." Gilbert connected his fever, as well as the lymphatic swellings associated with scrofula, or the king's evil, to an accident in the blacksmith's shop. This explanation of disease causation reflects prevailing beliefs about the transmuting, fluctuating nature of internal ailments. A bruised toe could trigger a series of processes that resulted in fever and, subsequently, the king's evil. This account also resonates with seventeenth-century conceptions of time and suffering: patients linked ailments to events that might have occurred years earlier. It was not farfetched to associate a bruised toe with fever, even months after the fact. While this petition certainly illustrates common understandings of illness onset and progression, it does so in ways that were congruent with Gilbert's aims. Rose presented her brother as a pitiful yet responsible man who was injured on the job and who exerted significant effort toward curing himself. He traveled to London to be touched by the king, a popular remedy for the evil, and he underwent a six-month course of surgical treatments.[22]

Chapter 1 outlines how patients in this period attributed ill health to six external factors that created temperature changes and, in turn, humoral obstructions and imbalances. While such explanations of illness onset were common among diarists and letter writers, only ten petitions in my sample cite any of the six nonnatural causes of illness. One man attributed poor health to the alternating hot and cold air in the mill where he worked. By contextualizing these temperature changes within his occupation rather than his day-to-day regimen, he successfully shifted responsibility from his lifestyle choices to the well-known hazards of his employment. Another petitioner, Hugh Harr, also noted the troubling effects of fluctuating temperatures. He was a servant who had lost the use of his legs while fighting in the army. He linked his injury both to the "coldnesse of the Ayre" and to "a stab in his thigh." Despite arriving home from service in a cart, he longed to regain the use of his legs and return to work. A year and a half later he had recovered enough to sign a yearlong contract with his previous master. His injuries, however, prevented him from keeping up with the work. He headed to Bath in search of a cure and later St. Bartholomew's Hospital in London, where he was deemed incurable and shown the door. Back home in his Essex parish, he was denied a monthly stipend by the overseers, so he pleaded to the justices in 1642 to overturn their decision.[23]

Of the ten petitions in my sample that mention the nonnaturals, eight target the emotions. A young apprentice named John Donald witnessed the physical effects of an intense emotional disturbance. His 1698 petition begins in a familiar way: by establishing his responsibility and work ethic. He was "seruiceable to the publick in which Employm[t] he behaueth himselfe to the good Content and satisfaccon of his Master." The remainder of the petition outlines Donald's inability to function independently, a condition he developed from sudden, intense fear. He awoke one night to find four men in disguise sneaking around the property where he worked. Convinced that the men threatened to destroy the mill, the twenty-year-old ran out of the house in nothing but a shirt. "Being sore affrighted," he ran straight into the river and "had like to haue destroyed himselfe in y[e] water, but was presently since which time he hath grown or neuer been sinceable [sensible], and now is not able to guide himselfe." Like so many contemporary petitions, Donald's account links debility to a work-related incident: it was the intense and sudden fear of losing the mill that led to his mental decline. The fact that he nearly lost his life only underlined the magnitude of his despair. The justices were persuaded and instructed his overseers to grant him a weekly stipend of eight pence. But he had to petition again a year later when the overseers decided to stop paying the stipend.[24]

In her work on the 1570 Norwich census, the historian Margaret Pelling found that census takers tended to document conditions they could confirm by inspection. These officials overlooked disorders that were based on self-perception or failed to threaten the capacity to work. The categories of illness recorded in pauper petitions reflect a similar trend. Rather than the internal disorders so common in writing by wealthier men and women, such as fluxes, aches, and colds, petitioners cited mostly external ailments that undeniably inhibited their day-to-day functioning: oozing sores, seizures, paralysis, and the like. More than three hundred petitioners in my sample suffered from lame, bruised, or broken limbs. Of this group, 58 percent were men, 37 percent were women, and 4 percent didn't specify their gender.[25] In many instances, petitioners' complaints affected their bodies in ways that poor law authorities could observe firsthand. When a shoemaker from Manchester submitted a plea for relief in 1651 on account of recurring fistulas, he highlighted what the poor law authorities could see for themselves: the lesions would "many tymes breakes out in some part . . . as now is to bee seene upon diuers fingers of both yo[r] peticon[rs] hands." This man was probably present as his petition was read, holding up his hands as undeniable proof of his condition. Those who endured internal, less visibly troubling disorders stressed their subsequent incapacity. Joan Langley's son had exceedingly violent headaches, a disorder that would not ordinarily justify parish relief. Langley's headaches, however, led to an observable, disabling condition: blindness. Likewise, a petitioner who had recurring fevers was careful to note that the ague had shifted into his leg, "whereof hee is become impotent and lame."[26] This pattern helps to explain the surprisingly few references to humoral sources of illness in petitions. It was not the decline of humoral theory within popular consciousness but the need to demonstrate dependency that compelled petitioners to define their ailments as external and incapacitating rather than internal and humoral.

Most petitioners did not cite a specific disorder but instead relied on descriptors such as infirm (128 petitions), weak (119 petitions), and impotent (57 petitions). Similar characterizations are prevalent in all types of illness narratives from the period, as patients commonly defined health according to their felt symptoms rather than to established disease categories. The term *lame* was particularly popular among petitioners because it did the work of conveying dependence.[27] Petitions noted how the claimant in question could "do nothing for her self" or "is not able to helpe himselfe further then hee is Carried." In 1633 a woman from Lancashire named Katherine Parke characterized her increasing immobility according to her shifting reliance on various objects. After using crutches for three years, she resorted to having others push her around in a wheelbarrow when her condition worsened. She petitioned for funds to finance a trip to the mineral springs on the outskirts of London in the hope that the healing waters would cure her limbs. Others conveyed their debility by describing their physical inability to travel to Quarter Sessions to present their cases.[28]

Several petitioners suffered from disorders that directly affected their trades: a spinner went blind, a teacher lost his voice, and a shoemaker injured his fingers. Prevailing gender roles structured these articulations of incapacity. Although a handful worked as midwives, teachers, or servants, very few of the 238 female petitioners here mentioned the nature of their work. Rather than define debility in occupational terms, female petitioners tended to highlight their struggles with everyday tasks. Twelve women, for instance, noted an inability to dress themselves, while others referred to the challenges of completing common household chores: one woman could "not soe much as pinn a pin on hir sleeue," while another "cannot hould her yourin [yarn]." Conversely, male petitioners tended to highlight an inability to endure the physical requirements of their work as farmers, tailors, blacksmiths, and miners. Some men referred vaguely to "hard labor & toyle," but many explained how ill health specifically hindered them from plying their trades. A young mason's apprentice, for instance, was so weak and ill that he was "noe waise able to . . . follow the Trade."[29]

Petitions further articulated debility by characterizing supplicants as pitiably as possible. One clerk played on the term *bedridden* to emphasize a claimant's state of decay: "Your poor pet[itioner] hath languished and layd In great misery and sicknesse bedd Rotten for three yeares." Others communicated dependency and desperation by defining their ailments as life threatening. Paupers described lying "at ye point of death," while many drew on stock language: "will perish for want of maintenance" is one such phrase. Some even stressed the moral responsibility of poor law authorities: "Unless the hand of charity be extended towards her relief . . . she must ineuitably perish."[30]

A similar strategy was to highlight the pauper's quite literally short-lived reliance on parish support. John Hindley suffered from open sores in his side in 1664. The gruesome disorder had afflicted him for more than a year, draining him of vitality and livelihood. He asked the poor law authorities for financial support so that he might live out his final days: "Take this his sad and deplorable condicon into your graue consideracons and direct some order out of this your Court to the Ouerseers of the said Townshipp, that they may be Compelled thereby to allow him some reasonable Sustenance in this his great distresse, Whoe is not likely (except god of his great mercy be released to change his Condicon) to be troublesome to them longe."[31] Hindley conveyed both the severity and the brevity of his need by defining his illness as incurable and fatal.

Others lay incapacitated for quite lengthy spans of time—in one instance for eleven years. Katherine Jackson was confined to her bed for four years "and hath been, by all her honest neighbours yt came to see her, often times supposed to be at the uery point to dy."[32] Rather than share her own perceptions and experiences, she confirmed the severity of her condition by taking the perspective of her "honest neighbours." Such characterizations of fatal, lengthy, and painful ailments did not enable individuals like Jackson and Hindley to negotiate distressed relationships or present themselves in pious terms, as they did for wealthier patients. These men and women were barely eking out a living, and the details of their dire conditions proved the enormity of their need.

Petitioners defined their conditions not only as severe and debilitating but as gruesomely, extraordinarily so. One woman was so weak she could not walk, "but creeps," while another could only "tumble out" of her house "of her hands & kneeds & hath beene soe for the space of twelufe weekes."[33] These women were characterized in dehumanizing ways—creeping like an animal and walking on hands and knees like a four-legged creature—to high-light their inability to function. Others played on the emotion of disgust. Richard Hoole, a poor man from Lancashire, described how his wife's face was "Eatten away with kancker moste lamentably to behould." Such dis-figuring ailments simultaneously evoked pity from poor law authorities and evidenced petitioners' inability to participate fully in society. There was an enduring association between marked bodies and inner virtue in early mod-ern England. Scars or deformities, most especially on the face, were external signifiers of internal decay. As a result, disfiguring diseases were forms of dis-ability, as they could prevent individuals from securing employment or drawing on social networks. A man from London with a canker on his face was so "loathsome" that "no one will imploy him." Petitioners could avoid the moral ramifications of physical deformity by placing their conditions within the context of labor and industry rather than the monstrous and mar-velous. An occupational context reminded readers that petitioners fell prey to misfortunes beyond their control. Pleading for aid from the parish was still socially marginalizing, but it lacked the connotations of sin and portent that early modern society mapped onto extraordinary bodies.[34]

In 1691 a couple from Cumbria explained that their parish overseer "did pretend yt we had 2 new calurd [colored] cowes." The overseer used this presumption to defend his decision to discontinue their weekly sti-pend. The couple petitioned to overturn his decision, explaining that they owned only one cow, "& if they take all we haue the cow excepted it will not pay her price." The couple looked to tangible, quantifiable indicators of their condition—a single cow—to prove their dependence, while their overseer did the same to justify cutting off their support. Material markers of poverty, much like debilitating disorders, provided visible proof of paupers' need. One woman could not even afford to clothe herself; she had to share her daughter's tattered garments. Several petitioners not only noted a lack of material possessions but detailed the process of losing them: "I haue pauned All that I haue." By pawning their household goods, petitioners provided quantifiable proof of their former lifestyles and current downfalls. Material loss allowed these men and women to present themselves as pitiable and also industrious and enabled them to do so in quantifiable terms. Dependency was an aberration in an otherwise self-sufficient existence. Sixty-seven petitioners here made reference to the material ramifications of ill health, almost equal numbers of men and women. About half received the relief they sought.[35]

Petitioners highlighted a loss of material wealth and also a "want of ffreinds." Jane Forster was a widow raising three small children, the youngest of whom was crippled. She herself was infirm and destitute, possessing "No Effects att all." Every member of an impoverished family like hers was typically consigned to work from an early age, as young as seven. Her appeal to Quarter Sessions was so convincing—the justices granted her an order for one shilling and six pence per week—because she was an ailing widow, alone responsible for raising three children who were unable to contribute to the family economy.[36] More than one hundred female petitioners in my sample characterized themselves as widows, a status that served as shorthand for a lack of familial support. Others listed children, neighbors, and spouses who were sick, disabled, or otherwise incapacitated as a way of demonstrating their social isolation and therefore inability to secure alternate means of support. The petition by Mary Grave that opens this chapter employs just such a strategy by noting the incapacity of her only daughter. Ellin Browne of Derbyshire was not a widow, although she described in detail how her husband was unable to provide financial support because he was imprisoned for unpaid debts. Her petition offered such an intricate overview of her husband's debts and subsequent absence that she only devoted two words to her own deteriorating condition: "diseased & Impotent." Forster, Grave, and Browne stressed their inability to access the networks of care that were so central to healing, as well as subsistence, in this period.[37]

The loss of much-needed social safety nets or the discovery that over-extended neighbors "begin to bee weary of the burthen" stirred up sentiments of charity and Christian obligation in the minds of readers. By detailing the toil and even subsequent poverty of their caretakers, petitioners proved their dependency and also provided positive models of generosity for parish offi-cials to emulate. If a poor neighbor could expend money, time, and energy, then a parish official likewise could perform a simple act of charity. The 1662 petition of Thomas Nalior, a Lancashire man who suffered from fever, paralysis, and sore, disabled limbs, illustrates how the charitable deeds of others could attest to the magnitude of a petitioner's condition. He "hath had nothinge but what pittifull neighbours haue sent him, and likewise now are willinge to be trobled to tooke to him & helpe him in this his loathsome condition onely a kinswoman of his hath out of natural affection thus farr beene wth him but she beinge of small estate unable to releeue him & greeue-inge to see his dayly miserie, is discouraged & almost wearied out."[38] The neighbors and relatives in this petition seem almost as pitiable as the peti-tioner himself, and their impoverishment threatened to unload more de-pendents on the parish. By noting the care of friends and family—and its limits—Nalior made a case for himself that implicated the needs of others.

Fellow parishioners validated petitioners' conditions in even more tan-gible ways: by signing their names. Groups of neighbors, friends, and church-wardens sometimes submitted petitions on behalf of individuals who were themselves too weak to petition. Others signed their names as proof that petitioners' conditions were well known in the community or, as one rector put it, "literally true." Medical testimony—mostly provided by surgeons, given the external nature of so many petitioners' ailments—served a similar pur-pose. Nicholas Knott hired a pair of surgeons, George and John Cloughe, in 1638 to treat a sore on his leg that reached seven inches deep. George cut into the wound with a penknife, "turn[ing] his hand round about in it which was uerie great payne unto mee and great Coste." Knott consulted the surgeons for three months, until he could stand again without help. He petitioned for relief because he had "growen soe weeke of it and soe full of payne that I am not able to worke withe it any longer, nor hardlie to goe on it." By providing an account of his prior attempt to treat the wound, he affirmed that his cur-rent debility was only the latest stage of a lengthy, severe, and expensive con-dition. The surgeons bore witness to the severity and pain of his ailment and to the cost of its cure.[39]

John Marten, a surgeon living and working in London, charitably treated an impoverished woman who had contracted venereal disease from her husband. Venereal disease was associated with illicit, intemperate behavior and most likely would have received an unfavorable response from poor law authorities. Not surprisingly, the patient requested relief from her overseers and was denied. Marten emphasized her innocence, referring to her as a "sober modest Woman." Like so many petitioners, he also characterized the pitiable, severe, and visible nature of her condition. She "made a shift to craul to my House, (being indeed scarce able to walk)" and had ulcers all over her body, one on her leg larger than the palm of a hand. Upon seeing "the fiery Botches all over her Face," Marten knew immediately that she was, so to speak, "poxt." The woman was "reduc'd to almost nothing but Skin and Bone; Stomachless and Feeble, and in short in such a miserable condition, that had not the Woman that came with her, had Compassion on her, and took her into her House, she must have died in the Street or a Ditch." By noting the patient's dependence on a compassionate neighbor, Marten drew on familiar modes of defining need and eliciting pity from readers. The patient knocked on his door after first seeking help from a hospital, spending all her money on surgeons, and unsuccessfully pleading for relief from her parish. Resigned to death, she had even tried to return to her home parish to live out her final days but was denied the privilege. When she approached a coach, its driver, upon seeing her condition and recognizing its cause, refused to take her. As Marten put it, she was "almost starv'd, and at her Wits end." He treated the woman for free, and she fully recovered without any disfigurement in just six weeks.[40]

The parallels between Marten's case and terse pauper petitions stem in part from Marten's charity. As the patient made her pitch to him, she occupied the same position of supplication and desperation as a petitioner pleading before poor law authorities. Perhaps she even appropriated the language of morality, debility, and despair from her unsuccessful petition. Another of Marten's patients explicitly employed the language of a petition in the final words of his letter to the surgeon: "and your Petitioner will ever Pray." Yet concerns about reputation also shaped Marten's account. His text resembles a medical treatise, but it is for the most part a lengthy advertisement promoting his wares and expertise. By recounting the extremity of the woman's condition, he highlighted the efficacy of his cure: "She recovered in six Weeks or less, to the admiration of all that knew her." And emphasizing her moral standing and the many ways she was denied help served to make Marten appear eminently compassionate: "I took pity on her, she being, as I was inform'd, an industrious Woman, and got the Distemper undeserv'd by the Brute her Husband."[41] Despite the genre of Marten's text and even the questionable veracity of his account, the parallels between his case and those of paupers pleading for relief suggest that early modern men and women drew on the formulations and expressions of petitions in a range of contexts.

Many of the findings here reflect patterns in similar types of writing from later periods. For instance, eighteenth- and nineteenth-century pauper letters emphasize authors' respectability and need and rely on the testimony of witnesses. Nineteenth-century paupers cited external, debilitating ailments, much like the petitioners here, and they continued to place their stories within the context of work and industry. Such continuities show that the rhetoric of supplication remained fairly consistent across time even as laws, beliefs, and concerns shifted.[42] For this reason alone, the terse petitions discussed here are significant. But these accounts also broaden our view of seventeenth-century illness. Themes that are central to narratives by wealthier patients, such as the religious significance of bodily suffering, break down in petitions. Paupers did not have the liberty to ruminate on the spiritual implications of ill health. They cited nonhumoral sources of illness and resulting disorders that were visible on the body, undeniably disabling, and at times extraordinarily gruesome. Petitioners also tended to highlight the material ramifications of illness, a concern almost nonexistent in writing by wealthier patients. While the rhetorical strategies of petitions surely account for many of these patterns, resulting narratives still have much to teach us about seventeenth-century perceptions of illness. Indeed, these heavily mediated legal documents cannot capture the full lived experiences of the laboring poor, but they can elucidate how the poor constructed and processed their experiences—how they expressed distress and articulated illness in ways that diverged from those of wealthy men and women.

In particular, economic circumstances compelled the sick poor to frame concerns also common to middling- and upper-status men and women in different ways. In petitions, the poor defined suffering in terms of incapacity rather than piety. They emphasized morality as a primary dimension of citizenship and industry rather than of lifestyle and religion. And they highlighted their pitiable social isolation as a means of evidencing need rather than settling soured relationships. Petitioners also repurposed familiar gendered scripts. They underscored their fortitude and self-sufficiency in order to convey industry, responsibility, and moral worth. And they displayed frailty and meekness in order to communicate the extent of their destitution. Embodying these seemingly contradictory qualities enabled paupers to fulfill a complex social role that required both diligence and dependence. When the body is a unit of labor and the ability to work fundamental to survival, illness acquires new meanings.

Conclusions

When I first began this project I was surprised to find little existing scholarship on early modern gender and illness. Other fields in the medical humanities, particularly medical anthropology and sociology, have more thoroughly explored men's and women's varying perceptions of the same bodily complaints. And historians working on later time periods, most notably the nineteenth century, have long examined the relationship between gender and health. Why was there nothing comparable for the earlier period? Part of the answer is found in the sources. It is difficult to unravel the subtle influences of gender on early modern patients' beliefs and behaviors by using the writing of practitioners. Chapter 1 examines the varied aims and writing practices of medical authors that can leave us guessing at the actual utterances and exchanges that transpired in clinical encounters. The answer also lies in the paucity of sex-specific diseases in early modern Europe, relative to later periods. By the nineteenth century, in contrast, sex-specific ailments were prevalent and had come to reify cultural beliefs about men and women. Diseases such as neurasthenia and hysteria were diagnosed disproportionately in women in the nineteenth century because of prevailing beliefs about the physical constitution of their bodies. Women were thought to be naturally frail, listless, and tender—traits that allegedly predisposed them to certain types of complaints. Such thinking caused women to view and respond to physical disorders in particular ways and came to justify their exclusion from various aspects of public life. Biology underpinned cultural assumptions about the "natural" inferiority of certain types of people. What it meant to be a patient was clearly marked in gendered terms.[1]

There were few sex-specific diseases in the seventeenth century aside from those associated with reproductive functions. The most common ailments that early modern patients cited were bruises, colds, convulsions, fevers, swellings, sores, numbness, cramps, gas, wounds, and stones. These complaints were neither associated with a particular sex nor explicitly understood in terms that reinforced men's and women's social roles, as they were two hundred years later. Yet the patterns analyzed throughout this book unveil the long historical roots of that nineteenth-century story—a tendency to validate and perpetuate gender inequality by naturalizing it in the body. Women's descriptions of falling instantly, mimetically ill in response to sudden emotional outbursts, for example, reflect assumptions about women's insufficient reason and ungovernable imaginations. Such views were so ingrained in early modern imaginations that they shaped women's explanations and perceptions of their bodily processes. Men too linked ill health to grief and sorrow. But the different ways men and women articulated the relationship between emotions and illness, discussed in chapter 3, reflected—and sustained—prominent beliefs about men's "natural" reason and women's lack of it. Sufferers projected the stereotypes encoded in medical views of the body, perpetuating those stereotypes in the process.

This troubling relationship between medicine and culture endures today. Cultural environments always shape knowledge production, often in imperceptible ways. And resulting knowledge in turn validates those invisible cultural assumptions.[2] This book looks beyond medical texts to show this process from the patient's point of view. Narratives of illness reveal how cultural stereotypes embedded in medical frameworks were digested, absorbed, and reproduced. Gendered explanations of the causes of sickness, responses to pain and suffering, and conceptions of the long road to recuperation reflect culturally produced beliefs about men and women, validating those beliefs in the lived experiences of the body.

This book shows how the gendered patterns in patients' writing were also products of religious convictions, economic status, and writing practices. Religion as it was lived and embodied informed how men and women alike viewed health and infirmity. Divine grace was felt in the body, as was anxiety about salvation. Believers experienced stirrings in their bowels and pricks in their hearts, and they felt how intense apprehension of God's judgment could exacerbate physical suffering, while acceptance of divine will eased it. Daily devotional acts, such as prayer and meditation, entailed a physical dimension that taught pious patients to view the vicissitudes of health and illness as barometers of spiritual ability. And devotional literature, including stories and images of martyrdom, provided conceptual frameworks for explaining the divine meanings of suffering, as well as a set of metaphors and models for physically responding to it. The men and women in this study looked to religion to make sense of illness over the course of the seventeenth century despite increased secularization. Belief in witchcraft, magic, possession, and the supernatural had all begun to wane by the end of the 1600s, and medical practitioners increasingly privileged natural remedies and explanations of illness over religious ones.[3] Yet the patient's perspective reveals the enduring power of religion in shaping ordinary understandings of illness, perhaps because so many individuals who chose to document their lives did so for spiritual purposes.

Glimpses into the lives of the sick poor offer scant evidence of these spiritual beliefs. Yet, like their wealthier counterparts, the poor were devout and relied on prevailing gendered and religious scripts to evaluate their bodies. They recounted the physical effects of intense emotional responses and were attuned to the social dimensions of ill health and recovery. But the sick poor articulated these beliefs and concerns—the topics of the preceding chapters of this book—in new ways. Impoverished men and women had to work hard to subsist, often in physically demanding trades, and they had to demonstrate morality and responsibility to win parish aid. They articulated debility in terms of able-bodiedness and need rather than piety and sin. Paupers cited types of ailments that varied from those in ego-literature, including many more disorders that were external, incapacitating, and disfiguring. Some suffered from less obviously debilitating ailments yet were careful to note how poor health put them in a position of economic peril. While few paupers attributed their physical disorders to humors, the handful that mentioned intense emotions or sudden temperature shifts—primary causes of ill health among wealthier patients—presented their illnesses in terms that deflected blame from themselves and placed causation squarely within the realm of occupational hazards. Finally, social relationships facilitated recovery from illness in tangible ways for men and women of all social ranks. Yet the impact of community relations on health took on new meanings when a poor family relied on parish administrators for subsistence. The poor highlighted their social isolation not only to express disappointments with relatives and to negotiate relationships but also to communicate the sheer magnitude of their need.

Such divergences among patients of assorted economic backgrounds stemmed partly from their varying forms of writing. Paupers certainly viewed illness in religious terms, but petitions, as sources, offer scant evidence of those beliefs. Imagined readers further determined the information that petitioners, healers, and wealthier patients chose to highlight, downplay, or omit. Writing played a crucial role in structuring stories of sickness, yet writing practices also intersected with gender to shape many of the patterns that this book outlines. For instance, accounting practices can begin to explain why so many male patients here quantified their illnesses. But the pattern also emerges in personal writing by men who were not keeping accounts, suggesting that the trend reflects prevailing representations of men's work and identities. Many men and women also employed the same writing practices yet, as the preceding chapters show, varied in their explanations of illness onset, responses to pain, and performances of suffering on the sickbed. Popular tropes could further shape constructions and even perceptions of physical distress differently for male and female writers. Finally, many of the individuals here were recording their experiences and also working through them. They were making sense of their lives and constructing a sense of themselves in the process. At first glance, Sarah Cowper's diary reads like an immense list of complaints. A closer look, however, reveals how writing provided a valuable means by which she coped with anxieties and came to terms with them. She herself recognized the benefits of this process: "To ease my spleen I straight go home and write."[4] Texts can tell us something about lived experiences, of course, but they also illuminate how economic circumstances, rhetorical strategies, religion, and gender could inform the perceptions of those experiences. Writing reveals the ways men and women made meaning of their lives. Physical infirmity—so frightening, prevalent, and spiritually and morally significant in the seventeenth century—offers a particularly rich site for recovering that work.

Many people today continue to believe that having a well-regulated lifestyle, or moderating the six nonnaturals, is central to maintaining health. Some strive to sleep a certain number of hours each night, to eat a balanced diet, or to exercise at least a few times a week. Many also cope with illness in ways that resonate with the efforts of men and women from the seventeenth century: by writing like Cowper, praying like Alice Thornton, or seeking alternative therapies like Samuel Pepys's lucky hare's foot. Yet the social occupies a diminished role for patients in the modern West, in stark contrast to its place in the lives of early modern men and women.[5] Friends and relatives visit loved ones in the hospital today, but sick visits are no longer a fundamental dimension of social relationships. For the most part, patients today suffer alongside immediate family members and hired health care workers or, in many instances, alone. Biomedical frameworks rather than social interactions underlie prevailing explanations of illnesses and their cures. In contrast, the social was at the core of early modern understandings and experiences of illness. Social interactions were a necessary component of negotiating diagnoses and administering cures. And the social was crucial to patients' explanations of illness onset, suffering, and recovery. Emotional responses to sullied relationships and vexing business transactions were common sources of ill health in the 1600s, while pity and compassion from friends and relatives facilitated recovery. This book shows how female patients stressed these interpersonal dimensions of suffering differently than their male counterparts did. Women tended to evaluate their ailments by looking to the bodies and opinions of others. Some fell instantly and severely sick in response to disturbing or otherwise problematic social interactions. And they viewed and performed suffering in ways that enabled them to mend thorny relationships. I am not suggesting that the men in this book were any less social than women. Indeed, some also attributed illness to emotional distress and observed the healing effects of others' affection. And many men viewed emotional disorders and debilitating pain within the context of occupational responsibilities and credit relations—inherently social realms. Both men and women understood the impact of the social on their bodies, but they articulated, emphasized, and experienced that relationship differently.

Perhaps the starkest disconnect between the stories here and our experiences today lies in the body itself. The bodies of seventeenth-century men and women do not always make sense to us. Blood could itch. Corrupt fluids oozed out through the pores of the skin. Coughing could shift internal fluids into entirely new parts of the body, and a headache might morph instantly into a kidney stone. We view corporeal processes quite differently than did early modern men and women. Yet historical accounts afford us a new perspective on our convictions and assumptions, on how we negotiate and narrate the landscape of illness and health today. By looking at stories of sickness from hundreds of years ago, we can see, perhaps with renewed clarity, how stereotypes or social norms have become embedded in our understandings of biology and in our own embodied experiences. Or how biomedical frameworks teach us to understand and therefore physically perceive ill health in particular ways—as an invading germ or a mutating cell rather than a corruption or obstruction. We begin to see more vividly how power relations can become inscribed in clinical relationships, determining who can speak and who can know. Situating our illness experiences in the words and mind-sets of seventeenth-century sufferers exposes the precious lessons of our own bodies.

Abbreviations

BL	British Library, London
CAC Carlisle	Cumbria Archive Centre, Carlisle
CAC Kendal	Cumbria Archive Centre, Kendal
CALS	Cheshire Archives and Local Studies, Chester
Chetham's	Chetham's Library, Manchester
Cowper, Daily Diary	Sarah Cowper, Daily Diary, MSS D/EP/F29–35, Hertfordshire Public Record Office, Hertford, reproduced in Amanda Vickery, ed., *Women's Language and Experience, 1500–1940* (Marlborough: Adam Matthew Publications, 1994), microfilm, part 1, reels 5–7. I cite MSS D/EP/F29–35 as vols. 1–7 respectively
DRO Exeter	Devon Record Office, Exeter
DRO Matlock	Derbyshire Record Office, Matlock
DWL	Dr. Williams's Library, London
ERO	Essex Record Office, Chelmsford
Folger	Folger Shakespeare Library, Washington DC
GA	Gloucestershire Archives, Gloucester
Huntington	Huntington Library, San Marino, CA
LA	Lancashire Archives, Preston
LMA	London Metropolitan Archives
RCP	Royal College of Physicians, London

Rich, Diary	Mary Rich, Diary, Add. MSS 27351–27355, British Library. I cite each manuscript by the last digit of its catalogue number, followed by the folio.
SRO	Somerset Record Office, Taunton
Thornton, Remembrances	Alice Wandesford Thornton, A Book of Remembrances, Microfilm MISC 326, Yale University, Sterling Memorial Library, New Haven, CT
WAAS	Worcestershire Archive and Archaeology Service, Worcester
Wellcome	Wellcome Library, London
WYAS	West Yorkshire Archive Service, Wakefield

Appendix A: Patients' Biographical Information

The following patients form the core of the analysis in this book. Longer entries are provided for patients whose narratives of illness are most detailed and abundant and who therefore serve as the central actors. Bibliographic references refer to manuscripts and publications that I consulted.

ANNESLEY, Arthur (1614–1686): Annesley was a politician, a nonconformist, and the first Earl of Anglesey. He lived in London and married Elizabeth Altham.

> Arthur Annesley, Diary, Add. MSS 18730, 40860, BL.

ARCHER, Isaac (1641–1700): Archer was a minister who preached in Cambridgeshire and Suffolk. He suffered from a speech impediment as a child and struggled with a stutter into adulthood, a challenge that he viewed as divine punishment for dishonorable behavior: "I was troubled at my stammering, for I found it somthing worse now . . . but I resolved to beare it patiently, and look upon it as the hand of God upon mee, for abusing my tongue." He conformed to the Church of England against his father's wishes in the early 1660s, which created a rift between them and deep emotional turmoil for Archer. The senior Archer expressed his disappointment most poignantly by largely writing his son out of his will. After his father's death in 1670, the distraught Archer pored over his father's private papers, comparing himself and his sins to those of his father and reliving their relationship through his father's words.[1]

> *Two East Anglian Diaries, 1641–1729: Isaac Archer and William Coe*, ed. Matthew Storey and David Dymond (Woodbridge: Boydell Press, 1994).

AUSTEN (Wilson), Katherine (1629–1683): The daughter of a London cloth merchant, she married Thomas Austen in 1645 and became widowed with three children in 1658.

Katherine Austen, Meditations in Prose and Verse (1664–1668), Add. MS 4454, BL.

BACON (Meautys), Lady Jane (1581–1659): Bacon lived in Suffolk and York-shire and married William Cornwallis and later Nathaniel Bacon.

The Private Correspondence of Jane Lady Cornwallis Bacon, 1613–1644, ed. Joanna Moody (Madison: Fairleigh Dickinson University Press, 2003).

BLUNDELL, Nicholas (1669–1737): Blundell was a Catholic landowner who lived in Lancashire.

The Great Diurnal of Nicholas Blundell, ed. J. J. Bagley and Frank Tyrer, 3 vols. (Liverpool: C. Tinling, 1968–1972).

CALVERLEY, Walter (1670–1749): He lived in Yorkshire and married Julia Blackett of Newcastle-upon-Tyne in 1707.

"Memorandum Book of Sir Walter Calverley, Bart," in *Yorkshire Diaries and Auto-biographies in the Seventeenth and Eighteenth Centuries,* ed. S. Margerison (Dur-ham: Andrews, 1886), 43–148.

CANNON, John (1684–1743): Cannon was a Somerset excise official, as well as a maltster, accountant, and schoolmaster. He married a domestic ser-vant, Susannah Deane, in 1714.

Manuscript Diary of John Cannon, Schoolmaster of Meare, Exciseman, Etc. (1684–1742), DD\SAS/C1193/4, SRO.

CLEGG, James (1679–1755): A Presbyterian minister, Clegg lived and worked in Derbyshire. He married Ann Champion (1682–1742) in 1704, and they went on to have nine children together; all but one survived to adulthood. To supplement the family income, Clegg moved his wife and children to a farm, Stoddart Hall, in 1713 and began working part-time as a physician. Following Champion's death, he married Sarah Eyre in 1744.

The Diary of James Clegg of Chapel-En-Le Frith, 1708–55, ed. Vanessa S. Doe, 3 vols. (Chesterfield: Derbyshire Record Society, 1978).

CLIFFORD, Anne (1590–1676): The Countess of Pembroke, Dorset, and Mont-gomery, Clifford was an Anglican whose personal writing details dis-putes over her inheritance. She married Richard Sackville, third Earl of Dorset, in 1609 and later Philip Herbert, Earl of Montgomery and fourth Earl of Pembroke.

The Diaries of Lady Anne Clifford, ed. D. J. H. Clifford (Wolfeboro Falls: Alan Sutton, 1990).

The Diary of Anne Clifford, 1616–1619: A Critical Edition, ed. Katherine O. Acheson (New York: Garland, 1995).

COE, William (1662–1729): Coe was an Anglican gentleman and farmer. He lived in Suffolk and married twice.

Isaac Archer and William Coe, *Two East Anglian Diaries, 1641–1729: Isaac Archer and William Coe*, ed. Matthew Storey and David Dymond (Woodbridge: Boydell Press, 1994).

CONWAY (Finch), Anne (1631–1679): Conway was a philosopher and intellectual who lived in London and Warwickshire. She was Anglican before converting to Quakerism. She married Edward Conway in 1651.

Conway Letters: The Correspondence of Anne, Viscountess Conway, Henry More, and Their Friends, 1642–1684, ed. Marjorie Hope Nicolson, revised ed. by Sarah Hutton (Oxford: Clarendon Press, 1992).

COWPER (Holled), Sarah (1644–1720): The daughter of a London merchant, Sarah Holled married William Cowper (1639–1706) in 1664. William was a lawyer and baronet, though his inheritance was rather paltry for his rank. In 1679 the family fortunes improved, with William becoming a member of Parliament for the borough of Hertford, where he sat until 1681 and then again from 1688 to 1700. The couple's two surviving sons, William and Spencer, further elevated the family's status by becoming lawyers, politicians, and, in William's case, an earl. While the two men raised the social status of the family, they also garnered unwanted attention when one was accused of murder and the other fathered two illegitimate children. Perhaps motivated by her son's murder trial in 1699, Cowper began keeping a diary the following year. Her writing fills more than twenty-three hundred manuscript pages and includes intimate accounts of her interactions with friends and acquaintances, her struggles for power with household servants, and her continual disappointments with family members.[2]

Sarah Cowper, Daily Diary, MSS D/EP/F29–35, Hertfordshire Public Record Office, Hertford, reproduced in Amanda Vickery, ed., *Women's Language and Experience, 1500–1940* (Marlborough: Adam Matthew Publications, 1994), microfilm, part 1, reels 5–7.

DAVIES, Rowland (1649–1721): Davies was a nonconformist clergyman healer from Cork; his family was from Hertfordshire but settled in Ireland. He married Elizabeth Stannard in 1674.

Journal of the Very Rev. Rowland Davies, LL.D., Dean of Ross (and Afterwards Dean of Cork), from March 8, 1688–9, to September 29, 1690, ed. Richard Caulfield (London: Printed for the Camden Society, 1858).

DELAVAL (Livingston), Elizabeth (1648?–1717): A member of a prominent Royalist family in Lincolnshire, she married Robert Delaval in 1670 and later Henry Hatcher. Delaval fled England when she was accused of conspiring with James II.

The Meditations of Lady Elizabeth Delaval, Written Between 1662 and 1671, ed. Douglas G. Greene (Gateshead: Northumberland Press, 1975).

D'EWES, Simonds (1602–1650): A gentleman and antiquary, D'Ewes lived in Suffolk. He married Anne Clopton and later Elizabeth Willoughby.

Simonds D'Ewes, Correspondence, Harleian MS 382, BL.

The Diary of Sir Simonds D'Ewes (1622–1624), ed. Elizabeth Bourcier (Paris: Didier, 1974).

DORMER (Cottrell), Anne (1648?–1695): Anne Dormer's staunchly Royalist parents fled the country during the civil war and left young Anne behind. She married Robert Dormer (c. 1628–1689) in 1668, and the two lived in London and Oxfordshire, where they had eleven children together. The details of her life are preserved in a series of letters she wrote from 1685 to 1691 to her sister, Lady Elizabeth Trumbull, expressing concerns about her troubled marriage and ever-weakening body.[3]

Trumbull Papers, Add. MS 72516, BL.

DUGARD, Lydia (1650–1675): Dugard lived in Warwickshire and London and married her cousin, the Anglican clergyman Samuel Dugard, in 1672.

Lydia Dugard (1650–1675), Autograph letters signed, to Samuel Dugard, MS X.d.477 (1–37), Folger.

EGERTON (Cavendish), Elizabeth (1626–1663): She married John Egerton in 1641 and thus became the Countess of Bridgewater.

Elizabeth Egerton, Countess of Bridgewater, Devotional Pieces, c. 1648–1663, Egerton MS 607, BL.

EVANS (Dawson), Anne (1696–post-1740): A nonconformist from Manchester, she married Roger Evans.

Anne Dawson, Diary (1721–1722), Add. MS 71626, BL.

EYRE, Adam (1614–1661): A Parliamentarian army officer from Yorkshire, Eyre married Susanna Mathewman in 1640.

"A Diurnall, or Catalogue of All My Accounts and Expences from the 1st of January, 1646–(7)," in *Yorkshire Diaries and Autobiographies in the Seventeenth and Eighteenth Centuries*, ed. H. J. Morehouse (Durham: Andrews, 1877), 1–118.

FANSHAWE (Harrison), Ann (1625–1680): She lived in London and married her second cousin, Richard Fanshawe, in 1644.

Anne Halkett and Ann Fanshawe, *The Memoirs of Anne, Lady Halkett, and Ann, Lady Fanshawe*, ed. John Loftis (Oxford: Clarendon Press, 1979).

FREKE, Elizabeth (1641–1714): Elizabeth Freke secretly married her cousin Percy Freke (c. 1643–1706) and had one child, Ralph. She moved between Ireland and her family estate in Norfolk several times and spent long spans of time visiting her sisters in London and Bristol. Freke used private writing to vent anxieties about her perilous financial situation and her ailing body. In her later years, she suffered from a chronic cough and asthma, an ailment known as tissick, and at times she was incapacitated for months on end. Her inventories of remedies and extensive recipe collections suggest that she produced significant quantities of medicines for both her own and her family's use.[4]

Freke Papers, Add. MSS 45718, 45719, BL.

The Remembrances of Elizabeth Freke, 1671–1714, ed. Raymond A. Anselment (Cambridge: Cambridge University Press, 2001).

HALKETT (Murray), Anne (1623–1699): Halkett was from London, though she spent much of her adult life in Scotland. She was an Anglican gentlewoman and Royalist who married Sir James Halkett in 1656.

Lady Anne Halkett: Selected Self-Writings, ed. Suzanne Trill (Aldershot: Ashgate, 2007).

The Memoirs of Anne, Lady Halkett, and Ann, Lady Fanshawe, ed. John Loftis (Oxford: Clarendon Press, 1979).

HARLEY (Conway), Brilliana (1598–1643): Harley was a nonconformist gentlewoman from Hertfordshire married to Sir Robert Harley.

Letters of the Lady Brilliana Harley, Wife of Sir Robert Harley, of Brampton Bryan, Knight of the Bath, ed. Thomas Taylor Lewis (London: Camden Society, 1854).

HARROLD, Edmund (1678–1721): Harrold was a Manchester wigmaker and book trader. He was Anglican and married four times.

Edmund Harrold, His Book of Remarks and Observations, 1712–16, MS Mun. A.2.137, Chetham's.

The Diary of Edmund Harrold, Wigmaker of Manchester, 1712–15, ed. Craig Horner (Aldershot: Ashgate, 2008).

HEYWOOD, Oliver (1629–1702): A Presbyterian minister from West Yorkshire, Heywood was ejected from office in 1662. He married Elizabeth Angier in 1655 and, following her death, Abigail Crompton in 1667.

The Rev. Oliver Heywood, B.A., 1630–1702: His Autobiography, Diaries, Anecdote and Event Books: Illustrating the General and Family History of Yorkshire and Lancashire, ed. J. Horsfall Turner, 4 vols. (Brighouse: A. B. Bayes, 1881–1885).

HOOKE, Robert (1635–1703): Hooke was a natural philosopher, surveyor, and member of the Royal Society in London.

The Diary of Robert Hooke, M.A., M.D., F.R.S., 1672–1680, Transcribed from the Original in the Possession of the Corporation of the City of London, ed. Henry W. Robinson and Walter Adams (London: Taylor and Francis, 1935).

ISHAM, Elizabeth (1609–1654): A single woman from Northamptonshire, Isham left behind a spiritual autobiography written around 1640.

Elizabeth Isham, My Booke of Rememenberance, MS RTCO1 (no. 62), Robert H. Taylor Collection, Princeton University Library, Princeton, NJ.

JEAKE, Samuel (1652–1699): Jeake lived and worked in Rye as a moneylender, investor, and trader of cloth, produce, and wool. He was extraordinarily well read for his middling rank, in part thanks to his father's extensive library. Jeake began keeping an astrological diary in 1666 in an attempt to link his life events to the heavens. He suffered from recurring fevers, a chronic affliction that enabled him to measure the accuracy of astrological principles by using his body as a testing ground. In 1680 he married Elizabeth Hartshorne, and they had six children, four of whom survived to adulthood.[5]

An Astrological Diary of the Seventeenth Century: Samuel Jeake of Rye, 1652–1699, ed. Michael Hunter and Annabel Gregory (Oxford: Clarendon Press, 1988).

JOLLY (also JOLLIE), Thomas (1629–1703): Jolly was a nonconformist pastor in Lancashire who was ejected from office in 1662 and imprisoned several times.

The Note Book of the Rev. Thomas Jolly, AD 1671–1693, ed. Henry Fishwick (Manchester: Chetham Society, 1894).

JOSSELIN, Ralph (1616–1683): He was a nonconformist minister and farmer from Essex.

The Diary of Ralph Josselin, 1616–1683, ed. Alan Macfarlane (London: Oxford University Press, 1976).

LISTER, Joseph (1627–1709): Lister was a nonconforming apprentice and servant from Yorkshire. He married Sarah Denton and had two children.

The Autobiography of Joseph Lister, of Bradford in Yorkshire, ed. Thomas Wright, Esq. M.A., F.S.A. (London: John Russell Smith, 1842).

LOWE, Roger (?–1679): Lowe was a nonconformist shopkeeper living in Lancashire. He also worked as an accountant, notary, and scribe. He married Emma Potter in 1668.

The Diary of Roger Lowe, of Ashton-in-Makerfield, Lancashire, 1663–74, ed. William L. Sachse (New Haven: Yale University Press, 1938).

MARTINDALE, Adam (1623–1686): A Presbyterian minister, Martindale lived in Cheshire and married Elizabeth Hall in 1646.

Adam Martindale, Autobiography, Add. MS 4239, BL.

The Life of Adam Martindale, ed. Richard Parkinson (Manchester: Chetham Society, 1845).

MOORE, Giles (1617–1679): Moore was a preacher from Sussex who married Susanne Luxford and had no children.

The Journal of Giles Moore, ed. Ruth Bird (Lewes: Sussex Record Society, 1971).

MORRIS, Claver (1659–1727): A physician in Dorset and Somerset, Morris married three times: Grace Green in 1685, Elizabeth Jeans in 1696, and Molly Bragge in 1703.

The Diary of a West County Physician, AD 1684–1726, ed. Edmund Hodhouse, M.D. (London: Simpkin Marshall, 1934).

NORTH (Montagu), Anne (1614–1681): Anne Montagu married the politician Dudley North in 1632. The couple lived in Essex and had ten children who lived to adulthood. Most of Anne's letters cited here were written to her son Francis North and her daughter Anne Foley.

North Papers, Add. MSS 32500, 32501, BL.

North Papers, HM 52322–52420, Huntington.

PASTON (North), Elizabeth (1647–1730): Paston was the daughter of Anne (Montagu) North and Dudley North. She married Sir Robert Wiseman and, after his death, William Paston, second Earl of Yarmouth. She had no children.

Paston Papers, Add. MSS 27447, 36988, BL.

PEPYS, Samuel (1633–1703): Pepys worked as an administrator for the navy and kept a diary from 1660 to 1669 that includes firsthand observations of the plague outbreak in 1665 and the London fire of 1666. He fastidiously documented his health, particularly the ups and downs of a lifelong battle with kidney stones. The diary is perhaps best known for its candid, detailed accounts of Restoration life, including Pepys's interactions with famous experimenters of the day and quarrels with his wife, Elizabeth St. Michel (1641–1669). He also documented his guilty pleasures, many of which he attempted to regulate, to no avail. For instance, he imposed fines on himself in order to resist attending the theater, although he used convoluted reasoning to justify breaking these vows: "My oath against going to plays doth not oblige me against this house because it was not then in being." He also documented his infidelities with maidservants and, for several years, with a woman named Betty Lane, who worked at a draper's stall in Westminster Hall. After a day of "sporting" with Lane and visiting a brothel but refusing to spend any money there, Pepys noted feeling "weary of the pleasure I have had today and ashamed to think of it."[6]

The Diary of Samuel Pepys: A New and Complete Transcription, ed. Robert Latham and William Matthews, 11 vols. (Berkeley: University of California Press, 1970–1983).

The Further Correspondence of Samuel Pepys 1662–1679, ed. J. R. Tanner (London: G. Bell and Sons, 1929).

The Private Correspondence and Miscellaneous Papers of Samuel Pepys, 1679–1703, ed. J. R. Tanner, 2 vols. (New York: Harcourt Brace, 1926).

PLEDGER, Elias (1665–?): Pledger was a nonconforming apothecary from Essex.

Elias Pledger, Diary, MS 28.4, DWL.

RICH (Boyle), Mary (1624–1678): Mary Rich, Countess of Warwick, lived in London and Essex, in the household of her father-in-law, Robert Rich. Her brother was the famous natural philosopher Robert Boyle and her sister the intellectual Katherine Jones, Lady Ranelagh. She married Charles Rich (1616–1673) in 1641, despite her father's initial opposition to the match. The couple had two children, one of whom died young. The other child, Charles, suffered from a sudden illness as a four-year-old, a frightening episode that deepened Rich's faith. By 1647, she had experienced a full spiritual conversion. She renounced the vanities of her youth and embraced a life of piety and meditation. Although Rich was a member of the Church of England, she was sympathetic to ministers who were ejected from their posts for refusing to conform to Anglicanism. Rich recorded her daily devotional exercises in more than thirteen hundred manuscript pages spanning from 1666 to 1677. She also wrote an autobiography and a book of meditations. Rich suffered continually from headaches and melancholy, which at times prevented her from completing her devotional routine. She often linked these infirmities to passionate arguments with her husband, who suffered from his own painful affliction, gout.[7]

Mary Rich, Diary, Autobiography (1625–1674), and Occasional Meditations (1663–1677), Add. MSS 27351–27357, BL.

RYDER, Dudley (1691–1756): Raised in Hackney, Middlesex, Ryder grew up to become a judge and chief justice of the King's Bench. We meet him here as a twenty-four-year-old law student at the Middle Temple in London. He enjoyed the pleasures of a bachelor's life in the city: dancing, dining at chophouses, chatting with friends in coffee shops, and pursuing women, however unsuccessfully. "I am the worst person in the world to entertain a lady in conversation," he lamented after a botched attempt at courtship. One wonders when he found the time to study.[8]

The Diary of Dudley Ryder, 1715–1716, ed. William Matthews (London: Methuen, 1939).

SAVAGE (Henry), Sarah (1664–1752): Savage hailed from Cheshire and Staffordshire. She was the daughter of the prominent nonconformist minister Philip Henry and the sister of Katherine Tylston. She married John Savage in 1687.

Henry Papers, Add. MS 42849, BL.

SPENCER (Sidney), Dorothy (1617–1684): The Countess of Sunderland, Spencer was raised in Kent and later resided in Northamptonshire. She married Henry, Lord Spencer, in 1639 and, following his death, Robert Smythe in 1652.

Sacharissa: Some Account of Dorothy Sidney, Countess of Sunderland, Her Family and Friends, 1617–1684, ed. Julia Cartwright (New York: Scribner, 1893).

STOCKTON, Owen (1630–1680): Stockton was a nonconformist minister who lived in Sussex and Suffolk. He married Elianor Rant in 1658.

Owen Stockton, Diary (1665–1677), MS 24.7, DWL.

STOUT, William (1665–1752): Stout was a Quaker grocer and ironmonger living in Lancashire. He never married.

The Autobiography of William Stout of Lancaster, 1665–1752, ed. J. D. Marshall (Manchester: Manchester University Press, 1967).

THORESBY, Ralph (1658–1725): Raised in an agricultural village near York, Thoresby moved to London at the age of eighteen to work as a merchant's apprentice. He also trained in Holland, and when he returned to England he settled in Leeds to take over his father's mercantile business. Finding little success at the cloth trade, Thoresby embarked on new pursuits as a topographer, surveyor, fellow of the Royal Society (elected in 1697), and antiquary. He published *The Topography of Leedes* in 1715 and *The History of the Church of Leedes* in 1724.

The Diary of Ralph Thoresby, FRS, Author of the Topography of Leeds (1677–1724), ed. Joseph Hunter, 2 vols. (London: Henry Colburn and Richard Bentley, 1830).

Letters Addressed to Ralph Thoresby, FRS, ed. W. T. Lancaster (Leeds: Thoresby Society, 1912).

THORNTON (Wandesford), Alice (1627–1707): Thornton was the daughter of the wealthy Anglicans Christopher and Alice Wandesford. Despite her anxieties about wedlock, she married William Thornton of Yorkshire (1624–1668) in 1651 and had nine children, three of whom survived to adulthood. She began compiling her life narrative in 1669, most likely in response to nasty rumors leveled against her and her daughter. These rumors seemed to originate from her niece and focused on Thornton's decision to marry her prepubescent daughter to a clergyman named Thomas Comber.[9]

The Autobiography of Mrs. Alice Thornton, ed. Charles Jackson, Surtees Society 62 (London: Andrews, 1875).

Alice Wandesford Thornton, A Book of Remembrances, Microfilm MISC 326, Yale University, Sterling Memorial Library, New Haven, CT.

TYLDESLEY, Thomas (1657–1715): Tyldesley is one of two Catholic men in this book. He was the grandson of an army officer of the same name, who fought for the king during the civil war and died in battle in 1651. Like his grandfather, Tyldesley was a wealthy landowner in Lancashire. His diary covers just a few years of his life, from 1712 to 1714, and focuses on gentlemanly pursuits such as fox hunting, entertaining friends, and enjoying elaborate meals. It also records an array of Tyldesley's health concerns, including gout, cramps, and the stone.

The Tyldesley Diary: Personal Records of Thomas Tyldesley (Grandson of Sir Thomas Tyldesley, the Royalist), During the Years 1712–13–14, ed. Joseph Gillow and Anthony Hewitson (Preston: A. Hewitson, 1873).

TYLSTON (Henry), Katherine (1665–1747): Tylston lived in Flintshire and Staffordshire. She was the daughter of the prominent nonconformist minister Philip Henry and the sister of Sarah Savage.

Henry Papers, Add. MS 42849, BL.

WALLINGTON, Nehemiah (1598–1658): Wallington was a London turner and devout Puritan who used self-writing to cope with deep anxieties about salvation. He married Grace Rampaigne.

Nehemiah Wallington, An Extract of the Passages of My Life (1654), V.a.436, Folger.

Nehemiah Wallington, Spiritual Diary of Nehemiah Wallington (1641–1643), Add. MS 40883, BL.

WECKHERLIN, Georg Rudolph (1584–1653): A government official and poet, Weckherlin was Lutheran and German by birth. He married Elizabeth Raworth in 1616.

Trumbull Papers, Add. MSS 72439, 72442, BL.

Appendix B: Pauper Petitions, 1623–1730

Total petitions: 648; from men: 342; from women: 238; from unspecified or couples: 68
Sources: CAC Carlisle, CAC Kendal, DRO Exeter, DRO Matlock, ERO, LA, LMA, SRO, WAAS, WYAS.

TABLE I. BODILY COMPLAINTS OF PETITIONERS

Complaint	Number of men	Percent of men	Number of women	Percent of women	Gender unspecified	Total number	Percent of total
Lame	125	36.5	75	31.5	13	213	32.9
Sick/sickness	66	19.3	79	33.2	7	152	23.5
Eye trouble	53	15.5	37	15.5	1	91	14
Limbs	19	5.6	16	6.7		35	5.4
Leg (broken/sore)	20	5.8	11	4.6		31	4.8
Arm (broken/sore)	13	3.8	11	4.6		24	3.7
Mental incapacity	10	2.9	10	4.2		20	3.1
Diseased	7	2	12	5		19	2.9
King's evil	10	2.9	8	3.4		18	2.8
Fever/ague	11	3.2	5	2.1		16	2.5
Bruised	6	1.8	5	2.1		11	1.7
Falling sickness	4	1.2	7	2.9		11	1.7
Running sores	7	2	0	0		7	1.1
Smallpox	3	0.9	2	0.8		5	0.8
Stone	3	0.9	2	0.8		5	0.8
Consumption	2	0.6	2	0.8		4	0.6
Melancholy	2	0.6	2	0.8		4	0.6
Swelling	1	0.3	3	1.3		4	0.6
Dropsy, cancer, canker, numbness						<4	<0.6

TABLE 2. OCCUPATIONS OF PETITIONERS

Occupation	Number	Percent of petitioners of the same gender
Men		
Worker/laborer	18	5.3
Husbandman/farmer	11	3.2
Tailor	6	1.8
Blacksmith	5	1.5
Yeoman	5	1.5
Clothier	4	1.2
Constable	4	1.2
Miner	4	1.2
Servant	4	1.2
Comber	3	0.9
Miller	3	0.9
Shoemaker	3	0.9
Mason	2	0.6
Parish clerk	2	0.6
Bellman	1	0.3
Carpenter	1	0.3
Cobbler	1	0.3
Curate	1	0.3
Joiner	1	0.3
Schoolmaster	1	0.3
Silk weaver	1	0.3
Stay maker	1	0.3
Tobacco maker	1	0.3
Usher	1	0.3
Watchman	1	0.3
Women		
Spinner	4	1.7
Servant	3	1.3
Midwife	1	0.4
Teacher	1	0.4

Notes

Introduction

1. Thornton, *Autobiography*, 83. The earliest use of the idiom "get cold feet," meaning "become cowardly or discouraged," is in Stephen Crane's 1893 novel *Maggie: A Girl of the Streets* (*Oxford English Dictionary Online*, s.v. "cold feet," n., at www.oed.com).
2. Thornton, *Autobiography*, 83, 77.
3. Pepys, *Diary*, 6:17, 167.
4. On this narrative of patient power, see Foucault, *The Birth of the Clinic;* Jewson, "Medical Knowledge and the Patronage System"; Jewson, "The Disappearance of the Sick Man from Medical Cosmology"; Porter, "The Patient's View"; Porter, "Lay Medical Knowledge in the Eighteenth Century"; Porter and Porter, *In Sickness and in Health;* Porter, ed., *Patients and Practitioners;* Porter and Porter, *Patient's Progress;* Fissell, *Patients, Power, and the Poor;* Pomata, *Contracting a Cure;* Beier, *Sufferers and Healers.*
5. Parsons, *The Social System.* For work by anthropologists and sociologists of medicine, see Lorber, *Gender and the Social Construction of Illness;* Bendelow, *Pain and Gender;* Martin, *The Woman in the Body.*
6. For a call for such a comparative approach, which is surprisingly absent among work on gender in the early modern period, see Ditz, "The New Men's History," 17.
7. Jane Shakerley to George Shakerley, July 6, 1701, DSS 1/5/60/37, CALS.
8. Scott, "The Evidence of Experience."
9. See Botonaki, "Seventeenth-Century Englishwomen's Spiritual Diaries"; M. Todd, "Puritan Self-Fashioning"; Mascuch, *Origins of the Individualist Self,* 55–131.

10. Lowe, *Diary,* 35; Walsham, *Providence in Early Modern England,* 19. On the problematic category of "Puritan" with regard to one individual, see Pollock, *With Faith and Physic,* esp. 57–67.

11. Valuable studies that draw on this kind of writing include Wear, "Puritan Perceptions of Illness"; Beier, *Sufferers and Healers;* Macfarlane, *The Family Life of Ralph Josselin;* Newton, *The Sick Child.*

12. See Wear, "Puritan Perceptions of Illness"; Beier, *Sufferers and Healers;* D. Harley, "Spiritual Physic"; D. Harley, "The Theology of Affliction"; Newton, *The Sick Child,* 130–137, 202–208; Howard, "Imagining the Pain and Peril"; Mutschler, "The Province of Affliction."

13. My approach here follows the pioneering work of David Hall: see *Worlds of Wonder.*

14. On self-writing by the middling sorts, see Amelang, *The Flight of Icarus.*

15. On these movements, see Debus, *Chemistry and Medical Debate;* Webster, *The Great Instauration;* Wear, *Knowledge and Practice.*

16. Several other historians of medicine also have argued for continuities in this period: see Newton, *The Sick Child,* 8, 74; Withey, *Physick and the Family,* 9; Wear, *Knowledge and Practice.*

17. This is not to say the pain of childbirth was insignificant: see, for example, Halkett, *Selected Self-Writings,* 6–7; Howard, "Imagining the Pain and Peril." On the social functions of early modern childbirth, see Wilson, "The Ceremony of Childbirth"; Pollock, "Childbearing and Female Bonding." On representations and treatment of women's health concerns, see Churchill, *Female Patients;* Dixon, *Perilous Chastity;* Smith, "Women's Health Care in England and France."

18. See, for instance, Foucault, *The Birth of the Clinic;* Jewson, "Medical Knowledge and the Patronage System"; Jewson, "The Disappearance of the Sick Man from Medical Cosmology."

19. Porter, "The Patient's View"; Porter, "Lay Medical Knowledge in the Eighteenth Century"; Porter and Porter, *In Sickness and in Health;* Porter, ed., *Patients and Practitioners;* Beier, *Sufferers and Healers;* Fissell, *Patients, Power, and the Poor;* Pomata, *Contracting a Cure.*

20. See the work cited in n. 19. For more recent scholarship that has been less attentive to gender, see Stolberg, *Experiencing Illness and the Sick Body;* Solomon, *Fictions of Well-Being.* For a few valuable studies that have provided assessments of gender difference, see Smith, "Women's Health Care in England and France," 90–131; Withey, *Physick and the Family,* 127, 129. See also K. Walker, "A Gendered History of Pain in England." For a focus

on men, see Smith, "The Body Embarrassed?" For important work on one or a few patients, see Porter, "The Patient's View"; Beier, *Sufferers and Healers;* Wear, "Puritan Perceptions of Illness"; Forster, "From the Patient's Point of View"; Rankin, "Duchess, Heal Thyself."

21. Duden, *The Woman Beneath the Skin,* esp. 106; Newton, *The Sick Child;* Smith, " 'An Account of an Unaccountable Distemper' "; Porter and Porter, *Patient's Progress,* 176.

22. Gowing, *Common Bodies;* Shepard, *Meanings of Manhood;* Foyster, *Manhood in Early Modern England;* Fletcher, *Gender, Sex, and Subordination;* Harvey, *Reading Sex in the Eighteenth Century.*

23. Gowing, *Common Bodies;* Gowing, "The Manner of Submission"; Fissell, *Vernacular Bodies.*

24. Allestree, *The Ladies Calling,* 81; Allestree, *The Whole Duty of Man,* 227. For a helpful overview of early modern gender ideals, see Shoemaker, *Gender in English Society,* 15–35.

25. Crooke, *Mikrokosmographia,* 276; Allestree, *The Ladies Calling,* 30. Chapter 3 of this book offers a fuller discussion of these views.

26. Mendelson and Crawford, *Women in Early Modern England,* 256–344; McIntosh, *Working Women in English Society;* Earle, "The Female Labour Market"; Hubbard, *City Women;* Gowing, *Domestic Dangers;* Gowing, *Common Bodies.*

27. Shepard, *Meanings of Manhood,* 93–126, 214–245. See also Yallop, "Representing Aged Masculinity"; Wiesner, "Wandervogels and Women"; Barker, "Soul, Purse and Family."

28. D. Ryder, *Diary,* 97, 117, 195, 205, 221, 244, 276, 295. On this point about a fairly clear set of virtues defining ideal womanhood versus multiple, conflicting notions of manhood, see Shepard, "Manhood, Patriarchy, and Gender." Patricia Crawford has offered compelling explanations for the prevalence and gendered nature of piety among upper-status women in this period, including the time such women had at their disposal for performing devotional duties, the lack of religious orders for women following the dissolution of the monasteries in the 1500s, and the allure of religion as a means for self-expression (*Women and Religion in England,* esp. 73–75).

29. Cowper, Daily Diary, 1:95. There is a significant body of scholarship on early modern writing and self-fashioning. Studies I have found helpful include Davis, *Women on the Margins;* Nussbaum, *The Autobiographical Subject;* Dragstra, Ottway, and Wilcox, eds., *Betraying Our Selves;* Eckerle and Dowd, eds., *Genre and Women's Life Writing.*

30. Appendix A provides biographical information for these fifty-two patients.

31. For a helpful overview of ego-literature, see Dekker, introduction to *Ego-documents and History*.

32. Edmund Harrold, His Book of Remarks and Observations, 1712–16, MS Mun. A.2.137, Chetham's; Thornton, *Autobiography*. Published editions of numerous seventeenth-century diaries are the products of similar nineteenth-century antiquarian projects. The British Library recently acquired two of Thornton's three notebooks, which were previously housed in private collections: Add. MS 88897/1–2, BL. The first of these two manuscripts has been published as Alice Thornton, *My First Booke of My Life*, ed. Raymond Anselment (Lincoln: University of Nebraska Press, 2014). I was unable to use Anselment's edition or the two manuscripts, which were only accessible after this book went to press. A fourth book, which Thornton probably used to compile the other three notebooks, is extant only on microfilm: Thornton, Remembrances.

33. Blundell, *The Great Diurnal;* see also Archer and Coe, *Two East Anglian Diaries*, 7. On Pepys, see Smyth, *Autobiography in Early Modern England*, 210. Compiling narratives from earlier notes could result in multiple, conflicting accounts of the same event: see Anselment, "Seventeenth-Century Manuscript Sources of Alice Thornton's Life"; Anselment, "Elizabeth Freke's Remembrances."

34. See Graham, "Women's Writing and the Self," 211. On the communal and public aspects of self-writing within godly communities, see Cambers, "Reading, the Godly, and Self-Writing."

35. For an example, see Ditz, "Shipwrecked; or, Masculinity Imperiled"; see also Schneider, *The Culture of Epistolarity*, 68–72. Quotes are from Henry More to Lady Anne Conway, May 10, 1659, in Conway, *Letters*, 157; Mary Butler, Countess of Arran, to Lady Mary (Legge) Goodricke, May 19, [1668], V.b.333(29), Folger.

36. *The Ladies' Compleat Letter Writer* (London, 1793), cited in Bound, "Writing the Self?," 9. On letter-writing guides, see Robertson, *The Art of Letter Writing;* Daybell, *Women Letter-Writers*, 18–23; Schneider, *The Culture of Epistolarity*, 22–74.

37. Stowe, "Singleton's Tooth," 328–329.

38. Hooke, *Diary*, 315; Clegg, *Diary*, 1:77; Samuel England, Notebook Containing Prescriptions and Case Notes, 1730–33, f. 300, MS 6, RCP.

Chapter 1. Curing and Caring for the Early Modern Body

1. Salmon, *Parateremata*, 192. On Salmon, see Wear, *Knowledge and Practice*, 438–439.

2. Salmon, *Parateremata*, 192; *Oxford English Dictionary Online*, s.v. "romantic," adjs. 2a, 2b, and 3, at www.oed.com. On his recipe for volatile laudanum, see Salmon, *Collectanea Medica*, 443.

3. Salmon, *Parateremata*, 387. On this narrative of patient power, see Foucault, *The Birth of the Clinic;* Jewson, "Medical Knowledge and the Patronage System"; Porter, "The Patient's View"; Porter, "Lay Medical Knowledge in the Eighteenth Century"; Porter and Porter, *In Sickness and in Health;* Porter, ed., *Patients and Practitioners;* Porter and Porter, *Patient's Progress;* Fissell, *Patients, Power, and the Poor;* Pomata, *Contracting a Cure;* Beier, *Sufferers and Healers.*

4. Lister, *Autobiography*, 43.

5. Pelling, "Compromised by Gender"; C. Crawford, "Patients' Rights and the Law of Contract"; Smith, "Reassessing the Role of the Family;" Siena, "The 'Foul Disease' and Privacy."

6. Pioneering scholarship on medical practice has tended to overlook gender, e.g., Duden, *The Woman Beneath the Skin;* Fissell, *Patients, Power, and the Poor;* Pomata, *Contracting a Cure;* Porter and Porter, *Patient's Progress,* esp. 176. A notable exception is Kassell, *Medicine and Magic*, esp. 160–170. On the ways biological sex differences such as lactation and menstruation could determine diagnoses and treatments, see Churchill, *Female Patients.*

7. Beckett, *Practical Surgery Illustrated and Improved*, 190.

8. H. Ryder, *Practical Chirurgery*, 73, 74.

9. On observations, see Pomata, "Sharing Cases"; Pomata, "Observation Rising"; Nutton, "Pieter van Foreest and the Plagues of Europe"; Nance, "Wondrous Experience as Text."

10. A competing argument was that menstruation purified women's blood: see P. Crawford, "Attitudes to Menstruation." On women's physiology and the humors, see Duden, *The Woman Beneath the Skin;* on aging, see Newton, *The Sick Child*, esp. 34–45.

11. Anne North to Francis North, Feb. 6, 1680, HM 52378, Huntington; Jane Hobson to Sir Hans Sloane, May 23, 1725, f. 233r, Sloane MS 4075, BL; John Warren to Francis Leicester, Feb. 2, 1729, DLT/C10/27, CALS; Cowper, Daily Diary, 1:117; George Colebrook, Letters on Medical Cases (c. 1690),

35, MS 206/4, RCP; Jeake (younger), *Astrological Diary*, 100. More recent scholarship has shifted away from viewing early modern health solely in terms of equilibrium: Stolberg, *Experiencing Illness and the Sick Body*, esp. 85–89, 126–135; Wear, *Knowledge and Practice*, 136–143; Kuriyama, "The Forgotten Fear of Excrement"; Pomata, *Contracting a Cure*, 129–139.

12. Jeake (younger), *Astrological Diary*, 126; Samuel Tufnell to William Holman, Feb. 4, 1725, D/Y 1/1/185/19, ERO.

13. Thoresby, *Diary*, 2:156–157. For a few examples of the phrase "it pleased God to visit me with," see Archer and Coe, *Two East Anglian Diaries*, 54, 76, 77; Lowe, *Diary*, 101; Anne Dormer to Elizabeth Trumbull, July 21, 1690, f. 217r, Add. MS 72516, BL; Mary Rich, Autobiography (1625–1674), f. 19v, Add. MS 27357, BL.

14. Pepys, *Diary*, 8:172; Hooke, *Diary*, 344. *Pole* was a euphemism for penis. Pepys makes too many references to colds to cite. For the instances mentioned here, see Pepys, *Diary*, 3:203, 247, 4:222, 380, 5:45, 76, 159, 277, 6:118, 8:387, 471. He also caught colds from washing his feet and removing his hat (7:172, 207, 5:277).

15. Wiseman, *Severall Chirurgicall Treatises*, 62; Pepys, *Diary*, 6:4, 5:260, 4:89, 8:388. Based on similar reasoning, patients complained that purges failed to work in cold weather; see, for example, Mary Jolliffe to Elizabeth Moreton, n.d., D340a/C19/1, GA.

16. Cowper, Daily Diary, 7:296. See also Rich, *Diary*, 4:f. 163r. Wind could have further negative effects on health: Cowper, Daily Diary, 3:28, 78, 4:315; Edward Stephens to Richard Stephens, 1676, f. 177v, Stowe MS 745, BL.

17. George Weckherlin to Elizabeth Trumbull, Dec. 4, 1638, f. 18r, Add. MS 72442, BL; F.W., *Warm Beere*, sig. ¶5v.

18. Jane Shakerley to Peter Shakerley, Oct. 6, 1700, DSS 1/3/175/13, CALS; Samuel England, Notebook Containing Prescriptions and Case Notes, 1730–33, f. 45, MS 6, RCP. Hot drinks that provoked sweats were also used as remedies. For a few additional examples of exercise as a cause of illness, see Katherine Paston to William Paston, n.d., f. 234, Add. MS 27447, BL; Mordecai Cary to James Jurin, June 1, 1733, f. 1, MS 6140, Wellcome; Manuscript Diary of John Cannon, Schoolmaster of Meare, Exciseman, Etc. (1684–1742), 242, 398, DD\SAS/C1193/4, SRO.

19. Lydia Dugard to Samuel Dugard, Sept. 1671, X.d.477(26), Folger. For examples of illness caused by sleep, see Anne Dormer to Elizabeth Trumbull, Nov. 3, [1688?], f. 192r, Add. MS 72516, BL; Rich, *Diary*, 1:f. 102v; Clegg,

Diary, 1:75, 82; Pepys, *Diary*, 6:287; Thomas Newhouse to Lady Knyvett, Feb. 15, 1611, f. 122, Egerton MS 2715, BL. Emotionally caused illness is the focus of chapter 3.

20. Katherine Paston to William Paston, [1625?], f. 38, Add. MS 36988, BL; Mordecai Cary to James Jurin, Nov. 20, 1734, f. 7, MS 6140, Wellcome. For the lamb example, see John Hurleston to Peter Shakerley, April 20, 1713, DSS 1/3/137/10, CALS. On milk clogs, see William Roberts to Lady Bell, May 8, 1626, f. 298, Egerton MS 2715, BL.

21. Matthew Moreton to Edward Moreton, Jan. 3, 1685, D340a/C18/6, GA.

22. Clegg, *Diary*, 1:94. On ghosts, see Thomas, *Religion and the Decline of Magic*, 587–606.

23. For example, five hundred of Richard Napier's patients believed they were bewitched: MacDonald, *Mystical Bedlam*, 107. See also Sawyer, " 'Strangely Handled in All Her Lyms' "; Petry, " 'Many Things Surpass Our Knowledge.' "

24. Livingston's writing is published under her married name: Delaval, *Meditations*, 77–79. Astrology offered another explanatory framework compatible with both spiritual and natural explanations of illness: Kassell, *Medicine and Magic;* Thomas, *Religion and the Decline of Magic*, 283–385.

25. J. Archer, *Secrets Disclosed, of Consumptions*, 56, 59; Digby, *A Late Discourse Made*, 9–10. For another sympathetic reaction involving urine and ash, see Fissell, *Patients, Power, and the Poor*, 20.

26. Quote is from the long title of Walwyn, *Physick for Families*. On these medical movements, see Debus, *Chemistry and Medical Debate;* Webster, *The Great Instauration;* Clericuzio, "From van Helmont to Boyle"; Wear, *Knowledge and Practice*, esp. 353–433, on the continued dominance of Galenism.

27. Archer and Coe, *Two East Anglian Diaries*, 165, 167. The poultice recipe is from Magdalen Coward, Book of Receipts, 1695, f. 10v, HM 88, Huntington. For an overview of early modern remedies, see Wear, *Knowledge and Practice*, 46–103; Fissell, *Patients, Power, and the Poor*, esp. 16–36.

28. Symcotts, *A Seventeenth-Century Doctor*, 57. On ailments resulting from blisters and plasters, see Sarah Long to Sir Hans Sloane, Dec. 31, 1737, f. 30r, Sloane MS 4076, BL; John Evelyn to his mother, Aug. 27, 1713, ff. 52–54, Add. MS 15949, BL; Mary Shirley, Lady Ferrers, to [?] Hinde, Dec. 2, 1730, f. 99v, Sloane MS 4066, BL; John Hale to Sir Hans Sloane, June 14, 1706, f. 201r, Sloane MS 4075, BL. Bloodletting and artificial wounds, known as *issues*, could result in sores, rashes, and dangerous swellings. For just a few examples, see Alexander Morgan, Medical Casebook (1714–1747), 27, MS 3631, Wellcome; Jone Ellyot to Sir Simonds D'Ewes,

March 16, f. 49, Harleian MS 382, BL; Wiseman, *Severall Chirurgicall Treatises*, 37–38; Eyre, "A Diurnall, or Catalogue of All My Accounts," 36.

29. Anne Dormer to Jack Dormer, Aug. 10, 1691, ff. 234r, 233v, Add. MS 72516, BL; Anne Dormer to Elizabeth Trumbull, Oct. 2, 1691, f. 235r, Add. MS 72516, BL. "On the gridiron" could mean in "a state of torment, persecution, or great uneasiness" (see *Oxford English Dictionary Online*, s.v. "gridiron," ns. 1a, 1b, and 2, at www.oed.com). Pepys noted similar effects in Lady Sandwich: "Drinking of the water at Tunbridge did almost kill her before she could with most violent physic get it out of her body again" (*Diary*, 6:152).

30. D. Ryder, *Diary*, 169, 170, 171.

31. Woolley, *The Accomplish'd Ladies Delight*. On household medicine, see Fissell, "The Marketplace of Print"; Pollock, *With Faith and Physic;* Leong, "Making Medicines"; Rankin, *Panaceia's Daughters;* Stine, "Opening Closets"; Smith, "The Relative Duties of a Man."

32. Manuscript Diary of John Cannon, Schoolmaster of Meare, Exciseman, Etc. (1684–1742), 101, DD\SAS\C1193/4, SRO.

33. D. Ryder, *Diary*, 227–228, 257.

34. Ibid., 257, 268, 233, 278.

35. Ibid., 196, 243–244, 276, 278, 282. On empirics, see Bynum and Porter, eds., *Medical Fringe and Medical Orthodoxy;* Porter, *Health for Sale*.

36. P. Bentham to J. Petiver, Nov. 18, 1709, ff. 80r–81v, and Nov. 22, 1709, ff. 87r–88r, Sloane MS 4077, BL. On Freke's medical practice and this point in particular, see Leong, "Making Medicines." For additional examples, see Symcotts, *A Seventeenth-Century Doctor*, 53, 54, 71–72; Fissell, *Patients, Power, and the Poor*, 37–39.

37. Quote in subhead ("Sent for a Surgeon") is from Richard Wilkes, Observations on Particular Cases of Patients (1731–1742), f. 65, MS 5005, Wellcome. Medical advertisement by Sarah Cornelius de Heusde, C.112.f.9(61), BL; medical advertisement by Mary Lucas, C.112.f.9(182), BL.

38. See Pelling, *Medical Conflicts;* Pelling, *The Common Lot*, esp. 179–202; Harkness, "A View from the Streets"; Munkhoff, "Searchers of the Dead"; Fissell, "Introduction: Women, Health, and Healing"; Broomhall, *Women's Medical Work*. For key studies on early modern medical practice, see Cook, *The Decline of the Old Medical Regime;* Pelling and Webster, "Medical Practitioners."

39. Moore, *Journal*, 124, 143, and also 122, 123, 128, 131, 132, 133, 134, 236, 238; Edmund Harrold, His Book of Remarks and Observations, 1712–16, f. 64r, and also ff. 3v, 4r, 5r, 46r, MS Mun. A.2.137, Chetham's.

40. Medical Diary and Account Book of John Westover of Wedmore (1685–1700), DD/X/HKN 1, SRO.

41. Sir Edmund King, M.D., Medical Papers and Collections, f. 94v, Sloane MS 1589, BL. On Ranelagh's life, see DiMeo, "Katherine Jones, Lady Ranelagh." For a similar example, see *General Observations and Prescriptions*.

42. On these points and on observations as a genre, see Pomata, *"Praxis Historialis,"* 127; Pomata, "Sharing Cases," esp. 214–215; Pomata, "Observation Rising." Some manuscript texts reveal authors' intentions to publish within the tradition of observations: Thomas Garlick, Praxis Chyrurgiae Rationalis, Sloane MS 2263, BL; Richard Wilkes, Observations on Particular Cases of Patients (1731–1742), MS 5005, Wellcome; James Molins, Medical treatise and receipts, Sloane MS 3293, BL; "Historia curarum," c. 1727–1736, D3549/20/1/7, GA; The Case Book of a General Practitioner (1726–1728), MS 7501, Wellcome.

43. On Colbatch's career, see Cook, "Sir John Colbatch and Augustan Medicine."

44. Colbatch, *A Treatise of the Gout*, xiv, 93, 89, 90; Colbatch, *Novum Lumen Chirurgicum*, 58; see also Colbatch, *A Treatise of the Gout*, 108; Colbatch, *Novum Lumen Chirurgicum*, 43, 46, 47, 79; Colbatch, *Four Treatises of Physick and Chirurgery*, 112. For similar examples, see Salmon, *Iatrica*, 134; Salmon, *Parateremata*, 44, 102; Rivière, *Four Books*, 41; Cam, *A Practical Treatise*, 156.

45. Dover, *The Ancient Physician's Legacy to His Country*, 108–110.

46. Sintelaer, *The Scourge of Venus and Mercury*, 303–305.

47. H. Ryder, *Practical Chirurgery*, 62. There are too many additional examples to cite. For a few, see H. Ryder, *New Practical Observations*, 26, 61, 62; Wiseman, *Severall Chirurgicall Treatises*, 21, 28, 32, 100, 110, 195; Colbatch, *Novum Lumen Chirurgicum*, 57; Stone, *A Complete Practice of Midwifery*, 3–4, 14–15, 24–25.

48. Wiseman, *Severall Chirurgicall Treatises*, 73; Bonet, *A Guide to the Practical Physician*, 588. Practitioners also blamed failed treatments on patients' refusals to undergo certain procedures: see Wiseman, *Severall Chirurgicall Treatises*, 31; H. Ryder, *Practical Chirurgery*, 52. There are too many examples of patients' self-treatments in case histories to cite. For a few, see Yonge, *Currus triumphalis, e Terebintho*, 75; Wiseman, *Severall Chirurgicall Treatises*, 18, 32, 40, 142.

49. Salmon, *Iatrica*, 390. For similar examples, see Wiseman, *Severall Chirurgicall Treatises*, 100; John Wright to William Briggs, M.D., April 24, 1681, f. 1r, Sloane MS 123, BL.

50. The Case Book of a General Practitioner (1726–1728), ff. 29v–30r, MS 7501, Wellcome; Sir Edmund King, M.D., Medical Papers and Collections, f. 247r, Sloane MS 1589, BL. See also Richard Wilkes, Observations on Particular Cases of Patients (1731–1742), f. 25, MS 5005, Wellcome; Samuel England, Notebook Containing Prescriptions and Case Notes, 1730–33, ff. 44v–45r, MS 5, RCP.

51. Margaret Ashburnham to Sir Hans Sloane, 1719, f. 280r–v, Sloane MS 4078, BL.

52. Cowper, Daily Diary, 5:2–3, 2:138. Cowper uses the phrase "ugly feeling" at 2:262, 4:366. On the therapeutic effects of sneezing, see also Hooke, *Diary*, 28.

53. *Medical Essays and Observations*, 274–275.

54. Lacroze, master of Eton, to Lady Yarmouth, Nov. 24, 1686, ff. 252–255, Add. MS 36988, BL.

55. George Colebrook, Letters on Medical Cases (c. 1690), 1, MS 206/4, RCP; Salmon, *Iatrica*, 10; Wiseman, *Severall Chirurgicall Treatises*, 391. See also Salmon, *Iatrica*, 92, 108; Sir Edmund King, M.D., Medical Papers and Collections, f. 138r, Sloane MS 1589, BL.

56. Sir William Petty, Papers, f. 254r, Add. MS 72891, BL; Rivière, *Four Books*, 25; Belloste, *The Hospital Surgeon*, 94; Bonet, *A Guide to the Practical Physician*, 82.

57. James, *A Medicinal Dictionary*, sig. 5G1r. The amputation is attributed to the Dutch physician Fredrik Rouysch and predates his death in 1731. For similar examples, see Colbatch, *Four Treatises of Physick and Chirurgery*, 48; Sir Edmund King, M.D., Medical Papers and Collections, April 23, 1689, f. 156r, Sloane MS 1589, BL.

58. Wiseman, *Severall Chirurgicall Treatises*, 241; Salmon, *Parateremata*, 50. For more examples, see Bonet, *A Guide to the Practical Physician*, 592; Clegg, *Diary*, 3:911.

59. Wiseman, *Severall Chirurgicall Treatises*, 56; Ward, *Diary*, 245. For more examples, see Thomas Garlick, Praxis Chyrurgiae Rationalis, f. 17v, Sloane MS 2263, BL; Silverman, *Tortured Subjects*, 143.

60. Rivière, *Four Books*, 53; Colbatch, *Four Treatises of Physick and Chirurgery*, 100; Joseph Binns, Medical Casebook (1633–1663), f. 25r, Sloane MS 153, BL; Samuel England, Notebook Containing Prescriptions and Case Notes, 1730–33, f. 47v, MS 5, RCP; Willis, *An Essay of the Pathology of the Brain*, 72. For additional examples of smelling, see Clegg, *Diary*, 1:31, 163; The Case Book of a General Practitioner (1726–1728), f. 30v, MS 7501, Wellcome; John Wright to William Briggs, M.D., Sept. 25, 1681, f.

7r, Sloane MS 123, BL; Sir William Petty, Papers, f. 254v, Add. MS 72891, BL; Wiseman, *Severall Chirurgicall Treatises*, 395. For examples of listening, see Petty, Papers, f. 270r; Wiseman, *Severall Chirurgicall Treatises*, 88. On physical evaluations, see Weisser, "Boils, Pushes, and Wheals."

61. Wiseman, *Severall Chirurgicall Treatises*, 31. For similar examples, see ibid., 18; Barbette, *A Treatise of the Plague*, appended to *The Chirurgical and Anatomical Works*, 42; Charles Kimberley, M.D., to Sir David Hamilton, May 22, n.d., f. 349v, Sloane MS 4075, BL. On female healers who specialized in treating intimate parts, see Wiseman, *Severall Chirurgicall Treatises*, 28; Siena, "The 'Foul Disease' and Privacy."

62. Pepys, *Diary*, 2:43.

63. Colbatch, *Four Treatises of Physick and Chirurgery*, 10; Rivière, *Four Books*, 226; Samuel England, Notebook Containing Prescriptions and Case Notes, 1730–33, f. 7r, MS 5, RCP. This discussion also draws on George Colebrook, Letters on Medical Cases (c. 1690), 3, MS 206/4, RCP; Medical Cases of Sir Hans Sloane, f. 135r, Sloane MS 4078, BL; Dubé, *The Poor Man's Physician and Surgeon*, 1–3; Wiseman, *Severall Chirurgicall Treatises*, 50. On poor patients, see Fissell, *Patients, Power, and the Poor.* On social status and medical treatment, see Churchill, "Bodily Differences?"

Chapter 2. Learning How to Be Ill

1. Livingston's writing is published under her married name: Delaval, *Meditations*, 75. I have found several similar instances of fruit-induced illness: Halkett and Fanshawe, *Memoirs*, 147–148; Clifford, *Diaries*, 22; Matthew Moreton to Edward Moreton, Jan. 3, 1685, D340a/C18/6, GA; Baxter, *Reliquiae Baxterianae*, 2, 10; Thornton, *Autobiography*, 54; Hooke, *Diary*, 308.

2. Saint Augustine, *Confessions*, 29.

3. Spiritual Diary of Nehemiah Wallington (1641–1643), f. 60v, Add. MS 40883, BL. On Wallington, see Seaver, *Wallington's World.* Two other historians have noted similar episodes and have separately suggested that the concern with fruit imitated Augustine's *Confessions:* Cooper, "Richard Baxter and His Physicians," 6–7; M. Todd, "Puritan Self-Fashioning," 247. Elizabeth Isham, who modeled her life narrative on Augustine's *Confessions,* also recounted an episode of fruit theft, though she did not fall ill after it; see Stephens, " 'My Cheefest Work,' " 198.

4. These men include Ralph Thoresby (*Diary*, 2:89), James Clegg (*Diary*, 1:117), Edmund Harrold (His Book of Remarks and Observations, 1712–16, f. 18r,

MS Mun. A.2.137, Chetham's), and Samuel Pepys, who compared himself to another man in a dream (*Diary*, 2:226).

5. Brilliana Harley to Edward Harley, Feb. 20, 1640, in Harley, *Letters*, 82; Hephzibah Parker and Mary Parker to Sir Hans Sloane, 1715, ff. 192–211, Sloane MS 4076, BL. See also Anne Dormer to Elizabeth Trumbull, Jan. 22, 1689, f. 216r, Add. MS 72516, BL.

6. Rich, Diary, 2:f. 31r, 1:ff. 54v–56r. For similar examples, see 1:f. 18v, 3:f. 200v.

7. Ibid., 2:f. 36r; Anne Dawson, Diary (1721–1722), f. 18v, Add. MS 71626, BL.

8. Katherine Austen, Meditations in Prose and Verse (1664–1668), f. 72r, Add. MS 4454, BL. On Austen's life, see Todd, "'I Do No Injury by Not Loving.'"

9. Henry More to Anne Conway, April 18, 1653, in Conway, *Letters*, 80; Anne Conway to Edward Conway, May 1, 1657, in ibid., 142. For additional examples, see Mrs. Carter to Sir Hans Sloane, Jan. 7, 1739, f. 294v, Sloane MS 4078, BL; Catharine Watson to Sir Hans Sloane, June 20, 1733, f. 38v, Sloane MS 4078, BL; Cowper, Daily Diary, 1:196. On observing others to evaluate remedies, see Dorothy Sidney to Henry Sidney, Sept. 2, 1679, in Sidney, *Sacharissa*, 218; Elizabeth Paston to Anne Foley, Feb. 12, 1715, f. 96, Add. MS 32501, BL; Catharine Watson to Sir Hans Sloane, n.d., ff. 289v–290r, Sloane MS 4061, BL; Cowper, Daily Diary, 1:263.

10. Freke, *Remembrances*, 69, 234, 235. I draw on both versions of Freke's account.

11. Freke, *Remembrances*, 251, 84, 85; see also 248–249.

12. See Mendelson and Crawford, *Women in Early Modern England*, 256–344; McIntosh, *Working Women in English Society;* Earle, "The Female Labour Market"; Sweet and Lane, eds., *Women and Urban Life;* Vickery, *The Gentleman's Daughter*, 127–160. On Dormer's servants, see Dormer to Elizabeth Trumbull, n.d., f. 176v, Add. MS 72516, BL.

13. Kathleen Brown and Mary Fissell together coined the term *body work*: see Brown, *Foul Bodies*, 5; Fissell, "Introduction: Women, Health, and Healing," 9.

14. Vives, *The Instruction of a Christen Woman*, 135, 139; Markham, *The English House-Wife*, 4; Thomas Tryon, *The Good Houswife Made a Doctor* (London: Printed by Andrew Sowle, [1685?]). English conduct books often reiterated Vives's gendered division of labor. See, for example, Clever and Dod, *A Godlie Forme of Householde Government*, 167.

15. On female authorship of recipes, see Rankin, *Panaceia's Daughters*, 71. On recipe collecting by men, see Leong, "Collecting Knowledge for the Family";

Withey, *Physick and the Family*, 143, 147–148. On the gendered nature of this domestic labor, see Herbert, *Female Alliances*, esp. 78–116. For additional recent scholarship on early modern recipes, see Leong, "Making Medicines"; Pennell, "Perfecting Practice?"; LeJacq, "The Bounds of Domestic Healing"; Dimeo and Pennell, eds., *Reading and Writing Recipe Books*.

16. Susannah Packe, Receipt Book, 1674, f. 79, V.a.215, Folger; Mary Hookes, Receipt Book, 1680, part 2, 18, Add. 931, Folger.

17. Elizabeth Hastings to Selina Hastings, Dec. 17, 1731, HA 4741, Huntington; Elizabeth Paston to Anne Foley, Feb. 12, 1715, Add. MS 32501, BL. This recipe for snail water draws on Kettilby, *A Collection of Above Three Hundred Receipts*, 127–128, 149. On the ways social relationships established recipes' credibility, see Leong and Pennell, "Recipe Collections and the Currency of Medical Knowledge."

18. Freke, *Remembrances*, 69.

19. Cowper, Daily Diary, 1:50, 55. See also 1:22, 50, 160, 214, 296, 2:34, 55, 6:216, 7:154, 271, 242, 271, 296, 307.

20. Ibid., 1:49, 31, 6:142. For similar stories about older women whose experiences echoed Cowper's anxieties, see 2:236, 3:7, 4:175, 5:174. On her fear of dying on June 29, see 1:106, 2:239, 3:93, 251, 4:75, 224, 371, 5:178–179, 6:142, 7:100. On fears of her servants poisoning her or her horses, see 1:17, 2:136. For just a few examples of her concerns about deceit, see 1:255, 3:68.

21. Jeake (younger), *Astrological Diary*, 120, 140, 141, 143. For melancholy, see 98, 132, 154, 193; for "noise in the ears," see 99.

22. Ibid., 108, 111, 181, 123, 91; see also 112, 116, 213. I have omitted astrological symbols from the quotations.

23. Thoresby, *Diary*, 2:317; Thomas Mort to Peter Shakerley, Jan. 15, 1713, DSS/1/3/157, CALS; Pepys, *Diary*, 5:260; 4:142. See also Pepys, *Diary*, 4:23, 142, 221, 222, 300, 320, 327, 330, 5:118, 236, 359, 6:4, 16, 51, 101; D. Ryder, *Diary*, 33; Ra. Wendon to [Lord Cholmondeley?], Jan. 15, 1680, DCH/L/58, CALS; Edmund Harrold, His Book of Remarks and Observations, 1712–16, f. 17v, MS Mun. A.2.137, Chetham's.

24. Jeake (younger), *Astrological Diary*, 121. There are too many examples of patients referring to their "old pain" to cite here. For a few, see Edward Dering, Journal (1675–1679), f. 37r, HM 55605, Huntington; Manuscript Diary of John Cannon, Schoolmaster of Meare, Exciseman, Etc. (1684–1742), 186, DD\SAS\C1193/4, SRO; Clegg, *Diary*, 2:357; Pepys, *Diary*, 1:1, 4:218, 369; Richard Humfrey to his wife, July 31, 1712, D/Y/1/1/107/1, ERO; Thomas Raworth to G. R. Weckherlin, June 1, 1635, f. 115r, Add. MS

72439, BL; Edmund Harrold, His Book of Remarks and Observations, 1712–16, f. 7r, MS Mun. A.2.137, Chetham's; Joseph Hill to Sir Hans Sloane, Nov. 13, 1738, f. 230v, Sloane MS 4075, BL; John Finch to Anne Conway, May 7, 1652, in Conway, *Letters,* 62.

25. Robert Herbert to Sir Hans Sloane, May 8, n.d., 219r, and Mary Herbert to Sir Hans Sloane, Sept. 8, n.d., 220v, Sloane MS 4075, BL.

26. Clegg, *Diary,* 1:114, 115. I have found more than thirty incidences of male patients observing or counting their stools: Jeake (younger), *Astrological Diary,* 108, 120, 142, 178, 181, 211; Thomas Meautys to Jane Bacon, Jan. 18, 1625, in Bacon, *Private Correspondence,* 126–127; Reynolds Calthorpe to Sir Hans Sloane, Aug. 1, 1719, f. 289, Sloane MS 4034, BL; Manuscript Diary of John Cannon, Schoolmaster of Meare, Exciseman, Etc. (1684–1742), 516, 441, DD\SAS/C1193/4, SRO; Tyldesley, *Diary,* 73, 74, 87, 134, 135; Morris, *Diary,* 72; Heywood, *Autobiography, Diaries, Anecdote and Event Books,* 4:275; D. Ryder, *Diary,* 269; George Colebrook, Letters on Medical Cases (c. 1690), 163, MS 206/4, RCP; Thomas Fane to Sir Hans Sloane, Aug. 26, 1732, f. 194v, Sloane MS 4077, BL. Perhaps Pepys devoted the most attention to his bowels of all the patients in this study: see *Diary,* 3:120, 4:153, 154, 202, 327–329, 358, 396, 5:153, 244, 7:207. Male authors also made many references to their urine—too many to cite here.

27. Katherine Shakerley to Elizabeth Shakerley, [1670], DSS/1/4/50/79, CALS. For women writing about their stools, see Catharine Watson to Sir Hans Sloane, May 2, n.d., f. 307r, Sloane MS 4061, BL; Watson to Sloane, n.d., ff. 57r–60v, Sloane MS 4078, BL; Ann Warner to Sloane, Sept. 5, 1724, f. 216r, Sloane MS 4077, BL.

28. D. Ryder, *Diary,* 29; Tomalin, *Samuel Pepys,* 209. On motives for diary keeping more generally, see Fothergill, *Private Chronicles,* 64–94.

29. See facsimile insert in Tyldesley, *Diary* (quotes are on 134, 135); Powell, *Diary,* 44. On this hybrid form of accounting and writing, see Harvey, *The Little Republic,* 88–98.

30. Edmund Harrold, His Book of Remarks and Observations, 1712–16, ff. 1v, 50r, 41v, 3v, 17v, 2v, MS Mun. A.2.137, Chetham's. *JC, JW,* and *RP* are the initials of friends and business acquaintances of Harrold's; Tarbock was a drinking partner. On Harrold's drunken rambles, see ff. 5v, 8r, 12v, 14v, 16r, 20v, 22v, 30r, 40r, 46v, 57v.

31. Lowe, *Diary;* Pepys, *Diary,* vol. 3.

32. Mayne, *Arithmetick Vulgar, Decimal, and Algebraical;* Lightbody, *Every Man His Own Gauger,* title page.

33. On women's economic dealings, see Shepard, "Manhood, Credit, and Patriarchy"; Muldrew, "'A Mutual Assent of Her Mind'?"; Vickery, *The Gentleman's Daughter,* 127–160; Hubbard, *City Women;* Botonaki, "Seventeenth-Century Englishwomen's Spiritual Diaries," which argues that some women appropriated the language of accounting in spiritual writing. On the point about girls' education and numeracy, see Earle, *The Making of the English Middle Class,* 161–162.

34. On accounting by merchants, see Vernon, *The Compleat Compting-House*; Colinson, *Idea rationaria*; Zahedieh, *The Capital and the Colonies,* esp. 86–90, 106–113; Harvey, *The Little Republic,* esp. 72–98.

35. On early modern women's medical experiments and production of knowledge in the home, see Leong and Rankin, eds., *Secrets and Knowledge;* Rankin, *Panaceia's Daughters;* Rankin, "Becoming an Expert Practitioner"; Hunter, "Women and Domestic Medicine"; Harkness, "Managing an Experimental Household."

36. Jeake (younger), *Astrological Diary,* 108, 211, 212; on his "Astrologicall Experiments Exemplified" and intellectual development, see 16, 40–50, 185, 194–195. Jeake (elder), *A Radical's Books,* provides a catalogue of his father's extensive library.

37. Pepys, *Diary,* 4:60 (see also 9:254); Cowper, Daily Diary, 2:55. The number 489 is Roy Porter's calculation in "The Patient's View," 177.

38. Bunyan, *Grace Abounding,* 43.

39. For the use of *quickening,* see Rich, Diary, 1:ff. 16r, 210r, 219v, 2:f. 68r, 3:f. 39r; Katherine Tylston, Devotional Journal (1718–1720), f. 128v, Add. MS 42849, BL; Elias Pledger, Diary, f. 38v, MS 28.4, DWL. For *barren,* see Nehemiah Wallington, An Extract of the Passages of My Life (1654), 221, 319, 394, V.a.436, Folger.

40. Rich, Diary, 2:f. 256v. On the spiritual influences of her husband's family, see ibid., 2:f. 246v, 5:f. 88v; Mendelson, *The Mental World of Stuart Women,* 80–110.

41. Rich, Diary, 1:ff. 189r, 189v, 190v.

42. Elias Pledger, Diary, f. 71v, MS 28.4, DWL; Rich, Diary, 3:f. 103r; Cowper, Daily Diary, 1:1. There are numerous additional examples: Rich, Diary, 1:ff. 39v, 57v, 68v–69r, 71r, 78r, 86v, 94r, 99r, 99v, 101r–103r, 104v, 119v, 152v, 154r, 182v, 190v, 202r, 208r, 226v, 239r, 245r, 282v, 285v, 2:ff. 3v, 11r, 11v, 54r–v,

127r, 173r, 179v, 206r, 208v, 255v, 285v–286v, 3:ff. 18v, 36v, 61v, 65v, 71v, 103r, 114r, 119r–120r, 151r, 160v, 161v–162r, 191v, 193r, 199r, 218r–v, 219v–321r, 4:ff. 10r, 24r–25v, 75r, 87r, 89r, 90r–v, 128v, 163r–164r, 5:ff. 57r, 87r, 116r, 130r; Pledger, Diary, f. 25r; Cowper, Daily Diary, 1:22, 2:123, 169, 218; Katherine Tylston, Devotional Journal (1718–1720), f. 122v, Add. MS 42849, BL; Heywood, *Autobiography, Diaries, Anecdote and Event Books*, 1:228, 3:121; D'Ewes, *Diary*, 71; Thoresby, *Diary*, 1:22; Archer and Coe, *Two East Anglian Diaries*, 60, 62; Sarah Savage, Devotional Journal, f. 87r, Add. MS 42849, BL; Elizabeth Egerton, Countess of Bridgewater, Devotional Pieces, c. 1648–1663, f. 89r, Egerton MS 607, BL.

43. 2 Corinthians 3:3; Psalms 51:17, 22:14. All Bible quotations are from the King James Version.

44. Rich, Diary, 4:f. 120v, 2:f. 219r; White, *A Way to the Tree of Life*, 151. I discovered White's text and quotation in Hambrick-Stowe, *The Practice of Piety*, 159. On Rich's use of tears as a means of repenting and receiving grace, see Anselment, "Mary Rich." On the spiritual effects of devotional reading, see Craik, *Reading Sensations*, esp. 11–34; Bryan, *Looking Inward*, esp. 105–144.

45. Heywood, *Autobiography, Diaries, Anecdote and Event Books*, 1:250, 256, See also similar accounts by Thomas Shepard and Cotton Mather, cited in Hambrick-Stowe, *The Practice of Piety*, 176. On the ways religious expression could challenge masculine norms, see Lindman, "Acting the Manly Christian."

46. Bynum, *Fragmentation and Redemption*, esp. 186–190, 119–150. On gender and the embodiment of devotion among Baptists, Methodists, and Quakers, see Lindman, *Bodies of Belief*, esp. 64–68; Mack, *Heart Religion in the British Enlightenment;* Tarter, "Quaking in the Light."

47. Owen Stockton, Diary (1665–1677), f. 59r, MS 24.7, DWL; Heywood, *Autobiography, Diaries, Anecdote and Event Books*, 1:227, 260; Archer and Coe, *Two East Anglian Diaries*, 57; Cowper, Daily Diary, 1:31, 2:82; Elias Pledger, Diary, ff. 33v, 37r, MS 28.4, DWL; Rich, Diary, 1:ff. 20r, 62v, 135v, 143v, 275v, 286r, 297r, 2:ff. 3v, 11v, 135r, 3:f. 38v, 4:ff. 10r, 24r, 90v, 108r, 164, 5:ff. 76, 81r, 116r; Baxter, *Reliquiae Baxterianae*, 5.

48. Rich, Diary, 4:ff. 26v, 163r–v. See also Lister, *Autobiography*, 29. For a different type of conflation of spiritual and physical weakness, see Sullivan, "The Watchful Spirit."

49. Mary Rich, Occasional Meditations (1663–1677), ff. 26r–27r, Add. MS 27356, BL.

50. See Mendelson, *The Mental World of Stuart Women*, 93–94; Beadle, *The Journal or Diary of a Thankful Christian*. Beadle lived in Rich's neighborhood, consulted with her, and dedicated his text to her parents-in-law.

51. Rich, Diary, 3:f. 160v, 5:f. 87r.

52. Kettlewell, *Death Made Comfortable*, 23.

53. Becon, *The Sycke Mans Salue*, 44; Taylor, *The Rule and Exercises of Holy Dying*, 63, 65.

54. Cowper, Daily Diary, 1:79, 200. See also 4:303.

55. Elizabeth (Stanley) Hastings, Commonplace Book, HM 15369, Huntington; Archer and Coe, *Two East Anglian Diaries*, 213.

56. Anne Dormer to Elizabeth Trumbull, July 20, n.d., f. 180r, Add. MS 72516, BL; Mary Rich, Occasional Meditations (1663–1677), f. 156v, Add. MS 27356, BL.

57. Taylor, *The Rule and Exercises of Holy Dying*, 70, 116; Kettlewell, *Death Made Comfortable*, 201–202. This prayer was compiled from Psalms 102:4–5, 38:3, 38:10, 102:3; Job 7:3–4.

58. Job 1:21; Patrick, *The Book of Job Paraphras'd*, 293; Cowper, Daily Diary, 2:212; Moore, *Journal*, 289. For additional comparisons to biblical figures, see Rich, Diary, 1:ff. 40r, 272r, 3:f. 167r; Thornton, *Autobiography*, 222; Thornton, Remembrances, 129; Salmon, *Iatrica*, 110.

59. Ambrose, *Redeeming the Time*, sig. Ar, 29; Walker, *Eureka, Eureka*, title page; Thoresby, *Diary*, 1:38, 53. Cowper's catalogue of books is reproduced in Kugler, *Errant Plagiary*, 205.

60. Becon, *The Sycke Mans Salue*, 11, 13.

61. Rich, Diary, 1:ff. 293r, 302r, 3:ff. 194v, 214v; see also 2:f. 35v. For her guilt about undutiful behavior, see 3:f. 202r. On instructing her servants, see, for example, 1:f. 258v.

62. Cowper, Daily Diary, 1:86.

63. Edmund Harrold, His Book of Remarks and Observations, 1712–16, f. 10r, MS Mun. A.2.137, Chetham's. See also Pepys, *Diary*, 8:324; Thornton, Remembrances, 137, 182, 186, 187–188, 189, 194; Thornton, *Autobiography*, 63–66, 137; Freke, *Remembrances*, 79, 244; D. Ryder, *Diary*, 117–118; Clegg, *Diary*, 3:915.

Chapter 3. Emotional Causes of Illness

1. Thornton, *Autobiography*, 52, 66.

2. Thoresby, *Diary*, 1:316, 324.

3. For selected scholarship on these topics, see Pollock, "Anger and the Negotiation of Relationships"; Broomhall, ed., *Emotions in the Household;* Payne, *With Words and Knives;* MacDonald, *"The Fearfull Estate of Francis Spira."* For more literary approaches, see Liliequist, ed., *A History of Emotions;* Paster, Rowe, and Floyd-Wilson, eds., *Reading the Early Modern Passions.*

4. See, for example, Porter and Porter, *In Sickness and in Health;* Porter, ed., *Patients and Practitioners;* Fissell, *Patients, Power, and the Poor;* Beier, *Sufferers and Healers;* Wear, *Knowledge and Practice.*

5. MacDonald, *Mystical Bedlam.* See also Rublack, "Fluxes"; Carrera, ed., *Emotions and Health;* Weisser, "Grieved and Disordered." Hannah Newton examines the emotions of sick children and their parents in *The Sick Child.*

6. Eustace, *Passion Is the Gale,* 481–486.

7. Lutz and White, "The Anthropology of Emotions." On the challenges of studying emotions throughout history, see Pollock, "Anger and the Negotiation of Relationships," esp. 589; Bourke, "Fear and Anxiety"; Rosenwein, "Worrying About Emotions in History."

8. Cowper, Daily Diary, 6:27; Walkington, *The Optick Glasse of Humors,* 51r.

9. Beckett, *Practical Surgery Illustrated and Improved,* 150. On the structures and functions of the souls and spirits, see Park, "The Organic Soul."

10. Burton, *The Anatomy of Melancholy,* 121. This discussion also draws on 30–40, 122–128.

11. Thornton, *Autobiography,* 33; see also Thornton, Remembrances, 22. Isaac Archer attributed a similar process to drinking cold water: Archer and Coe, *Two East Anglian Diaries,* 54–55. For an example of emotions activating a dormant disease, see Cowper, Daily Diary, 3:209.

12. Harris, *The Divine Physician,* 81; Alberti, "Emotions in the Early Modern Medical Tradition." By the eighteenth century, patients were articulating these same beliefs within a framework of nerves: Stolberg, *Experiencing Illness and the Sick Body,* 187–190.

13. Bright, *A Treatise of Melancholie,* 144, 154, 157, 158; Lister, *Autobiography,* 43. On the bodily effects of fear, see Gentilcore, "The Fear of Disease"; Wear, "Fear, Anxiety and the Plague." See also Ja[ne?] Grundy, Feb. 12, 1694, DDKE/9/131/51, LA.

14. For references to spirits, see Anne Dormer to Elizabeth Trumbull, May 16, [1691?], f. 230v, Add. MS 72516, BL; Cowper, Daily Diary, 1:209, 313, 2:171, 262, 3:59, 5:229, 6:132, 143, 7:48. For accounts of emotions or illness within

the heart, see Anne Dormer to Jack Dormer, Aug. 10, 1691, f. 234v, Add. MS 72516, BL; Anne Dormer to Elizabeth Trumbull, May 16, [1691?], f. 230v; Thornton, *Autobiography*, 83, 175; Katherine Tylston, Devotional Journal (1718–1720), f. 122r, Add. MS 42849, BL; Pepys, *Diary*, 4:117; Thoresby, *Diary*, 1:44; Rich, Diary, 4:f. 24r; Rich, Autobiography (1625–1674), f. 32r, Add. MS 27357, BL; Archer and Coe, *Two East Anglian Diaries*, 181; *Medical Essays and Observations*, 353–354.

15. Thornton, *Autobiography*, 149, 173; alternate version in Thornton, Remembrances, 92, 136. For additional examples, see Thornton, *Autobiography*, 52, 67, 92, 118. *Sounding* meant "swooning."

16. Rich, Diary, 3:f. 215r; Delaval, *Meditations*, 75; Halkett and Fanshawe, *Memoirs*, 191; John Sharp to Andrew Fountain, April 15, 1701, D3549/6/1/F16, GA.

17. Elizabeth Trumbull to William Trumbull, Oct. 18, 1622, f. 18r, Add. MS 72425, BL. I have found seventeen women who described illness onset in this way. See citations above and below, as well as Cowper, Daily Diary, 7:342; Rich, Diary, 3:ff. 76, 208v, 216v–217r; Rich, Autobiography (1625–1674), ff. 26r, 35v, Add. MS 27357, BL; Sidney, *Sacharissa*, 103; Elizabeth Hastings to Selina Hastings, Countess of Huntington, Aug. 9, 1728, HA 4726, Huntington; Jane Shakerley to George Shakerley, n.d., DSS/1/5/60/43, CALS; Evelyn, *Diary*, 145–146; Archer and Coe, *Two East Anglian Diaries*, 150, 156, 158, 159, 181; Anne Dormer to Elizabeth Trumbull, Aug. 12, [1689?], f. 204r, Add. MS 72516, BL; Thornton, Remembrances, 115; Katherine Tylston, Devotional Journal (1718–1720), f. 122r, Add. MS 42849, BL; Elizabeth Isham, My Booke of Rememenberance, ff. 17r, 22r, MS RTCO1 (no. 62), Robert H. Taylor Collection, Princeton University Library, cited from unpublished transcription by Isaac Stephens. I have also found twelve similar examples by female patients in writing by healers.

18. Anne Dormer to Elizabeth Trumbull, May 30, 16[86?], f. 162r, Add. MS 72516, BL; Rich, Diary, 1:f. 221v; Freke, *Remembrances*, 81, 82, and alternate version on 247. See also Anne Dormer to Elizabeth Trumbull, Sept. 20, 1690, f. 225v, Add. MS 72516, BL; Clegg, *Diary*, 1:119; Archer and Coe, *Two East Anglian Diaries*, 150, 164; Catharine Watson to Sir Hans Sloane, n.d., f. 59r, Sloane MS 4078, BL. Grief could also impede recovery: see Freke, *Remembrances*, 234.

19. Roger North to Robert Foley, Dec. 31, 1691, f. 139, Add. MS 32500, BL. See also Pepys, *Diary*, 3:11; Sidney, *Sacharissa*, 103; Mary Rich, Autobiography

(1625–1674), ff. 18v–19r, Add. MS 27357, BL; Edward Clarke to his father, Dec. 21, 1671, DD\SF/7/1/15, SRO.

20. Talbor, *Pyretologia*, 36; Lowe, *Diary*, 76, 77. For additional examples of charms in personal writing, see Pepys, *Diary*, 6:177; Cowper, Daily Diary, 1:301–302, 4:261.

21. 2 Corinthians 3:2–3; Cowper, Daily Diary, 1:82. On charms, healing, and religious language, see Thomas, *Religion and the Decline of Magic*, 177–184.

22. See Thomas, *Religion and the Decline of Magic*, 502–512.

23. Quarter Sessions Bundles, 1653, Q/SBa 2/85, ERO. On speech and witch-craft accusations, see Purkiss, "Women's Stories of Witchcraft"; Stavreva, "Fighting Words."

24. Cowper, Daily Diary, 6:273–274; see also 1:3, 18, 72, 117, 128, 137, 247, 2:112, 221, 3:293–294.

25. Rich, Diary, 3:f. 192v. Rev. Thomas Woodroffe's annotations on the diary suggest that Charles Rich called his wife a whore. For additional examples of harmful words inducing illness, see ibid., 1:ff. 140v, 177v, 182v, 2:ff. 124v, 127r, 132r, 3:ff. 86r, 116r, 148v, 194v; Christiana Hastings to her brother, the Earl of Huntington, Sept. 20–21, 1672, HA 4680, Huntington; Cowper, Daily Diary, 1:64, 76, 204, 219, 3:61, 293, 4:361, 6:3, 142, 273–274, 293, 7:3, 88, 274, 307; Anne Dormer to Elizabeth Trumbull, June 22, [1687?], f. 166r, n.d., ff. 190v, 191v, July 21, 1690, f. 220r, Add. MS 72516, BL; Dorothy Spencer, Countess of Sunderland, to an unnamed lady, June 29, [after 1630], Add. 764, Folger; Harcourt, "Occasional Memoirs, Prayers and Lists of Mercies," 179; Katherine Austen, Meditations in Prose and Verse (1664–1668), f. 72r, Add. MS 4454, BL; George Weckherlin to Elizabeth Trumbull, Nov. 26, 1644, f. 104r, Add. MS 72442, BL; Anne Dawson, Diary (1721–1722), f. 40v, Add. MS 71626, BL; Mrs. Carter to Sir Hans Sloane, Jan. 7, 1739, f. 294v, Sloane MS 4078, BL; Freke, *Remembrances*, 93; Thornton, *Autobiography*, 49–50; Archer and Coe, *Two East Anglian Diaries*, 115.

26. Gowing, *Domestic Dangers;* Shepard, *Meanings of Manhood*, 152–173. On slander, see also Bound, "'An Angry and Malicious Mind'?"; Hindle, "The Shaming of Margaret Knowsley."

27. Gouge, *Of Domesticall Duties*, 284.

28. Thornton, Remembrances, 135; Thornton, *Autobiography*, 166, 167; see also Thornton, Remembrances, 118. For additional examples of gossip-induced illness, see Cowper, Daily Diary, 2:33, 4:109, 306; Freke, *Remembrances*, 255–256.

29. Thornton, *Autobiography*, 235; Thornton, Remembrances, 131, 120–121; Thornton, *Autobiography*, 222.

30. Thornton, *Autobiography*, 222; Thornton, Remembrances, 121; Thornton, *Autobiography*, 237, 224. *Larum* had the same meaning as *alarm* but could also mean "a call to arms" upon an enemy's approach: *Oxford English Dictionary Online*, s.v. "larum," n. 1a, at www.oed.com.

31. Thoresby, *Diary*, 1:44; Hamilton, *Diary*, 62; Arthur Annesley, Diary, f. 5r, Add. MS 40860, BL. See also Thoresby, *Diary*, 1:32; Pepys, *Diary*, 3:213, 8:129; Barlow, *Journal*, 1:112.

32. Clegg, *Diary*, 1:106; Pepys, *Diary*, 8:526; Thoresby, *Diary*, 1:316. See also Thornton, *Autobiography*, 160. Lisa Wynne Smith has also noted a connection between men's emotions and commercial concerns in "Women's Health Care in England and France," 107–108.

33. Henry Sturmy to John Sturmy, Feb. 9, 1702, D2375/F11, GA. See also George Weckherlin to Elizabeth Trumbull, July 16, 1645, f. 117r, Add. MS 72442, BL; Jeake (younger), *Astrological Diary*, 182, 193; Pepys, *Diary*, 1:111, 2:56, 6:186, 287, 7:288, 9:62; Thornton, *Autobiography*, 81; Lowe, *Diary*, 28.

34. Anne Dormer to Elizabeth Trumbull, July 28, n.d., f. 189v, Add. MS 72516, BL; Cowper, Daily Diary, 5:95.

35. D. Ryder, *Diary*, 90, 91, 339.

36. Lowe, *Diary*, 70; Pepys, *Diary*, 5:176. See also D. Ryder, *Diary*, 38, 119.

37. Bright, *A Treatise of Melancholie*, 143–144.

38. Cowper, Daily Diary, 2:183. Elizabeth Delaval similarly noted, "My passion's and my sences have resisted my reason and led my will captive" (*Meditations*, 26).

39. Thornton, *Autobiography*, 137; Thornton, Remembrances, 64; Pepys, *Diary*, 4:227. For additional examples of emotions causing miscarriages, see Thornton, *Autobiography*, 50, 136, 140; Thornton, Remembrances, 57; Archer and Coe, *Two East Anglian Diaries*, 153; D. Ryder, *Diary*, 166; Beata Pope to Frances North, July 23, [1670s], HM 521397, Huntington.

40. Thornton recorded the details of this episode only in her manuscript account. Quotes are in Thornton, Remembrances, 57–59; Thornton, *Autobiography*, 140. On the maternal imagination, see Fissell, *Vernacular Bodies*, esp. 207–211; Huet, *Monstrous Imagination*.

41. Park, *Secrets of Women*, 66–76, esp. 73. On philosophical and religious debates about vision in early modern Europe, see Clark, *Vanities of the Eye*.

42. Ward, *Diary*, 92; Nicholas Culpeper, *Culpeper's Last Legacy* (London, 1655), 65, cited in Wear, "Fear, Anxiety and the Plague," 357. The remedy

for hand swellings is in Oglander, *A Royalist's Notebook*, 220. On this world view, see Ashworth, "Natural History and the Emblematic World View."

43. Mary Rich, Autobiography (1625–1674), f. 35v, Add. MS 27357, BL; Cowper, Daily Diary, 7:27; Freke, *Remembrances*, 85. See also Anne Dormer to Elizabeth Trumbull, July 21, 1690, f. 220r, Add. MS 72516, BL.

44. Jane Shakerley to George Shakerley, Aug. 15, 1697, DSS/1/5/60/6, CALS; Lydia Dugard to Samuel Dugard, Nov. 26, 1667, X.d.477(10), Folger. For additional examples, see Jane Shakerley to George Shakerley, July 6, 1701, DSS/1/5/60/37, CALS; Brilliana Harley to Edward Harley, April 29, 1639, in Harley, *Letters*, 47; John Finch to Anne Conway, April 9, 1653, in Conway, *Letters*, 78; George Weckherlin to Elizabeth Weckherlin, July 2, 1645, f. 102r, Add. MS 72439, BL; Lydia Dugard to Samuel Dugard, March 22, 1668, X.d.477(13), Folger.

45. Elizabeth Poley to her brother [Richard D'Ewes?], 1641, f. 205, Harleian MS 382, BL; Lydia Dugard to Samuel Dugard, Oct. 3, 1668, X.d.477(15), Folger. There are too many examples of this trend to cite here. For a few, see Mary Fleetwood to George Shakerley, May 4, 1702, DSS/1/5/16/14, CALS; Anne Dormer to William Trumbull, n.d., f. 239r, Add. MS 72516, BL; Mary Leke, Countess of Scarsdale, to the Countess of Huntington, Oct. 24, 1682, HA 8214, Huntington. Some individuals were literal about this kind of relational recovery. Anne Archer, for instance, recovered in tandem with her son: "Upon his mending, she began to be better" (Archer and Coe, *Two East Anglian Diaries*, 150).

46. Marshall, *John Locke, Toleration and Early Enlightenment Culture*, 281–311. For examples from individuals in this study, see Cowper, Daily Diary, 1:88; Archer and Coe, *Two East Anglian Diaries*, 116.

47. Lydia Dugard to Samuel Dugard, March 25, 1672, X.d.477(31), Folger; Cowper, Daily Diary, 1:79, 2:96. See also Lydia Dugard to Samuel Dugard, Dec. 1670, X.d.477(21), Folger; Cowper, Daily Diary, 1:97, 123, 2:109, 186, 275, 5:47, 155–156, 7:343.

48. D. Ryder, *Diary*, 349; Thoresby, *Diary*, 1:4–5. For a dream similar to Ryder's, see Pepys, *Diary*, 6:232.

49. Pepys, *Diary*, 4:140, 158, 157, 173, 229; see also 278.

50. Thornton, *Autobiography*, 262.

51. Harris, *The Divine Physician*, 61; George Tonstall, M.D., to John Thoresby, 1677, f. 143r, Stowe MS 745, BL.

52. Katherine Tylston, Devotional Journal of 1718–1720, f. 122r, Add. MS 42849, BL.

53. Mordecai Cary to James Jurin, June 1, 1733, f. 1, MS 6140, Wellcome; see also Cary to Jurin, July 28, 1733, f. 4, ibid. For similar descriptions of scampering animals, see Medical Diary and Account Book of John Westover of Wedmore (1685–1700), f. 75v, DD/X/HKN 1, SRO; Bonet, *A Guide to the Practical Physician*, 46.

54. Anne Shakerley to George Shakerley, n.d., DSS/1/5/57/32, CALS. This paragraph also draws on Cowper, Daily Diary, 1:204, 219; Anne Dormer to Elizabeth Trumbull, May 16, [1691?], f. 230v, Add. MS 72516, BL; Freke, *Remembrances*, 68; Rich, Diary, 3:ff. 216r, 220r; Rich, Autobiography (1625–1674), f. 32r, Add. MS 27357, BL; Giffard, *Life and Correspondence*, 334.

55. Jone Elyott to her father, Aug. 28, 1630, f. 7r, Harleian MS 382, BL.

Chapter 4. Suffering on the Sickbed

1. Cowper, Daily Diary, 1:197.

2. Ibid., 200, 201.

3. On Cowper's life, see Kugler, *Errant Plagiary*.

4. Porter and Porter, *In Sickness and in Health*, 192. On the "sick role," see Parsons, *The Social System*, 436–439; Porter and Porter, *In Sickness and in Health*, 187–200; Withey, *Physick and the Family*, 123–140; Mutschler, "The Province of Affliction."

5. Arthur Annesley, Diary (1673–1684), f. 5v, Add. MS 18730, BL; Rich, Diary, 4:f. 46r. On sick visits, see Beier, *Sufferers and Healers*, 245–249; Stolberg, *Experiencing Illness and the Sick Body*, 53–55.

6. On Rich's tears of repentance, see Anselment, "Mary Rich," esp. 338, 343.

7. Rich, Diary, 5:f. 168r; see also 1:ff. 293r, 302r–v. For similar examples, see ibid., 1:ff. 217r, 276r, 3:f. 200v, 4:f. 46r, 5:ff. 166v, 168r; Anne Dawson, Diary (1721–1722), f. 39v, Add. MS 71626, BL.

8. Freke, *Remembrances*, 77, 242; Wright, *The Passions of the Minde*, 102–103. On the healthful influences of cheerfulness, love, and friendship, see Rublack, "Fluxes," esp. 3–4; Solomon, "Non-natural Love"; Yallop, *Age and Identity in Eighteenth-Century England*, 83–105; Wear, "Fear, Anxiety and the Plague."

9. Charleton, *A Natural History of the Passions*, 108; M. Burges to Edward Clarke, Sept. 16, 1695, DD\SF/7/1/33, SRO; Thomas Knyvett to Katherine Knyvett, Nov. 11, 1637, in Knyvett, *Letters*, 91. For additional examples, see Lister, *Autobiography*, 44; Thornton, Remembrances, 131; Thornton, *Autobiography*, 124; Elizabeth Paston to Anne Foley, April 26, 1695, f. 156r,

Add. MS 32500, BL; Jone Ellyot to her brother, Feb. 24, [1640s?], f. 27r, Harleian MS 382, BL; Anne Dormer to Elizabeth Trumbull, July 21, 1690, f. 221v, March 10, n.d., f. 174v, Sept. 10, n.d., f. 168v, MS 72516, BL; Cowper, Daily Diary, 1:291. For letters and interactions characterized as cordials, see Lucy Davis Hastings to the Earl of Huntington, March 30, 1673, HA 5795, Huntington; Thornton, Remembrances, 133; Cowper, Daily Diary, 7:8; chapter 3.

10. Cowper, Daily Diary, 3:58; Anne Dormer to Elizabeth Trumbull, Sept. 20, 1690, ff. 223v, 224r, Add. MS 72516, BL. See also Cowper, Daily Diary, 1:206, 3:86, 293–294; Archer and Coe, *Two East Anglian Diaries*, 76.

11. Rich, Diary, 3:ff. 215v, 216r, 221v. For additional examples, see Brilliana Harley to Edward Harley, March 22, 1638, in Harley, *Letters*, 33; Lister, *Autobiography*, 29.

12. Cowper, Daily Diary, 1:205–206, 202, 3:297. Visitors spent two to three hours with Thomas Tyldesley during his sick days: Tyldesley, *Diary*, 35, 79, 123.

13. Cowper, Daily Diary, 1:282, 283, 227.

14. Ibid., 42–43, 17, 185.

15. Freke, *Remembrances*, 198. For the example from Cowper, see Daily Diary, 3:218.

16. Freke, *Remembrances*, 71, 72; see also 236–237.

17. Ibid., 76, 69, 191; alternate versions are on 241, 235, 280; see also 52, 73, 77–78, 97–98, 190. For additional complaints about insufficient pity, see Cowper, Daily Diary, 1:196, 7:336; Thornton, *Autobiography*, 150, 166–167; Thornton, Remembrances, 92; Blundell, *The Great Diurnal*, 1:52; Anne Dormer to Elizabeth Trumbull, July 28, n.d., f. 189v, Add. MS 72516, BL. On death rituals, see Houlbrooke, *Death, Religion, and the Family;* Houlbrooke, ed., *Death, Ritual, and Bereavement;* Brady, "'A Share of Sorrows.'"

18. Freke, *Remembrances*, 67, 157, 129, 229; see also 73, 76, 77, 93, 158, 191, 196, 234, 235, 238, 242, 255–256, 279, 287.

19. Thornton, *Autobiography*, 166–167; Halkett and Fanshawe, *Memoirs*, 137; Clifford, *Diary*, 117. For additional examples, see Thornton, *Autobiography*, 87–88, 96, 142, 153; Cowper, Daily Diary, 1:21.

20. Calverley, "Memorandum Book," 43, 64; Pepys, *Diary*, 7:137; Arthur Annesley, Diary (1673–1684), ff. 31v, 104r, Add. MS 18730, BL. For examples of chronic ailments, see also Lowe, *Diary*, 101; Jeake (younger), *Astrological Diary*, esp. 88, 98, 107; Calverley, "Memorandum Book," 50; Archer and Coe, *Two East Anglian Diaries*, 213.

21. Lowe, *Diary*, 22; Jane Shakerley to George Shakerley, March 1702, DSS/1/5/60/50, CALS. There are numerous additional examples; for a few, see Archer and Coe, *Two East Anglian Diaries*, 119, 157, 161, 162, 163; Clegg, *Diary*, 1:18; Owen Stockton, Diary (1665–1677), f. 78, MS 24.7, DWL; Ezekiel Rogers to Lady Barrington, Sept. 28, n.d., f. 240, Egerton MS 2644, BL; John Doulben to [?], Jan. 29, 1646, DSS/1/2/2/1, CALS.

22. Thoresby, *Diary*, 2:390, 391, 392. For another writer who evaluated the progression of illness according to her ability to attend religious services, see Cowper, Daily Diary, 3:28.

23. Thoresby, *Diary*, 2:83. For similar examples, see ibid., 194, 299, 386; Arthur Annesley, Diary (1673–1684), ff. 84v, 111v, Add. MS 18730, BL; Rich, Diary, 2:f. 246r; Clegg, *Diary*, 1:44, 132, 180, 2:350, 376; Cowper, Daily Diary, 1:62, 3:196, 4:29, 7:189. On birthdays, see also Hambrick-Stowe, *The Practice of Piety*, 174.

24. Fissell, *Patients, Power, and the Poor*, 34–35. On this religious world view and its link to conceptions of time, see Hall, *Worlds of Wonder*, 213–238.

25. Cowper, Daily Diary, 1:221, 222, 235, 28–29, 2:128; see also 1:17, 45.

26. D. Ryder, *Diary*, 213.

27. Cowper, Daily Diary, 1:197, 200, 178, 254; Mary (Levinge) Shirley, Countess Ferrers, to Mary Shirley, Feb. 22, 1730, HA 10832, Huntington.

28. For the women, see citations above; also Elizabeth Poley to Sir Simonds D'Ewes, n.d., f. 180, Harleian MS 382, BL; Halkett and Fanshawe, *Memoirs*, 74; Margaret Shappard to Sarah Say, [1730s], Say Papers, 12.107(129), DWL; Anne Underwoode to her husband, 1617, f. 183, Egerton MS 2644, BL; Katherine Austen, Meditations in Prose and Verse (1664–1668), f. 61r, Add. MS 4454, BL; Thornton, *Autobiography*, 85, 149; Thornton, Remembrances, 92; Rich, Diary, 3:f. 228r, 4:f. 163r; Cowper, Daily Diary, 3:80. For the men, see William Jessop to Ann Hulton, Feb. 4, 1664, DDHU 47/6, LA; Arthur Annesley, Diary (1673–1684), f. 70v, Add. MS 18730, BL; John Finch to Anne Conway, Nov. 30, 1653, in Conway, *Letters*, 89; Davies, *Journal*, 32–33.

29. Davies, *Journal*, 32–33.

30. Cowper, Daily Diary, 1:202; Henry More to Anne Conway, June 2, 1653, in Conway, *Letters*, 82.

31. Francis Conway to Edward Conway, Jan. 23, 1668, in Conway, *Letters*, 292. Similarly, Anne North described how a child in her family "fetch't her breath so short as if she had been dying" (North to Anne Foley, Nov. 8, 1680, f. 50, Add. MS 32500, BL).

32. Powell, *Diary*, 44; Morris, *Diary*, 55; Jeake (younger), *Astrological Diary*, 136. For additional examples from men, see Manuscript Diary of John Cannon, Schoolmaster of Meare, Exciseman, Etc. (1684–1742), 180, 214, DD\SAS/C1193/4, SRO; Henry More to Anne Conway, Dec. 10, 1653, in Conway, *Letters*, 91; Archer and Coe, *Two East Anglian Diaries*, 213; Edward Stephens to Richard Stephens, 1676, f. 117r, Stowe MS 745, BL; Thoresby, *Diary*, 1:327; Clegg, *Diary*, 1:114, 3:915; Heywood, *Autobiography, Diaries, Anecdote and Event Books*, 1:169, 4:141; Lister, *Autobiography*, 29, 44.

33. Archer and Coe, *Two East Anglian Diaries*, 154.

34. Freke, *Remembrances*, 75, 189; see also 61, 69, 79, 81, 93, 157, 191, 200, 276. Alternate versions of these episodes are on 240, 278, 229, 235, 244, 252–253, 256, 280. For similar examples from women, see Thornton, *Autobiography*, 11, 33, 83, 96, 132–133, 141–142, 149, 153, 235; Thornton, Remembrances, 10, 30, 43, 121; Halkett and Fanshawe, *Memoirs*, 74, 137; Anna Meautys to Jane Lady Cornwallis Bacon, March 2, 1641, in Bacon, *Private Correspondence*, 264; Cowper, Daily Diary, 1:202; Clifford, *Diary*, 117; Sarah Savage, Devotional Journal, f. 88v, Add. MS 42849, BL; Katherine Austen, Meditations in Prose and Verse (1664–1668), f. 62r, Add. MS 4454, BL; Mary Tuke to Mrs. Evelyn, 1693, ff. 130–131, Add. MS 15949, BL.

35. Archer and Coe, *Two East Anglian Diaries*, 139. For another example, see Blundell, *The Great Diurnal*, 1:71. I have found numerous similar instances in medical observations and letters to physicians—too many to cite here. A few include "She thought she shd dye euery hour," The Case Book of a General Practitioner (1726–1728), f. 36r, MS 7501, Wellcome; "She would often say, That nothing could equal that pain but the pangs of Death," Salmon, *Iatrica*, 134; "She would often cry out she should dye," Salmon, *Parateremata*, 44; "She was in her own thoughts a dying all that day," Silas Bradbury to Sir Hans Sloane, May 29, 1719, f. 247, Sloane MS 4034, BL.

36. Thornton, *Autobiography*, 152, 153; Thornton, Remembrances, 102–103.

37. Thornton, *Autobiography*, 153, 141, 142. Similarly, in 1654 Thornton explained how her "deare mother and aunt and friends did not expect my life," and in 1665 she described "beeing soe weake . . . that all gave me for dead" (92, 149). For additional examples, see Clifford, *Diary*, 117; Freke, *Remembrances*, 61, 93, 229, 256; Halkett and Fanshawe, *Memoirs*, 137; Anna Meautys to Jane Lady Cornwallis Bacon, March 2, 1641, in Bacon, *Private Correspondence*, 264. Men made this move too: see Manuscript Diary of John Cannon, Schoolmaster of Meare, Exciseman, Etc. (1684–1742), 214, DD\SAS/C1193/4, SRO; Morris, *Diary*, 55; Thoresby, *Diary*, 1:327; Clegg,

Diary, 3:915; Heywood, *Autobiography, Diaries, Anecdote and Event Books*, 4:141.

38. Mary Beth Rose has made similar assertions about Thornton in particular, suggesting that the Yorkshire gentlewoman chose affliction as "a projection of her desired self": "Gender, Genre, and History," 261. See also George, *Women in the First Capitalist Society*, 168–179; Beier, *Sufferers and Healers*, 211–241.

39. Freke, *Remembrances*, 79, 253; see also 92–93, 256. On the two versions of Freke's diary and her self-fashioning, see Anselment, "Elizabeth Freke's Remembrances."

40. Lowe, *Diary*, 57.

41. Owen Stockton, Diary (1665–1677), f. 46r, MS 24.7, DWL; Sarah Savage, Devotional Journal, f. 88v, Add. MS 42849, BL; see also Rich, Diary, 1:f. 18v.

42. Lister, *Autobiography*, 28, 29.

43. Ibid., 29. On suffering and deliverance, see Howard, "Imagining the Pain and Peril"; Anselment, "The Deliverance of Alice Thornton"; Rose, "Gender, Genre, and History," 245–278.

44. Cowper, Daily Diary, 1:274; see also 244.

45. Pepys, *Diary*, 4:332.

46. Tyldesley, *Diary*, 74.

47. Pepys, *Diary*, 2:207, 35, 4:202, 5:150, 3:26; see also 5:157.

48. Lady Rhoda Delves to the Countess of Huntington, July 5, 1728, HA 2213, Huntington; Ezekiel Rogers to Lady Joan Barrington, Sept. 28, n.d., f. 240, Egerton MS 2644, BL.

49. Pe[ter] Burweek to Grace, Countess of Eglinton, July 22, 1692, X.d.428(150), Folger; Blundell, *The Great Diurnal*, 1:40; William Burrell to Sir Hans Sloane, July 19, 1725, f. 28r, Sloane MS 4048, BL; Alexander Gawne to Sir James [Montagu?], 1708, f. 185r, Add. MS 61607, BL. On spas, see Porter, ed., *The Medical History of Waters and Spas;* Hembry, *The English Spa;* Herbert, "Gender and the Spa."

50. Philip Gawdy to his brother, n.d., f. 43r, Add. MS 27395, BL.

51. George Rudolph Weckherlin to Elizabeth Trumbull, Dec. 9, 1639, ff. 40r–41v, Feb. 17, 1639, f. 49r–v, May 10, 1642, f. 82v, Add. MS 72442, BL; Anne Shakerley to George Shakerley, May 22, [early 1700s], DSS/1/5/57/3, CALS; Blundell, *The Great Diurnal*, 2:92; Arthur Annesley, Diary (1673–1684), f. 9v, Add. MS 18730, BL. There are too many additional examples of patients who named the sources of their remedies to cite.

52. Smith, "Reassessing the Role of the Family." See also C. Crawford, "Patients' Rights and the Law of Contract."

53. James Molins, Medical treatise and receipts, f. 244r, Sloane MS 3293, BL; Wiseman, *Severall Chirurgicall Treatises*, 397. For a few (of many more) additional examples, see George Colebrook, Letters on Medical Cases (c. 1690), May 15, 1702, 158, MS 206/4, RCP; Symcotts, *A Seventeenth-Century Doctor*, 73; Wiseman, *Severall Chirurgicall Treatises*, 195. See also Louis-Courvoisier and Pilloud, "Consulting by Letter"; Churchill, *Female Patients*, 57–63.

54. Douglas, *A Short Account of Mortifications*, 17, 7.

55. Colbatch, *A Treatise of the Gout*, 99.

56. Cowper, Daily Diary, 1:291–292, quoting Proverbs 17:22.

57. Yallop, *Age and Identity*, 83–105.

58. Halkett and Fanshawe, *Memoirs*, 137.

Chapter 5. Perceptions of Pain

1. Pepys, *Diary*, 5:150.

2. Ibid., 3:136, 4:218, 7:207, 5:312, 7:406, 5:329. For additional examples of these self-evaluations, see 1:163, 164, 2:241, 5:162, 167.

3. Ibid., 2:60, 5:100. On the operation, see ibid., 10:173–176; Tomalin, *Samuel Pepys*, 59–63. On early modern lithotomy, see Cook, *Trials of an Ordinary Doctor*, 76–105. On his special case for the stone, see Pepys, *Diary*, 5:247.

4. Pepys, *Diary*, 2:226, 8:303; Pepys to John Jackson, April 8, 1700, in Pepys, *Private Correspondence and Miscellaneous Papers*, 1:316.

5. Pepys, *Diary*, 2:87.

6. Cohen, "The Animated Pain of the Body," 39. This initial section of the chapter builds on pioneering work by Lisa Smith, "'An Account of an Unaccountable Distemper,'" and Lisa Silverman, *Tortured Subjects*, 133–151. For examples of Cohen's point, see Rey, *The History of Pain;* Mann, ed., *The History of the Management of Pain;* Hinnells and Porter, eds., *Religion, Health and Suffering;* De Moulin, "A Historical-Phenomenological Study of Bodily Pain." More recent work has begun to remedy the skewed focus that Cohen highlighted: see Bending, *The Representation of Bodily Pain;* Hide, Bourke, and Mangion, eds., "Perspectives on Pain"; Moscoso, *Pain;* Van Dijkhuizen and Enenkel, eds., *The Sense of Suffering;* K. Walker, "A Gendered History of Pain in England."

7. Lisa Silverman has suggested that pain took on positive spiritual meaning only after medical interventions failed to alleviate it. See *Tortured Subjects*, 133.

8. Using patient-healer correspondence, Lisa Smith has argued that gender did not inform patients' experiences of pain: see " 'An Account of an Unaccountable Distemper.' " Phyllis Mack and Sharon Howard offer valuable studies of pious women that explore how the roles of wives, mothers, and nurses mediated perceptions of pain: Mack, *Heart Religion in the British Enlightenment*, 171–218; Howard, "Imagining the Pain and Peril."

9. Mordecai Cary to James Jurin, 1733–1734, ff. 1–7, MS 6140, Wellcome. Quotes are from July 28, 1733, f. 4. For another comparison of pain to darts, see Mrs. Carter to Sir Hans Sloane, Jan. 7, 1739, f. 294v, Sloane MS 4078, BL.

10. Mordecai Cary to James Jurin, 1733–1734, ff. 1–7, MS 6140, Wellcome.

11. Henry Ireton to Sir Hans Sloane, June 20, 1709, ff. 304r, 304v, Sloane MS 4075, BL.

12. Ibid., ff. 305r, 303r, 303v; Henry Ireton to Sir Hans Sloane, June 22, 1709, f. 308r, Sloane MS 4075, BL. Katherine Shakerley of Hulme demonstrated a similar awareness of her internal body when she wrote that "I haue som tims a pane in my side . . . it lies in the kednes": Shakerley to Elizabeth Shakerley, Feb. 26, 1670, DSS 1/4/50/73, CALS.

13. Pepys, *Diary*, 1:219.

14. Cowper, Daily Diary, 7:271, 174, 244, 209, 261. See also 154, 242. These examples further illustrate the gender differences that chapter 2 outlines.

15. Sir William Petty, Papers, ff. 228, 254v, Add. MS 72891, BL; [?] Jones to Arthur Price, May 12, 1735, f. 296, Sloane MS 4077, BL; The Case Book of a General Practitioner (1726–1728), f. 36r, MS 7501, Wellcome; Robert Thomlinson to his brother Richard, March 14, 1720, f. 273r, Sloane MS 4077, BL; Arthur Price to Sir Hans Sloane, Dec. 12, 1734, f. 301, Sloane MS 4077, BL; [Sir Hans Sloane?], Mr. Lovetts Case, f. 47, Sloane MS 4076, BL; Bonet, *A Guide to the Practical Physician*, 568; Charlotte Seymour to Sir Hans Sloane, Nov. 27, n.d., f. 65v, Sloane MS 4078, BL; Blundell, *The Great Diurnal*, 1:102.

16. George Weckherlin to Elizabeth Trumbull, Dec. 29, 1639, f. 40r, July 16, 1647, f. 162r, Add. MS 72442, BL; Symcotts, *A Seventeenth-Century Doctor*, 90.

17. Colbatch, *A Treatise of the Gout*, 127. The two other instances I have found are not by patients. A physician described his patient's back pains as "not

inferior to those of a woman in trauell" (George Colebrook, Letters on Medical Cases [c. 1690], 38, MS 206/4, RCP), and Elizabeth Isham noted being so sick that "one which saw me said it might be as painfull as a womans trauell" (My Booke of Rememenberance, f. 17r, MS RTCO1 [no. 62], Robert H. Taylor Collection, Princeton University Library, cited from unpublished transcription by Isaac Stephens).

18. Colbatch, *A Treatise of the Gout*, 127; Mary Shirley, Lady Ferrers, to [?] Hinde, 1732, f. 99v, Sloane MS 4066, BL; Morris, *Diary*, 86. This discussion also draws on Cowper, Daily Diary, 1:178; Adam Martindale, Autobiography, f. 84v, Add. MS 4239, BL. There are too many additional examples to cite here. For a small sample, see Sir Edmund King, M.D., Medical Papers and Collections, f. 270r, June 12, [16]85, Sloane MS 1589, BL; George Colebrook, Letters on Medical Cases (c. 1690), 143, MS 206/4, RCP; *General Observations*, 3.

19. George Colebrook, Letters on Medical Cases (c. 1690), 95, MS 206/4, RCP.

20. Cowper, Daily Diary, 4:25. For additional examples of pain causing fever, see Thornton, *Autobiography*, 166; Pepys, *Diary*, 7:210; Jeake (younger), *Astrological Diary*, 145; Salmon, *Iatrica*, 108.

21. Mary Parker and Hephzibah Parker to Sir Hans Sloane, 1715–1716, ff. 192–211, Sloane MS 4076, BL. Quotes are from Sept. 19, 1716, f. 195, Jan. 3, n.d., f. 198.

22. Bonet, *A Guide to the Practical Physician*, 502; Samuel England, Notebook Containing Prescriptions and Case Notes, 1730–33, f. 325, MS 6, RCP. On manipulating the body to guide internal substances, see Thomas Howard to Sir Hans Sloane, July 27, 1698, f. 104r, Sloane MS 4037, BL; Pepys, *Diary*, 4:332; Grizel Mainwaring to the Duchess of Marlborough, Aug. 6, 1712, ff. 166–167, Add. MS 61461, BL.

23. Anne North to Francis North, May 2, 1680, HM 52379, Huntington.

24. Magdalen Coward, Book of Receipts, 1695, 61r, 12v, 17r, HM 88, Huntington.

25. Willis, *Pharmaceutice Rationalis*, 144–148; Woodman, *Medicus Novissimus*, 58. On the role of pain in medical encounters, see Weisser, "Boils, Pushes, and Wheals"; chapter 1. On alleviating pain, see Porter, "Western Medicine and Pain"; Moscoso, *Pain*, 117–123; Cohen, *The Modulated Scream*, 87–112.

26. Cowper, Daily Diary, 3:162; see also 1:284, 3:91. For examples of pain inhibiting spiritual meditation, see ibid., 1:197, 7:335; Heywood, *Autobiography, Diaries, Anecdote and Event Books*, 1:228; chapter 2 of this book. On

the scriptural origins of accepting physical suffering, see Knott, *Discourses of Martyrdom in English Literature*, 28–29; Van Dijkhuizen, "Partakers of Pain."

27. Thoresby, *Diary*, 1:211, 2:185, 410. For an example of the memory of pain, see Delaval, *Meditations*, 80.

28. Taylor, *The Rule and Exercises of Holy Dying*, 95. On *ars moriendi* and pain, see Mayhew, "Godly Beds of Pain."

29. Elizabeth Egerton, Countess of Bridgewater, Devotional Pieces, c. 1648–1663, f. 36v, Egerton MS 607, BL; Richard Carpenter to John Trevelyan, March 24, 1620, DD\WO/55/7/47–1, SRO. For additional examples of sufferers who responded to pain with passive endurance, resigned to God's will, see Thornton, *Autobiography*, 86; Anne Conway to Henry More, May 24, 1664, in Conway, *Letters*, 224.

30. Sherlock, *A Practical Discourse Concerning Death*, 67; Blaise Pascal, *Prière pour demander à Dieu le bon usage des maladies*, quoted in translation in Rey, *The History of Pain*, 101.

31. *The Jesuit Relations*, 162, 164. Jogues survived this episode but died from a similar ordeal four years later. On flagellants, see Silverman, *Tortured Subjects*, 8.

32. Thoresby, *Diary*, 1:467; Jeake (younger), *Astrological Diary*, 92; Pepys, *Diary*, 9:284; Rich, Diary, 1:f. 38r. There is an immense amount of literature on Foxe's text, officially titled *Actes and Monuments of These Latter and Perillous Dayes* and first published in 1563. More recent studies include Knott, *Discourses of Martyrdom;* King, *Foxe's "Book of Martyrs";* Highley and King, *John Foxe and His World;* Mueller, "Pain, Persecution, and the Construction of Selfhood."

33. Cowper, Daily Diary, 4:11; Freke, *Remembrances*, 196; Behn, *Oroonoko*, 77. On the influences of Foxe and judicial torture, see also Howard, "Imagining the Pain and Peril." Catholics too looked to a discourse of martyrdom to ascribe spiritual meaning to pain: see Hanson, "Torture and Truth in Renaissance England"; Dillon, *The Construction of Martyrdom*.

34. This discussion draws on Sharon Howard's astute reading of the passage in "Imagining the Pain and Peril," esp. 370, 377. For the quote from Thornton, see her *Autobiography*, 95, and Remembrances, 114.

35. George Colebrook, Letters on Medical Cases (c. 1690), 81, MS 206/4, RCP; unaddressed and unsigned notes relating to medical treatments and symptoms, July 1699, DLT/4996/32/13, CALS; Dr. James Keill to Sir Hans Sloane, July 1709, f. 1v, Sloane MS 4042, BL. See also Walwyn,

Physick for Families, 67. For similar language in accounts of children's suffering, see Newton, *The Sick Child*, 193–195. On torture and pain in early modern France, see Silverman, *Tortured Subjects*.

36. Heywood, *Autobiography, Diaries, Anecdote and Event Books*, 1:254.

37. Sintelaer, *The Scourge of Venus and Mercury*, sig. A9r–v; 206. A slightly different version of this image is the frontis of Stephen Blankaart's *Venus Belegert en Ontset* (Amsterdam: Timotheus ten Hoorn, 1685). Sintelaer uses the language of martyrdom throughout his text, referring to the "Mercurial Rack" and to venereal patients as "martyrs of Venus."

38. Anne Dormer to Elizabeth Trumbull, March 10, [1682?], f. 175r, June 22, [1687?], ff. 165v, 166r, July 20, n.d., f. 181v, Add. MS 72516, BL. Dormer also wrote that she was always "watching and endeauouring to guess right and so my mind is eternally upon the rack" (Dec. 10, 16[88?], f. 213v, Add. MS 72516, BL).

39. On medieval views of martyrs' heroic endurance, see Cohen, "The Animated Pain of the Body," 44–45. Cohen has more recently argued that the impassivity of medieval martyrs gradually gave way to an emphasis on physical suffering in an attempt to relate to Christ: *The Modulated Scream*, 227–249.

40. Foxe, *Actes and Monuments*, 1449. David Hall offers an example from early New England of a Baptist who, in imitation of Foxe's martyrs, claimed to feel no pain when he was whipped for his beliefs. Following his punishment, he told the magistrates, "You have struck me as with roses" (*Worlds of Wonder*, 188). On the differences between the suffering of early Christian and sixteenth-century Marian martyrs, see Knott, "John Foxe and the Joy of Suffering."

41. An Account of the Lady Lucy, 1675, ff. 4–5, V.a.166, Folger.

42. Archer and Coe, *Two East Anglian Diaries*, 151–152; Heywood, *Life of John Angier*, 115. For similar accounts, see Archer and Coe, *Two East Anglian Diaries*, 159, 160; Thornton, *Remembrances*, 150–151; Thornton, *Autobiography*, 174; Halkett, *Selected Self-Writings*, 32. Elizabeth Isham likened her sister to a martyr twice, once when she exhibited exceeding joy despite her "greatest extremity of paine": My Booke of Rememenberance, ff. 22r, 6r, RTCO1 (no. 62), Robert H. Taylor Collection, Princeton University Library, cited from unpublished transcription by Isaac Stephens.

43. Salmon, *Iatrica*, 6; Miscellanea XII, f. 2v, MS 805, Wellcome.

44. Grace Nettleton to Francis Leicester, Jan. 21, 1726, DLT/C10/96, CALS. See also Thornton, *Autobiography*, 23; Rich, Diary, 3:ff. 205v–206r, 207r,

211v–212r; Halkett, *Selected Self-Writings*, 48; Frances Cottrell to Sir W. Trumbull and Lady Trumbull, July 10, [1710], f. 122, Add. MS 72518, BL. On physicians' opposition to anesthesia in the 1800s, see Pernick, *A Calculus of Suffering*, esp. 43.

45. Thornton, *Autobiography*, 107, 106, 108; Thornton, Remembrances, 31–34. Wandesford quoted Psalms 42:14–15 and 43:5–6. Thornton's account of her sister's death is quite similar: see *Autobiography*, 50–51.

46. Anne Dormer to Elizabeth Trumbull, Sept. 20, 1690, f. 223r, Nov. 8, n.d., f. 206r, Add. MS 72516, BL. Pious men displayed similar Christian virtues: see, for example, Wagstaffe, *A Letter out of Suffolk*.

47. Archer and Coe, *Two East Anglian Diaries*, 160.

48. Cowper, Daily Diary, 1:178; Lady Francis Clifton to Anne Conway, Oct. 3 and Oct. 17, 1678, in Conway, *Letters*, 443.

49. Thornton, *Autobiography*, 63, 64, 65; Thornton, Remembrances, 24.

50. Anne Dormer to Elizabeth Trumbull, n.d., f. 177r, Add. MS 72516, BL.

51. D. Ryder, *Diary*, 119, 285, 141–142; see also 258.

52. Stout, *Autobiography*, 91; Clegg, *Diary*, 1:108; Manuscript Diary of John Cannon, Schoolmaster of Meare, Exciseman, Etc. (1684–1742), 516, DD\SAS/C1193/4, SRO; Pepys, *Diary*, 7:37. For additional examples, see Tyldesley, *Diary*, 66; Jeake (younger), *Astrological Diary*, 206; Heywood, *Autobiography, Diaries, Anecdote and Event Books*, 1:169; Jolly, *Note Book*, 57. I have also found numerous examples in writing to and from healers. A few include David Hamilton to Sir Hans Sloane, May 2, n.d., f. 103r, Sloane MS 4059, BL; Henry Downing to Sir Hans Sloane, July 19, 1726, f. 73v, Sloane MS 4075, BL.

53. Sir Humphrey Mildmay, Diary (July 3, 1633–July 9, 1652), 21, W.b.600, Folger; Tyldesley, *Diary*, 157; Archer and Coe, *Two East Anglian Diaries*, 157.

54. Foxe, *Actes and Monuments*, 1209. Of the 358 martyrs in Foxe's book, 48 were women: see Hickerson, *Making Women Martyrs*.

55. Tyldesley, *Diary*, 64, 65, 66, 67, 75.

56. Ibid., 70, 71, 62, 63, 76.

57. For important scholarship that focuses on pain within an early modern medical context primarily using writing by healers, see Porter and Porter, *In Sickness and in Health*, 97–132; Stolberg, *Experiencing Illness and the Sick Body*, 27–32; Sawyer, "Patients, Healers, and Disease," 476–481; Silverman, *Tortured Subjects*, 133–151; Smith, " 'An Account of an Unaccountable Distemper' "; K. Walker, "A Gendered History of Pain in England."

For literary and textual representations of pain, see many of the valuable contributions to Van Dijkhuizen and Enenkel, eds., *The Sense of Suffering*.

58. In the introduction to their edition of his diary, Robert Latham and William Matthews suggest that Pepys's religious affiliation was purely political: Pepys, *Diary*, 1:cxx. On the Catholic baptism, see 7:329; on attending mass, see 2:102, 3:202.

59. Ibid., 4:318, 5:62.

60. Ibid., 9:337, 338, 370–371. For the other instance on which Elizabeth Pepys threatened to convert to Catholicism, see 5:92.

Chapter 6. Illness Narratives by the Poor

1. QSP/158/14, LA.

2. Ibid.; Cowper, Daily Diary, 1:55; DD\SE/45/1/87, SRO. For Hugh Sexey's charity in Somerset, I cite the reference numbers on the documents, which differ from those in the catalogue. Selling the bed was a common formulation: see also Q/SBb 23/5, ERO; MJ/SP/1711/09/23, LMA.

3. On hospitals, see Fissell, *Patients, Power, and the Poor;* Siena, *Venereal Disease, Hospitals and the Urban Poor;* Lawrence, *Charitable Knowledge;* Barry and Jones, *Medicine and Charity Before the Welfare State*. On pauper letters, see Snell, *Annals of the Labouring Poor;* Bailey, " 'Think Wot a Mother Must Feel' "; Sharpe, "Survival Strategies and Stories"; S. King, " 'Stop This Overwhelming Torrent of Destiny' "; Sokoll, *Essex Pauper Letters*. Steven King has attributed the wealth of sources for the later period to multiple factors, including but not limited to demographic changes, migration, and urbanization: "Voices of the Poor in the Long Eighteenth Century," xliv.

4. Of the petitions I examined, twenty-six refer to begging, all from these areas. On the geographical variations of poor relief, see S. King, *Poverty and Welfare in England*. The analysis in this chapter is based on petitions from the following archives: Cumbria Archive Centre in Carlisle, Cumbria Archive Centre in Kendal, Derbyshire Record Office, Devon Record Office, Essex Record Office, Lancashire Archives, London Metropolitan Archives, Somerset Record Office, West Yorkshire Archive Service, and Worcestershire Archive and Archaeology Service.

5. Exceptions here include petitioners seeking charitable gifts from Hugh Sexey's Hospital in Bruton, Somerset, and eight petitioners applying for admission to St. Thomas' Hospital and St. Bartholomew's Hospital in Lon-

don. I have found few differences in the rhetoric among petitions asking for charitable gifts, stipends from overseers, or admission to hospitals, despite the varying laws governing each. On these overlaps, see Fissell, *Patients, Power, and the Poor,* 99; Hindle, *On the Parish?,* 162. On hospital petitions, see Gray, "The Experience of Old Age"; Stein, *Negotiating the French Pox,* 123–136; Outhwaite, "'Objects of Charity.'" On petitions to poor law authorities, see Fessler, "The Official Attitude Towards the Sick Poor"; Hindle, *On the Parish?,* 405–428; Boulton, "Going to the Parish"; Withey, *Physick and the Family,* 179–190.

6. Q/SBa 2/82, ERO.

7. MJ/SP/1688/10/001, LMA. For this nineteenth-century example, see Sokoll, "Writing for Relief," 105. For additional examples from the 1600s, see Q/SB/2/1342, DRO Matlock; Q/SB/2/1346, DRO Matlock; Q/11/18/13, CAC Carlisle.

8. QSB/1/162/62, LA.

9. DD\SE/45/1/34, SRO; QSP/126/14, LA. Several historians have acknowledged paupers' tendency to embellish their stories to evoke sympathy: see P. Crawford, *Parents of Poor Children,* 27; Sokoll, *Essex Pauper Letters,* 68; Hudson, "Arguing Disability," 106; King and Tomkins, eds., *The Poor in England,* 17.

10. P76/JS1/124/11, LMA; P92/SAV/764, LMA. For a few additional examples of petitioners who emphasized their lengthy residence in the parish and their record of contributing to poor relief, see Q/11/34/3, CAC Carlisle; QSP/52/18, LA; DD\SE/45/1/46, SRO; Q/SPET/1/127, SRO.

11. Slack, *Poverty and Policy,* 17; Fissell, "The 'Sick and Drooping Poor'"; Fissell, *Patients, Power, and the Poor,* 3, 97–101.

12. QS1/14/4/6/4, WYAS; Q/SBb 32/22, ERO; DD\SE/45/1/4, SRO; Q/SPET/1/35, SRO; QSP/256/9, LA. For additional examples, see QSP/217/18, LA; QSP/123/14, LA; QSP/52/18, LA; QSB/1/202/81, LA; Q/11/7/16, CAC Carlisle; P92/SAV/777, LMA. For similar findings, see Hindle, *On the Parish?,* 383–386.

13. DD\SE/45/1/73, SRO; Q/11/46/43, CAC Carlisle. The charity granted Smart five shillings; Boradale's sum is lost. On the compromised masculinity of poor fathers, see P. Crawford, *Parents of Poor Children;* Bailey, "'Think Wot a Mother Must Feel,'" 9. On markers of manhood among nonhouseholding men, see Shepard, *Meanings of Manhood,* 186–195.

14. Q/11/8/17, CAC Carlisle; DD\SE/45/1/51, SRO; 1718 A-1/PO12, DRO Exeter. *Crazy* here means frail or weak. Patricia Crawford has found

a similar trend among poor mothers who listed the number of children they raised as a badge of public worth: *Parents of Poor Children*, 248.

15. Q/11/14/16, CAC Carlisle. See also Q/11/149/13, CAC Carlisle; QS1/14/8/6/9, WYAS.

16. Slack, *Poverty and Policy*, 25. For an overview of the above-defined categories, see Slack, *The English Poor Law;* Slack *Poverty and Policy*, 17–36.

17. On old age and poor relief, see Pelling, *The Common Lot*, 134–154; Ottaway, *The Decline of Life;* Botelho, *Old Age and the English Poor Law.*

18. Cowper, Daily Diary, 1:309; Freke, *Remembrances*, 157; P92/SAV/786, LMA. See also QSP/1089/6, LA. On the meanings of accidents in early modern England, see Porter, "Accidents in the Eighteenth Century." Other causes of ill health among petitioners included assault, bites from mad dogs, and emotions.

19. Q/11/28/22, CAC Carlisle; QS1/22/2/6/13, WYAS; Q/11/59/27, CAC Carlisle; MJ/SP/1708/05/03, LMA.

20. Pepys, *Diary*, 2:56, 4:71, 6:186, 7:168; Elias Pledger, Diary, f. 45v, MS 28.4, DWL. See also Jeake (younger), *Astrological Diary*, 182; Archer and Coe, *Two East Anglian Diaries*, 60; Sir Henry Goodricke to his son Savile, Feb. 8, 1639, V.b.333(1), Folger.

21. Edward Browne to Archbishop Sharp, June 19, 1695, D3549/6/1/B33, GA; Clegg, *Diary*, 1:18, 25, 76, 82, 84, 122–123, 2:361, 365, 372. On the physical toll of preaching, see also Thoresby, *Diary*, 1:350; Archer and Coe, *Two East Anglian Diaries*, 162; Heywood, *Autobiography, Diaries, Anecdote and Event Books*, 1:237; Robert Thomlinson to his brother Richard, 1720, ff. 271r, 273r, Sloane MS 4077, BL.

22. 1/1/155/88, WAAS. On this point about time, see chapter 4.

23. P76/JS1/125/5, LMA; Q/SBa 2/47, ERO.

24. Q/11/45/23, CAC Carlisle; Q/11/49/6, CAC Carlisle.

25. Pelling, *The Common Lot*, 85. Appendix B provides a full list of petitioners' complaints. An exception to my point about external ailments seems to be the 152 petitioners who cited "sickness," but even they tended to use this term in combination with words that signified a visible or disabling condition, such as *lame* or *infirm*.

26. QSP/52/18, LA; 1/1/153/70, WAAS; QSP/171/14, LA. See also QSP/126/14, LA.

27. Several historians have noted the prevalence of the term *lame* among the laboring poor: Fessler, "The Official Attitude Towards the Sick Poor," 97;

Pelling, *The Common Lot*, 72–73; Gray, "The Self-Perception of Chronic Physical Incapacity," 135.

28. Q/11/158/34, CAC Carlisle; Q/SB/2/640b, DRO Matlock; QSB/1/118/47, LA. There are too many additional examples to cite. For a few, see QSB/1/79/59, LA; Q/11/87/1, CAC Carlisle. For petitioners who could not get to court on account of illness, see Q/11/158/35, CAC Carlisle; Q/SB/2/319, DRO Matlock.

29. 1718 A-1/PO30, DRO Exeter; QSP/135/1, LA; Q/11/119/11, CAC Carlisle; QSB/1/266/65, LA; Q/SB/2/1346, DRO Matlock; DD\SE/45/1/43, SRO; Q/11/5/16, CAC Carlisle. For a full list of petitioners' occupations, see appendix B.

30. QSP/63/19, LA; P76/JS1/124/13B, LMA; DD\SE/45/1/57, SRO. Some noted fatal ailments to justify the need for life-saving treatment: Q/11/97/30, CAC Carlisle; Q/11/115/15, CAC Carlisle.

31. QSP/260/4, LA.

32. Q/11/96/8, CAC Carlisle. For examples of incredibly lengthy illnesses, see P92/SAV/750, LMA; DD\SE/45/1/79, SRO; Q/11/73/43, CAC Carlisle; Q/11/157/5, CAC Carlisle; Q/11/115/15, CAC Carlisle; Q/11/36/10, CAC Carlisle; QSP/101/3, LA; QSP/176/20, LA.

33. QSP/79/18, LA; QSP/215/21, LA.

34. QSP/270/2, LA; MJ/SP/1703/01/13, LMA; see also QSP/240/12, LA; QS1/55/2/6, WYAS. Some petitioners were born impaired, including the majority of the twenty here who cited "distraction," an early modern term for mental incapacity. On physical deformity and its meanings, see Pelling, "Appearance and Reality"; Fissell, *Vernacular Bodies*, 64–69; Fissell, *Patients, Power, and Poor*, 29–33.

35. Q/11/18/13, CAC Carlisle; Q/11/104/8, CAC Carlisle. For additional examples, see Q/SB/2/1346, DRO Matlock; DD\SE/45/1/13, SRO; QSP/176/20, LA; P76/JS1/124/12, LMA; DRO/002/E/04/002, LMA. The emphasis on selling material possessions also reflects a law that required paupers to forfeit their rights to property upon receiving parish relief (Hindle, *On the Parish?*, 78).

36. Q/11/59/2, CAC Carlisle; Q/11/128/16, CAC Carlisle.

37. Q/SB/2/1352, DRO Matlock. A substantial number of petitioners similarly noted a lack of friends or family to support them—too many to cite here. For a few, see Q/SB/2/327, DRO Matlock; Q/11/74/4, CAC Carlisle; Q/11/31/24, CAC Carlisle. Some petitioners asked for help after

exhausting their resources on ailing family members: see Q/11/156/2, CAC Carlisle; Q/11/96/9, CAC Carlisle.

38. QSB/1/118/48, LA; QSP/223/19, LA.

39. Q/11/67/21, CAC Carlisle; QSB/1/195/78, LA. See also QSP/63/24, LA.

40. Marten, *A Treatise of All the Degrees*, 154–155. On hospitals and treatment for impoverished venereal patients, see Siena, *Venereal Disease, Hospitals and the Urban Poor*.

41. Marten, *A Treatise of All the Degrees*, 155; quote from the patient's letter is on 225.

42. On these patterns in later sources, see Sharpe, "Survival Strategies and Stories"; Sharpe, "'The Bowels of Compation'"; S. King, "'Stop This Overwhelming Torrent of Destiny.'"

Conclusions

1. On this history, see Smith-Rosenberg and Rosenberg, "The Female Animal"; Smith-Rosenberg, *Disorderly Conduct;* Delamont and Duffin, eds., *The Nineteenth-Century Woman*. Some historians link the origins of these views of women's bodies to fundamental changes in conceptions of sex difference that developed in the late 1700s. Prior to this moment, so the argument goes, men and women were thought to differ only by a matter of degrees, not through and through. Fundamental distinctions between the sexes were only fully realized in the late eighteenth century, when political theorists, philosophers, and anatomists began looking to incommensurable sex differences to naturalize women's exclusion from civic and political roles. See Laqueur, *Making Sex;* Schiebinger, "Skeletons in the Closet."

2. On the reciprocal relationship between culture and science, see especially Martin, "The Egg and the Sperm."

3. Mortimer, *The Dying and the Doctors;* Thomas, *Religion and the Decline of Magic*. On the sustained roles of religion and morality in shaping medical theories and physicians' self-presentations, see Sumich, *Divine Doctors and Dreadful Distempers*.

4. Cowper, Daily Diary, 1:51.

5. Some non-Western modern cultures do view illness in socially embedded ways that resonate with early modern accounts. See, for example, Livingston, *Debility and the Moral Imagination in Botswana;* Janzen and Arkinstall, *The Quest for Therapy in Lower Zaire*.

Appendix A

1. Archer and Coe, *Two East Anglian Diaries*, 88. On Archer's life, see 1–27; on his father's will, see 123, 186–187.
2. On Cowper's life, see Kugler, *Errant Plagiary*, which links the trial to Cowper's diary writing on 3. On the scandals surrounding Cowper's sons, see Knights, *The Devil in Disguise*.
3. Mary E. O'Connor, "Dormer [née Cottrell], Anne," in *Oxford Dictionary of National Biography*, ed. H. C. G. Matthew and Brian Harrison (Oxford: Oxford University Press, 2004), at www.oxforddnb.com. See also Mendelson, "Neighbourhood as Female Community"; O'Connor, "Interpreting Early Modern Woman Abuse."
4. On Freke's health and medical work, see Leong, "Making Medicines"; Anselment, "'The Wantt of Health.'"
5. See Jeake (younger), *Astrological Diary*, 1–81. For the elder Jeake's library, see Jeake (elder), *A Radical's Books*.
6. Pepys, *Diary*, 4:128–129, 5:220. On Pepys's life, see Tomalin, *Samuel Pepys*.
7. On Rich, see Palgrave, *Mary Rich;* Mendelson, *The Mental World of Stuart Women;* Wray, "[Re]constructing the Past."
8. D. Ryder, *Diary*, 90; David Lemmings, "Ryder, Sir Dudley," in *Oxford Dictionary of National Biography*, ed. H. C. G. Matthew and Brian Harrison (Oxford: Oxford University Press, 2004), at www.oxforddnb.com.
9. See Anselment, "The Deliverance of Alice Thornton"; Anselment, "'My First Booke of My Life'"; George, *Women in the First Capitalist Society*, 168–179.

Bibliography

Manuscript Sources

BRITISH LIBRARY, LONDON

Arthur Annesley, Diary, Add. MSS 18730 (1673–1684), 40860 (1671–1675)

Katherine Austen, Meditations in Prose and Verse (1664–1668), Add. MS 4454

Barrington Papers, Egerton MS 2644

Joseph Binns, Medical Casebook, Sloane MS 153

Blenheim Papers, Add. MSS 61461, 61607

William Briggs, Correspondence, Sloane MS 123

Anne Dawson, Diary (1721–1722), Add. MS 71626

Dering Correspondence, Stowe MS 745

Simonds D'Ewes, Correspondence, Harleian MS 382

Elizabeth Egerton, Countess of Bridgewater, Devotional Pieces, c. 1648–1663, Egerton MS 607

Evelyn Correspondence, Add. MS 15949

Freke Papers, Add. MSS 45718, 45719

Thomas Garlick, Praxis Chyrurgiae, Sloane MS 2263

Gawdy Correspondence, Add. MS 27395, Egerton MS 2715

Henry Papers, Add. MS 42849

Sir Edmund King, M.D., Medical Papers and Collections, Sloane MS 1589

Adam Martindale, Autobiography, Add. MS 4239

James Molins, Medical treatise and receipts, Sloane MS 3293

North Papers, Add. MSS 32500, 32501

Paston Papers, Add. MSS 27447, 36988

Sir William Petty, Papers, Add. MS 72891

Mary Rich, Diary, Autobiography (1625–1674), and Occasional Meditations (1663–1677), Add. MSS 27351–27357

Hans Sloane Correspondence, Sloane MSS 4034, 4037, 4042, 4048, 4059, 4061, 4066, 4075–4078
Trumbull Papers, Add. MSS 72425, 72439, 72442, 72516, 72518
Nehemiah Wallington, Spiritual Diary of Nehemiah Wallington (1641–1643), Add. MS 40883

CHESHIRE ARCHIVES AND LOCAL STUDIES, CHESTER
Cholmondeley Papers, DCH
Leicester-Warren Papers, DLT
Shakerley Correspondence, DSS

CHETHAM'S LIBRARY, MANCHESTER
Edmund Harrold, His Book of Remarks and Observations, 1712–16, MS Mun. A.2.137

CUMBRIA ARCHIVE CENTRE, CARLISLE
Quarter Session Rolls, Q/11

CUMBRIA ARCHIVE CENTRE, KENDAL
Westmorland Quarter Sessions, WQ/SR/1–99

DERBYSHIRE RECORD OFFICE, MATLOCK
Session Papers, Q/SB/2

DEVON RECORD OFFICE, EXETER
Holy Trinity Parish Petitions, 1718 A-1/PO9–33

DR. WILLIAMS'S LIBRARY, LONDON
Elias Pledger, Diary, MS 28.4
Say Papers, MS 12.107
Owen Stockton, Diary (1665–1677), MS 24.7

ESSEX RECORD OFFICE, CHELMSFORD
Holman Manuscripts, D/Y/1
Sessions Bundles, Q/SBa, Q/SBb

FOLGER SHAKESPEARE LIBRARY, WASHINGTON DC

An Account of the Lady Lucy, 1675, V.a.166

Cavendish-Talbot Papers, X.d.428

Lydia Dugard (1650–1675), Autograph letters signed, to Samuel Dugard, X.d.477

Goodricke Papers, V.b.333

Mary Hookes, Receipt Book, 1680, Add. 931

Sir Humphrey Mildmay, Diary (July 3, 1633–July 9, 1652), W.b.600

Susannah Packe, Receipt Book, 1674, V.a.215

Sunderland Correspondence, Add. 764

Nehemiah Wallington, An Extract of the Passages of My Life (1654), V.a.436

GLOUCESTERSHIRE ARCHIVES, GLOUCESTER

Lloyd-Baker Papers, D3549

Moreton Correspondence, D340a/C

Sturmy Correspondence, D2375

HUNTINGTON LIBRARY, SAN MARINO, CA

Magdalen Coward, Book of Receipts, 1695, HM 88

Edward Dering, Journal (1675–1679), HM 55605

Elizabeth (Stanley) Hastings, Commonplace Book, HM 15369

Hastings Papers, HA

North Papers, HM 52322–52420

LANCASHIRE ARCHIVES, PRESTON

Hulton Correspondence, DDHU 47/1–33

Kenyon Correspondence, DDKE/9

Quarter Sessions Petitions, QSP

Quarter Sessions Recognizance Rolls, QSB/1

LONDON METROPOLITAN ARCHIVES

Middlesex Sessions of the Peace, MJ/SP

Petition for Poor Relief, Saint Mary, Staines: Surrey, DRO/002/E/04/002

Saint James, Clerkenwell, Parish Records, P76/JS1/124/1–22, P76/JS1/125/1–16

Saint Saviour's, Southwark, Parish Records, P92/SAV/749–786

ROYAL COLLEGE OF PHYSICIANS, LONDON

George Colebrook, Letters on Medical Cases (c. 1690), MS 206/4

Samuel England, Notebook Containing Prescriptions and Case Notes, 1730–33, MSS 5–6

SOMERSET RECORD OFFICE, TAUNTON

John Cannon, Manuscript Diary of John Cannon, Schoolmaster of Meare, Exciseman, Etc. (1684–1742), DD\SAS\C1193\4

Petitions to Hugh Sexey's Hospital, DD\SE\45\1–2

Quarter Sessions Petitions, Q/SPET/1

Sanford Family Correspondence, DD\SF

Trevelyan Papers, DD\WO

John Westover, Medical Diary and Account Book of John Westover of Wedmore (1685–1700), DD/X/HKN 1

WELLCOME LIBRARY, LONDON

Cary Correspondence, MS 6140

The Case Book of a General Practitioner (1726–1728), MS 7501

Miscellanea XII, MS 805

Alexander Morgan, Medical Casebook, MS 3631

Richard Wilkes, Observations on Particular Cases of Patients (1731–1742), MS 5005

WEST YORKSHIRE ARCHIVE SERVICE, WAKEFIELD

West Riding Quarter Sessions Rolls, QS1

WORCESTERSHIRE ARCHIVE AND ARCHAEOLOGY
SERVICE, WORCESTER

Quarter Sessions Rolls, QSP 1/1

YALE UNIVERSITY, STERLING MEMORIAL LIBRARY,
NEW HAVEN, CT

Alice Wandesford Thornton, A Book of Remembrances, Microfilm MISC 326

OTHER: TRANSCRIPTIONS/REPRODUCTIONS OF MANUSCRIPTS

Sarah Cowper, Daily Diary, MSS D/EP/F29–35, Hertfordshire Public Record Office, Hertford. Reproduced in Amanda Vickery, ed., *Women's Language and Experience, 1500–1940*, microfilm, part 1, reels 5–7. Marlborough: Adam Matthew Publications, 1994.

Elizabeth Isham, My Booke of Rememenberance, MS RTCO1 (no. 62), Robert H. Taylor Collection, Princeton University Library, Princeton, NJ. Cited from unpublished transcription by Isaac Stephens.

Printed Primary Sources

Allestree, Richard. *The Ladies Calling*. Oxford: Printed at the Theater, 1673.

———. *The Whole Duty of Man Laid Down in a Plain Way for the Meanest Reader*. London: Printed for T. Garthwait, 1659.

Ambrose, Isaac. *Redeeming the Time: A Sermon Preached at Preston in Lancashire, January 4th, 1657, at the Funerall of the Honourable Lady, the Lady Margaret Houghton*. London: Printed by T.C. for Nath. Webb and William Grantham, 1658.

Archer, Isaac, and William Coe. *Two East Anglian Diaries, 1641–1729: Isaac Archer and William Coe*. Ed. Matthew Storey and David Dymond. Woodbridge: Boydell Press, 1994.

Archer, John. *Secrets Disclosed, of Consumptions*. London: Printed for the author, 1684.

Augustine, Saint. *Confessions*. Ed. Henry Chadwick. Oxford: Oxford University Press, 1998.

Bacon, Jane Cornwallis. *The Private Correspondence of Jane Lady Cornwallis Bacon, 1613–1644*. Ed. Joanna Moody. Madison: Fairleigh Dickinson University Press, 2003.

Barbette, Paul. *The Chirurgical and Anatomical Works of Paul Barbette, M.D., Practitioner at Amsterdam*. London: Printed by J. Darby, 1672.

Barlow, Edward. *Barlow's Journal of His Life at Sea in King's Ships, East and West Indiamen and Other Marchantmen from 1659 to 1703*. Ed. Basil Lubbock. 2 vols. London: Hurst and Blackett, 1934.

Baxter, Richard. *Reliquiae Baxterianae; or, Mr. Richard Baxter's Narrative of the Most Memorable Passages of His Life and Times*. Vol. 1. London: Printed for T. Parkhurst, J. Robinson, F. Lawrence, and F. Dunton, 1696.

Beadle, John. *The Journal or Diary of a Thankful Christian*. London: Printed by E. Cotes for Tho. Parkhurst, 1656.

Beckett, William. *Practical Surgery Illustrated and Improved*. London: Printed for E. Curll, 1740.

Becon, Thomas. *The Sycke Mans Salue Wherin the Faithfull Christians May Learne Both How to Behaue Them Selues Paciently and Thankefully, in the Tyme of Sickenes*. London: Iohn Day, 1561.

Behn, Aphra. *Oroonoko; or, The Royal Slave*. 1688. Reprint: New York: W. W. Norton, 1997.

Belloste, Augustin. *The Hospital Surgeon*. London: Printed for J. and B. Sprint, J. Nicholson, A. Bell, and R. Smith, 1713.

Blundell, Nicholas. *The Great Diurnal of Nicholas Blundell*. Ed. J. J. Bagley and Frank Tyrer. 3 vols. Liverpool: C. Tinling, 1968–1972.

Bonet, Théophile. *A Guide to the Practical Physician*. London: Printed for Thomas Flesher, 1684.

Bright, Timothie. *A Treatise of Melancholie Containing the Causes Thereof, and Reasons of the Strange Effects It Worketh in Our Minds and Bodies*. London: Thomas Vautrollier, 1586.

Bunyan, John. *Grace Abounding to the Chief of Sinners; or, A Brief and Faithful Relation of the Exceeding Mercy of God in Christ, to His Poor Servant John Bvnyan*. London: Printed by George Larkin, 1666.

Burton, Robert. *The Anatomy of Melancholy, What It Is: With All the Kindes, Causes, Symptomes, Prognostickes, and Seuerall Cures of It*. Oxford: Printed by Iohn Lichfield and Iames Short for Henry Cripps, 1621.

Calverley, Sir Walter. "Memorandum Book of Sir Walter Calverley, Bart." In *Yorkshire Diaries and Autobiographies in the Seventeenth and Eighteenth Centuries*, ed. S. Margerison, 43–148. Durham: Andrews, 1886.

Cam, Joseph. *A Practical Treatise; or, Second Thoughts on the Consequences of the Venereal Disease*. London: Printed for the author, 1724.

Charleton, Walter. *A Natural History of the Passions*. London: Printed for R. Wellington, and E. Rumball, 1701.

Clegg, James. *The Diary of James Clegg of Chapel-En-Le Frith, 1708–55*. Ed. Vanessa S. Doe. 3 vols. Chesterfield: Derbyshire Record Society, 1978.

Clever, Robert, and John Dod. *A Godlie Forme of Householde Government for the Ordering of Private Families*. London: Printed for Thomas Man, 1612.

Clifford, Anne. *The Diaries of Lady Anne Clifford*. Ed. D. J. H. Clifford. Wolfeboro Falls: Alan Sutton, 1990.

———. *The Diary of Anne Clifford, 1616–1619: A Critical Edition*. Ed. Katherine O. Acheson. New York: Garland, 1995.

Colbatch, John. *Four Treatises of Physick and Chirurgery*. London: Printed by J.D. for Daniel Brown, 1698.

———. *Novum Lumen Chirurgicum; or, A New Light of Chirurgery*. London: Printed for D. Brown, 1698.

———. *A Treatise of the Gout: Wherein Both Its Cause and Cure Are Demonstrably Made Appear*. London: Printed for Daniel Brown and Roger Clavel, 1697.

Colinson, Robert. *Idea rationaria; or, The Perfect Accomptant, Necessary for All Merchants and Trafficquers.* Edinburgh: Printed by David Lindsay, James Kniblo, Josua van Solingen, and John Colmar, 1683.

Conway, Anne. *Conway Letters: The Correspondence of Anne, Viscountess Conway, Henry More, and Their Friends, 1642–1684.* Ed. Marjorie Hope Nicolson, revised ed. by Sarah Hutton. Oxford: Clarendon Press, 1992.

Crooke, Helkiah. *Mikrokosmographia: A Description of the Body of Man.* London: Printed by W. Iaggard, 1618.

Davies, Rowland. *Journal of the Very Rev. Rowland Davies, LL.D., Dean of Ross (and Afterwards Dean of Cork), from March 8, 1688–9, to September 29, 1690.* Ed. Richard Caulfield. London: Printed for the Camden Society, 1858.

Delaval, Elizabeth. *The Meditations of Lady Elizabeth Delaval, Written Between 1662 and 1671.* Ed. Douglas G. Greene. Gateshead: Northumberland Press, 1975.

D'Ewes, Simonds. *The Diary of Sir Simonds D'Ewes (1622–1624).* Ed. Elizabeth Bourcier. Paris: Didier, 1974.

Digby, Kenelm. *A Late Discourse Made . . . Touching the Cure of Wounds.* London: Printed by J.G., 1664.

Douglas, John. *A Short Account of Mortifications, and of the Surprizing Effect of the Bark, in Putting a Stop to Their Progress, &c.* London: Printed for John Nourse, 1732.

Dover, Thomas. *The Ancient Physician's Legacy to His Country, Being What He Has Collected in Forty-Nine Years Practice.* London: Printed for the Relict of the late R. Bradly, F.R.S., 1733.

Dubé, Paul. *The Poor Man's Physician and Surgeon.* London: Printed for T. Newborough, T. Leigh, and D. Midwinter, 1704.

Evelyn, John. *The Diary of John Evelyn.* Ed. E. S. DeBeer. Oxford: Clarendon Press, 1955.

Eyre, Adam. "A Diurnall, or Catalogue of All My Accounts and Expences from the 1st of January, 1646–(7)." In *Yorkshire Diaries and Autobiographies in the Seventeenth and Eighteenth Centuries,* ed. H. J. Morehouse, 1–118. Durham: Andrews, 1877.

Foxe, John. *Actes and Monuments of These Latter and Perillous Dayes, Touching Matters of the Church.* London: Printed by Iohn Daye, 1576.

Freke, Elizabeth. *The Remembrances of Elizabeth Freke, 1671–1714.* Ed. Raymond A. Anselment. Cambridge: Cambridge University Press, 2001.

General Observations and Prescriptions in the Pra[c]tice of Physick. London: Printed for W. Mears, J. Brown, and T. Woodward, 1715.

Giffard, Martha. *Martha, Lady Giffard, Her Life and Correspondence (1664–1722): A Sequel to the Letters of Dorothy Osborne.* Ed. Julia G. Longe. London: George Allen and Sons, 1911.

Gouge, William. *Of Domesticall Duties.* London: Printed by George Miller for Edward Brewster, 1634.

Halkett, Anne. *Lady Anne Halkett: Selected Self-Writings.* Ed. Suzanne Trill. Aldershot: Ashgate, 2007.

Halkett, Anne, and Ann Fanshawe. *The Memoirs of Anne, Lady Halkett, and Ann, Lady Fanshawe.* Ed. John Loftis. Oxford: Clarendon Press, 1979.

Hamilton, David. *The Diary of Sir David Hamilton, 1709–1714.* Ed. Philip Roberts. Oxford: Clarendon Press, 1975.

Harcourt, Anne. "Occasional Memoirs, Prayers and Lists of Mercies, c. 1649–61." In *The Harcourt Papers,* ed. E. W. Harcourt, 1:169–199. Oxford, 1876.

Harley, Brilliana. *Letters of the Lady Brilliana Harley, Wife of Sir Robert Harley, of Brampton Bryan, Knight of the Bath.* Ed. Thomas Taylor Lewis. London: Camden Society, 1854.

Harris, John. *The Divine Physician, Prescribing Rules for the Prevention and Cure of Most Diseases, as Well of the Body, as the Soul.* [London?]: Printed for George Rose by Nath. Brook and Will. Whitwood, 1676.

Harrold, Edmund. *The Diary of Edmund Harrold, Wigmaker of Manchester, 1712–15.* Ed. Craig Horner. Aldershot: Ashgate, 2008.

Heywood, Oliver. *Oliver Heywood's Life of John Angier, Together with Angier's Diary, and Extracts from His "An Helpe to Better Hearts."* Ed. Ernest Axon. Manchester: Chetham Society, 1937.

———. *The Rev. Oliver Heywood, B.A., 1630–1702: His Autobiography, Diaries, Anecdote and Event Books: Illustrating the General and Family History of Yorkshire and Lancashire.* Ed. J. Horsfall Turner. 4 vols. Brighouse: A. B. Bayes, 1881–1885.

Hooke, Robert. *The Diary of Robert Hooke, M.A., M.D., F.R.S., 1672–1680, Transcribed from the Original in the Possession of the Corporation of the City of London.* Ed. Henry W. Robinson and Walter Adams. London: Taylor and Francis, 1935.

James, Robert. *A Medicinal Dictionary.* London: Printed for T. Osborne, 1743.

Jeake, Samuel (elder). *A Radical's Books: The Library Catalogue of Samuel Jeake of Rye, 1623–90.* Ed. Michael Hunter, Giles Mandelbrote, Richard Ovenden, and Nigel Smith. Woodbridge: D. S. Brewer, 1999.

Jeake, Samuel (younger). *An Astrological Diary of the Seventeenth Century: Samuel Jeake of Rye, 1652–1699.* Ed. Michael Hunter and Annabel Gregory. Oxford: Clarendon Press, 1988.

The Jesuit Relations: Natives and Missionaries in Seventeenth-Century North America. Ed. Allan Greer. Boston: Bedford/St. Martin's, 2000.

Jolly, Thomas. *The Note Book of the Rev. Thomas Jolly, AD 1671–1693.* Ed. Henry Fishwick. Manchester: Chetham Society, 1894.

Kettilby, Mary. *A Collection of Above Three Hundred Receipts in Cookery, Physick and Surgery.* London: Printed for Richard Wilkin, 1714.

Kettlewell, John. *Death Made Comfortable; or, The Way to Dye Well: Consisting of Directions for an Holy and an Happy Death.* London: Printed for Robert Kettlewell, 1695.

Knyvett, Thomas. *The Knyvett Letters, 1620–1644.* Ed. Bertram Schofield. London: Constable, 1949.

Letters Addressed to Ralph Thoresby, FRS. Ed. W. T. Lancaster. Leeds: Thoresby Society, 1912.

Lightbody, James. *Every Man His Own Gauger.* London: Printed for G.C., 1695.

Lister, Joseph. *The Autobiography of Joseph Lister, of Bradford in Yorkshire.* Ed. Thomas Wright, Esq., M.A., F.S.A. London: John Russell Smith, 1842.

Lowe, Roger. *The Diary of Roger Lowe, of Ashton-in-Makerfield, Lancashire, 1663–74.* Ed. William L. Sachse. New Haven: Yale University Press, 1938.

Markham, Gervase. *The English House-Wife.* London: Printed for Hannah Sawbridge, 1683.

Marten, John. *A Treatise of All the Degrees and Symptoms of the Venereal Disease.* London: Printed for S. Crouch, N. Crouch, J. Knapton, W. Hawes, P. Varenne, C. King, and J. Isted, 1707.

Mayne, John. *Arithmetick Vulgar, Decimal, and Algebraical.* London: Printed for J.A., 1675.

Medical Essays and Observations. Vol. 1. Edinburgh: Printed by T. and W. Ruddimans for Mr. William Monro, 1733.

Moore, Giles. *The Journal of Giles Moore.* Ed. Ruth Bird. Lewes: Sussex Record Society, 1971.

Morris, Claver. *The Diary of a West County Physician, AD 1684–1726.* Ed. Edmund Hodhouse, M.D. London: Simpkin Marshall, 1934.

Oglander, John. *A Royalist's Notebook: The Commonplace Book of Sir John Oglander, Kt., of Nunwell.* Ed. Francis Bamford. London: Constable, 1936.

Patrick, Simon. *The Book of Job Paraphras'd by Symon Patrick.* London: E. Flesher for R. Royston, 1679.

Pepys, Samuel. *The Diary of Samuel Pepys: A New and Complete Transcription.* Ed. Robert Latham and William Matthews. 11 vols. Berkeley: University of California Press, 1970–1983.

————. *The Further Correspondence of Samuel Pepys, 1662–1679,* ed. J. R. Tanner (London: G. Bell and Sons, 1929).

————. *The Private Correspondence and Miscellaneous Papers of Samuel Pepys, 1679–1703.* Ed. J. R. Tanner. 2 vols. New York: Harcourt Brace, 1926.

Powell, Walter. *The Diary of Walter Powell of Llantilio Crossenny in the County of Monmouth, Gentleman, 1603–1654.* Bristol: J. Wright, 1907.

Rivière, Lazare. *Four Books of That Learned and Renowned Doctor, Lazarus Riverius, Containing Five Hundred and Thirteen Observations or Histories of Famous and Rare Cures.* London: Printed by John Streater, 1672.

Ryder, Dudley. *The Diary of Dudley Ryder, 1715–1716.* Ed. William Matthews. London: Methuen, 1939.

Ryder, Hugh. *New Practical Observations in Surgery.* London: Printed for James Partridge, Stationer to His Royal Highness Prince George of Denmark, 1685.

————. *Practical Chirurgery: Being a Methodical Account of Divers Eminent Observations, Cases, and Cures.* London: Printed for John Taylor and Sam Holford, 1689.

Salmon, William. *Collectanea Medica, the Country Physician.* London: Printed for John Taylor, 1703.

————. *Iatrica; seu, Praxis Medendi, the Practice of Curing: Being a Medicinal History of Above Three Thousand Famous Observations in the Cure of Diseases.* London: Printed for To. Dawks and Langley Curtiss, 1681.

————. *Parateremata; or, Select Physical and Chyrurgical Observations.* London: Printed for Thomas Passinger and John Richardson, 1687.

Sherlock, William. *A Practical Discourse Concerning Death.* London: Printed for W. Rogers, 1689.

Sidney, Dorothy. *Sacharissa: Some Account of Dorothy Sidney, Countess of Sunderland, Her Family and Friends, 1617–1684.* Ed. Julia Cartwright. New York: Scribner, 1893.

Sintelaer, John. *The Scourge of Venus and Mercury.* London: Printed for G. Harris, 1709.

Stone, Sarah. *A Complete Practice of Midwifery: Consisting of Upwards of Forty Cases or Observations in That Valuable Art.* London: Printed for T. Cooper, 1737.

Stout, William. *The Autobiography of William Stout of Lancaster, 1665–1752.* Ed. J. D. Marshall. Manchester: Manchester University Press, 1967.

Symcotts, John. *A Seventeenth-Century Doctor and His Patients: John Symcotts, 1592?–1662*. Ed. F. N. L. Poynter and W. J. Bishop. Vol. 31. Bedfordshire: Bedfordshire Historical Record Society, 1951.

Talbor, Robert. *Pyretologia, a Rational Account of the Cause and Cure of Agues*. London: Printed for R. Robinson, 1672.

Taylor, Jeremy. *The Rule and Exercises of Holy Dying: In Which Are Described the Means and Instruments of Preparing Our Selves, and Others Respectively, for a Blessed Death*. London: Printed by Roger Norton for Richard Royston, 1670.

Thoresby, Ralph. *The Diary of Ralph Thoresby, FRS, Author of the Topography of Leeds (1677–1724)*. Ed. Joseph Hunter. 2 vols. London: Henry Colburn and Richard Bentley, 1830.

Thornton, Alice. *The Autobiography of Mrs. Alice Thornton*. Ed. Charles Jackson. Surtees Society 62. London: Andrews, 1875.

Tyldesley, Thomas. *The Tyldesley Diary: Personal Records of Thomas Tyldesley (Grandson of Sir Thomas Tyldesley, the Royalist), During the Years 1712–13–14*. Ed. Joseph Gillow and Anthony Hewitson. Preston: A. Hewitson, 1873.

Vernon, John. *The Compleat Compting-House; or, The Young Lad Taken from the Writing-School, and Fully Instructed, by Way of Dialogue, in All the Mysteries of a Merchant*. Dublin: Printed for G. Grierson, 1719.

Vives, Juan Luis. *The Instruction of a Christen Woman*. 1529. Trans. Richard Hyrde. Ed. Virginia Walcott Beauchamp, Elizabeth Hageman, and Margaret Miskell. Urbana: University of Illinois Press, 2002.

W., F. *Warm Beere; or, A Treatise Wherein Is Declared by Many Reasons, That Beere So Qualified Is Farre More Wholsome then That Which Is Drunke Cold*. Cambridge: Printed by R.D. for Henry Overton, 1641.

Wagstaffe, Thomas. *A Letter out of Suffolk to a Friend in London, Giving Some Account of the Last Sickness and Death of Dr. William Sancroft*. London, 1694.

Walker, Anthony. *Eureka, Eureka: The Virtuous Woman Found, Her Loss Bewailed, and Character Examined in a Sermon Preached at Felsted in Essex, April 30, 1678, at the Funeral of . . . Mary, Countess Dowager of Warwick*. London: Printed for Nathanael Ranew, 1678.

Walkington, Thomas. *The Optick Glasse of Humors; or, The Touchstone of a Golden Temperature; or, The Philosophers Stone to Make a Golden Temper*. London: Imprinted by Iohn Windet for Martin Clerke, 1607.

Walwyn, William. *Physick for Families*. London: Printed by J.R., 1681.

Ward, John. *Diary of the Rev. John Ward, A.M., Vicar of Stratford-upon-Avon, Extending from 1648 to 1679*. Ed. Charles Severn. London: Henry Colburn, 1839.

White, John. *A Way to the Tree of Life Discovered in Sundry Directions for the Profitable Reading of the Scriptvres*. London: Printed by M.F. for R. Royston, 1647.

Willis, Thomas. *An Essay of the Pathology of the Brain and Nervous Stock*. London: Printed by J.B. for T. Dring, 1681.

———. *Pharmaceutice Rationalis; or, An Exercitation of the Operations of Medicines in Humane Bodies*. London: Printed for Thomas Dring, Charles Harper, and John Leigh, 1679.

Wiseman, Richard. *Severall Chirurgicall Treatises*. London: Printed by E. Flesher and J. Macock for R. Royston and B. Took, 1676.

Woodman, Philip. *Medicus Novissimus; or, The Modern Physician*. London: Printed by J.H. for Chr. Comingsby, 1712.

Woolley, Hannah. *The Accomplish'd Ladies Delight in Preserving, Physick, Beautifying and Cookery*. London: Printed for Benjamin Harris, 1684.

Wright, Thomas. *The Passions of the Minde*. London: Printed by V[alentine] S[immes] for W. B[urre], 1601.

Yonge, James. *Currus triumphalis, e Terebintho; or, An Account of the Many Admirable Vertues of Oleum Terebinthine*. London: Printed for J. Martyn, Printer to the Royal Society, 1679.

Secondary Sources

Alberti, Fay Bound. "Emotions in the Early Modern Medical Tradition." In *Medicine, Emotion and Disease, 1700–1950*, ed. Alberti, 1–21. Houndmills: Palgrave Macmillan, 2006.

Amelang, James S. *The Flight of Icarus: Artisan Autobiography in Early Modern Europe*. Stanford: Stanford University Press, 1998.

Anselment, Raymond A. "The Deliverance of Alice Thornton: The Re-creation of a Seventeenth-Century Life." *Prose Studies* 19 (1996): 19–36.

———. "Elizabeth Freke's Remembrances: Reconstructing a Self." *Tulsa Studies in Women's Literature* 16 (1997): 57–75.

———. "Mary Rich, Countess of Warwick, and the Gift of Tears." *Seventeenth Century* 22 (2007): 336–357.

———. " 'My First Booke of My Life': The Apology of a Seventeenth-Century Gentry Woman." *Prose Studies* 24 (2001): 1–14.

———. "Seventeenth-Century Manuscript Sources of Alice Thornton's Life." *Studies in English Literature* 45 (2005): 135–155.

————. "'The Wantt of Health': An Early Eighteenth-Century Self-Portrait of Sickness." *Literature and Medicine* 15, no. 2 (1996): 225–243.

Ashworth, William B., Jr. "Natural History and the Emblematic World View." In *Reappraisals of the Scientific Revolution*, ed. David C. Lindberg and Robert S. Westman, 303–332. Cambridge: Cambridge University Press, 1990.

Bailey, Joanne. "'Think Wot a Mother Must Feel': Parenting in English Pauper Letters, c. 1760–1834." *Family and Community History* 13 (2010): 5–19.

Barker, Hannah. "Soul, Purse and Family: Middling and Lower-Class Masculinity in Eighteenth-Century Manchester." *Social History* 33 (2008): 12–35.

Barry, Jonathan, and Colin Jones. *Medicine and Charity Before the Welfare State.* New York: Routledge, 1991.

Beier, Lucinda McCray. *Sufferers and Healers: The Experience of Illness in Seventeenth-Century England.* London: Routledge, 1987.

Bendelow, Gillian. *Pain and Gender.* Harlow: Prentice Hall, 2000.

Bending, Lucy. *The Representation of Bodily Pain in Late Nineteenth-Century English Culture.* Oxford: Clarendon Press, 2000.

Botelho, L. A. *Old Age and the English Poor Law, 1500–1700.* Woodbridge: Boydell Press, 2004.

Botonaki, Effie. "Seventeenth-Century Englishwomen's Spiritual Diaries: Self-Examination, Covenanting, and Account Keeping." *Sixteenth Century Journal* 30 (1999): 3–21.

Boulton, Jeremy. "Going to the Parish: The Parish Pension and Its Meaning in the London Suburbs, 1640–1724." In *Chronicling Poverty: The Voices and Strategies of the English Poor, 1640–1840.* Ed. Tim Hitchcock, Peter King, and Pamela Sharpe, 19–46. Houndmills: Macmillan Press, 1997.

Bound, Fay. "'An Angry and Malicious Mind'? Narratives of Slander at the Church Courts of York, c. 1660–c. 1760." *History Workshop Journal* 56 (2003): 59–77.

————. "Writing the Self? Love and the Letter in England, c. 1660–c. 1760." *Literature and History* 11 (2002): 1–19.

Bourke, Joanna. "Fear and Anxiety: Writing about Emotion in Modern History." *History Workshop Journal* 55 (2003): 111–133.

Brady, Andrea. "'A Share of Sorrows': Death in the Early Modern English Household." In *Emotions in the Household, 1200–1900*, ed. Susan Broomhall, 185–202. New York: Palgrave Macmillan, 2007.

Broomhall, Susan. *Women's Medical Work in Early Modern France.* Manchester: Manchester University Press, 2004.

————, ed. *Emotions in the Household, 1200–1900.* New York: Palgrave Macmillan, 2007.

Brown, Kathleen M. *Foul Bodies: Cleanliness in Early America.* New Haven: Yale University Press, 2009.

Bryan, Jennifer. *Looking Inward: Devotional Reading and the Private Self in Late Medieval England.* Philadelphia: University of Pennsylvania Press, 2008.

Bynum, Caroline Walker. *Fragmentation and Redemption: Essays on Gender and the Human Body in Medieval Religion.* New York: Zone Books, 1991.

Bynum, W. F., and Roy Porter, eds. *Medical Fringe and Medical Orthodoxy, 1750– 1850.* London: Croom Helm, 1987.

Cambers, Andrew. "Reading, the Godly, and Self-Writing in England, circa 1580–1720." *Journal of British Studies* 46 (2007): 796–825.

Carrera, Elena, ed. *Emotions and Health, 1200–1700.* Leiden: Brill, 2013.

Churchill, Wendy D. "Bodily Differences? Gender, Race, and Class in Hans Sloane's Jamaican Medical Practice, 1687–1688." *Journal of the History of Medicine and Allied Sciences* 60 (2005): 391–444.

————. *Female Patients in Early Modern Britain: Gender, Diagnosis, and Treatment.* Burlington: Ashgate, 2012.

Clark, Stuart. *Vanities of the Eye: Vision in Early Modern European Culture.* Oxford: Oxford University Press, 2007.

Clericuzio, Antonio. "From van Helmont to Boyle: A Study of the Transmission of Helmontian Chemical and Medical Theories in Seventeenth-Century England." *British Journal for the History of Science* 26 (1993): 303–334.

Cohen, Esther. "The Animated Pain of the Body." *American Historical Review* 105, no. 1 (2000): 36–68.

————. *The Modulated Scream: Pain in Late Medieval Culture.* Chicago: University of Chicago Press, 2009.

Cook, Harold J. *The Decline of the Old Medical Regime in Stuart London.* Ithaca: Cornell University Press, 1986.

————. "Sir John Colbatch and Augustan Medicine: Experimentalism, Character and Entrepreneurialism." *Annals of Science* 47 (1990): 475–505.

————. *Trials of an Ordinary Doctor: Joannes Groenevelt in Seventeenth-Century London.* Baltimore: Johns Hopkins University Press, 1994.

Cooper, Tim. "Richard Baxter and His Physicians." *Social History of Medicine* 20 (2007): 1–20.

Craik, Katharine A. *Reading Sensations in Early Modern England.* New York: Palgrave, 2007.

Crawford, Catherine. "Patients' Rights and the Law of Contract in Eighteenth-Century London." *Social History of Medicine* 13 (2000): 381–410.

Crawford, Patricia. "Attitudes to Menstruation in Seventeenth-Century England." *Past and Present* 91 (1981): 47–73.

———. *Parents of Poor Children in England, 1580–1800.* Oxford: Oxford University Press, 2010.

———. *Women and Religion in England, 1500–1720.* London: Routledge, 1993.

Davis, Natalie Zemon. *Women on the Margins: Three Seventeenth-Century Lives.* Cambridge, MA: Harvard University Press, 1995.

Daybell, James. *Women Letter-Writers in Tudor England.* Oxford: Oxford University Press, 2006.

Debus, Allen G. *Chemistry and Medical Debate: Van Helmont to Boerhaave.* Canton: Science History Publications, 2001.

Dekker, Rudolf. Introduction to *Egodocuments and History: Autobiographical Writing in Its Social Context Since the Middle Ages,* ed. Dekker, 7–20. Hilversum: Verloren, 2002.

Delamont, Sara, and Lorna Duffin, eds. *The Nineteenth-Century Woman: Her Cultural and Physical World.* London: Croom Helm, 1978.

De Moulin, Daniel. "A Historical-Phenomenological Study of Bodily Pain in Western Man." *Bulletin of the History of Medicine* 48 (1974): 540–570.

Dillon, Anne. *The Construction of Martyrdom in the English Catholic Community, 1535–1603.* Aldershot: Ashgate, 2002.

DiMeo, Michelle. "Katherine Jones, Lady Ranelagh (1615–91): Science and Medicine in a Seventeenth-Century Englishwoman's Writing." PhD diss., University of Warwick, 2009.

DiMeo, Michelle, and Sara Pennell, eds. *Reading and Writing Recipe Books, 1550–1800.* Manchester: Manchester University Press, 2013.

Ditz, Toby L. "The New Men's History and the Peculiar Absence of Gendered Power: Some Remedies from Early American History." *Gender and History* 16, no. 1 (2004): 1–35.

———. "Shipwrecked; or, Masculinity Imperiled: Mercantile Representations of Failure and the Gendered Self in Eighteenth-Century Philadelphia." *Journal of American History* 81 (1994): 51–80.

Dixon, Laurinda S. *Perilous Chastity: Women and Illness in Pre-Enlightenment Art and Medicine.* Ithaca: Cornell University Press, 1995.

Dragstra, Henk, Sheila Ottway, and Helen Wilcox, eds. *Betraying Our Selves: Forms of Self-Representation in Early Modern English Texts.* New York: St. Martin's Press, 2000.

Duden, Barbara. *The Woman Beneath the Skin: A Doctor's Patients in Eighteenth-Century Germany*. Cambridge, MA: Harvard University Press, 1991.

Earle, Peter. "The Female Labour Market in London in the Late Seventeenth and Early Eighteenth Centuries." *Economic History Review* 42 (1989): 328–353.

———. *The Making of the English Middle Class: Business, Society, and Family Life in London, 1660–1730*. London: Methuen, 1989.

Eckerle, Julie A., and Michelle M. Dowd, eds. *Genre and Women's Life Writing in Early Modern England*. Aldershot: Ashgate, 2007.

Eustace, Nicole. *Passion Is the Gale: Emotion, Power, and the Coming of the American Revolution*. Chapel Hill: University of North Carolina Press, 2008.

Fessler, Alfred. "The Official Attitude Towards the Sick Poor in Seventeenth-Century Lancashire." *Transactions of the Historic Society of Lancashire and Cheshire* 102 (1950): 85–113.

Fissell, Mary E. "Introduction: Women, Health, and Healing in Early Modern Europe." *Bulletin of the History of Medicine* 82 (2008): 1–17.

———. "The Marketplace of Print." In *Medicine and the Market in England and Its Colonies, c. 1450–c. 1850*, ed. Mark Jenner and Patrick Wallis, 108–132. Houndmills: Palgrave Macmillan, 2007.

———. *Patients, Power, and the Poor in Eighteenth-Century Bristol*. Cambridge: Cambridge University Press, 1991.

———. "The 'Sick and Drooping Poor' in Eighteenth-Century Bristol and Its Regions." *Social History of Medicine* 2 (1989): 35–58.

———. *Vernacular Bodies: The Politics of Reproduction in Early Modern England*. Oxford: Oxford University Press, 2004.

Fletcher, Anthony. *Gender, Sex, and Subordination in England, 1500–1800*. New Haven: Yale University Press, 1995.

Forster, Elborg. "From the Patient's Point of View: Illness and Health in the Letters of Liselotte von der Pfalz (1652–1722)." *Bulletin of the History of Medicine* 60 (1986): 297–320.

Fothergill, Robert A. *Private Chronicles: A Study of English Diaries*. London: Oxford University Press, 1974.

Foucault, Michel. *The Birth of the Clinic: An Archaeology of Medical Perception*. Trans. A. M. Sheridan Smith. New York: Vintage Books, 1975.

Foyster, Elizabeth A. *Manhood in Early Modern England: Honour, Sex, and Marriage*. New York: Longman, 1999.

Gentilcore, David. "The Fear of Disease and the Disease of Fear." In *Fear in Early Modern Society*, ed. William G. Naphy and Penny Roberts, 184–208. Manchester: Manchester University Press, 1997.

George, Margaret. *Women in the First Capitalist Society: Experiences in Seventeenth-Century England*. Urbana: University of Illinois Press, 1988.

Gowing, Laura. *Common Bodies: Women, Touch, and Power in Seventeenth-Century England*. New Haven: Yale University Press, 2003.

———. *Domestic Dangers: Women, Words, and Sex in Early Modern London*. Oxford: Clarendon Press, 1996.

———. "The Manner of Submission: Gender and Demeanour in Seventeenth-Century London." *Cultural and Social History* 10 (2013): 25–45.

Graham, Elspeth. "Women's Writing and the Self." In *Women and Literature in Britain, 1500–1700*, ed. Helen Wilcox, 209–233. Cambridge: Cambridge University Press, 1996.

Gray, Louise. "The Experience of Old Age in the Narratives of the Rural Poor in Early Modern Germany." In *Power and Poverty: Old Age in the Pre-industrial Past*, ed. Susannah R. Ottaway, L. A. Botelho, and Katharine Kittredge, 107–124. Westport: Greenwood Press, 2002.

———. "The Self-Perception of Chronic Physical Incapacity Among the Labouring Poor: Pauper Narratives and Territorial Hospitals in Early Modern Rural Germany." PhD diss., University of London, 2001.

Hall, David D. *Worlds of Wonder, Days of Judgment: Popular Religious Belief in Early New England*. Cambridge, MA: Harvard University Press, 1990.

Hambrick-Stowe, Charles E. *The Practice of Piety: Puritan Devotional Disciplines in Seventeenth-Century New England*. Chapel Hill: University of North Carolina Press, 1982.

Hanson, Elizabeth. "Torture and Truth in Renaissance England." *Representations* 34 (1991): 53–84.

Harkness, Deborah E. "Managing an Experimental Household: The Dees of Mortlake and the Practice of Natural Philosophy." *Isis* 88 (1997): 247–262.

———. "A View from the Streets: Women and Medical Work in Elizabethan London." *Bulletin of the History of Medicine* 82 (2008): 52–85.

Harley, David. "Spiritual Physic, Providence and English Medicine, 1560–1640." In *Medicine and the Reformation*, ed. Ole Peter Grell and Andrew Cunningham, 101–117. London: Routledge, 1993.

———. "The Theology of Affliction and the Experience of Sickness in the Godly Family, 1650–1714: The Henrys and the Newcomes." In *Religio Medici: Medicine and Religion in Seventeenth-Century England*, ed. Ole Peter Grell and Andrew Cunningham, 273–292. Aldershot: Scolar Press, 1996.

Harvey, Karen. *The Little Republic: Masculinity and Domestic Authority in Eighteenth-Century Britain*. Oxford: Oxford University Press, 2012.

———. *Reading Sex in the Eighteenth Century: Bodies and Gender in English Erotic Culture.* Cambridge: Cambridge University Press, 2004.

Hembry, Phyllis M. *The English Spa, 1560–1815: A Social History.* London: Athlone Press, 1990.

Herbert, Amanda E. *Female Alliances: Gender, Identity, and Friendship in Early Modern Britain.* New Haven: Yale University Press, 2014.

———. "Gender and the Spa: Space, Sociability and Self at British Health Spas, 1640–1714." *Journal of Social History* 43 (2009): 361–383.

Hickerson, Megan L. *Making Women Martyrs in Tudor England.* Houndmills: Palgrave Macmillan, 2005.

Hide, Louise, Joanna Bourke, and Carmen Mangion, eds. "Perspectives on Pain." Special issue, *19: Interdisciplinary Studies in the Long Nineteenth Century* 15 (2012).

Highley, Christopher, and John N. King, *John Foxe and His World.* Aldershot: Ashgate, 2002.

Hindle, Steve. *On the Parish? The Micro-politics of Poor Relief in Rural England, c. 1550–1750.* Oxford: Clarendon Press, 2004.

———. "The Shaming of Margaret Knowsley: Gossip, Gender and the Experience of Authority in Early Modern England." *Continuity and Change* 9 (1994): 391–419.

Hinnells, John R., and Roy Porter, eds. *Religion, Health and Suffering.* London: Kegan Paul International, 1999.

Houlbrooke, Ralph. *Death, Religion, and the Family in England, 1480–1750.* Oxford: Clarendon Press, 1998.

———, ed. *Death, Ritual, and Bereavement.* London: Routledge, 1989.

Howard, Sharon. "Imagining the Pain and Peril of Seventeenth-Century Childbirth: Travail and Deliverance in the Making of an Early Modern World." *Social History of Medicine* 16 (2003): 367–382.

Hubbard, Eleanor. *City Women: Money, Sex, and the Social Order in Early Modern London.* Oxford: Oxford University Press, 2012.

Hudson, Geoffrey L. "Arguing Disability: Ex-Servicemen's Stories in Early Modern England." In *Medicine, Madness and Social History,* ed. Roberta Bivins and John Pickstone, 105–117. Basingstoke: Palgrave Macmillan, 2007.

Huet, Marie-Hélène. *Monstrous Imagination.* Cambridge, MA: Harvard University Press, 1993.

Hunter, Lynette. "Women and Domestic Medicine: Lady Experimenters, 1570–1620." In *Women, Science and Medicine, 1500–1700: Mothers and Sisters of the Royal Society*, ed. Sarah Hutton and Hunter, 89–107. Stroud: Sutton Publishing, 1997.

Janzen, John M., and William Arkinstall. *The Quest for Therapy in Lower Zaire.* Berkeley: University of California Press, 1978.

Jewson, Nicholas. "The Disappearance of the Sick Man from Medical Cosmology, 1770–1870." *Sociology* 10 (1976): 225–44.

———. "Medical Knowledge and the Patronage System in Eighteenth Century England." *Sociology* 8 (1974): 369–385.

Kassell, Lauren. *Medicine and Magic in Elizabethan London: Simon Forman: Astrologer, Alchemist, and Physician.* Oxford: Clarendon Press, 2005.

King, John N. *Foxe's "Book of Martyrs" and Early Modern Print Culture.* Cambridge: Cambridge University Press, 2006.

King, Steven. *Poverty and Welfare in England, 1700–1850: A Regional Perspective.* Manchester: Manchester University Press, 2000.

———. "'Stop This Overwhelming Torrent of Destiny': Negotiating Financial Aid at Times of Sickness Under the English Old Poor Law, 1800–1840." *Bulletin of the History of Medicine* 79 (2005): 238–241.

———. "Voices of the Poor in the Long Eighteenth Century." In *Narratives of the Poor in Eighteenth-Century Britain,* ed. Alysa Levene, xxxiii–liv. London: Pickering and Chatto, 2006.

King, Steven, and Alannah Tomkins, eds. *The Poor in England, 1700–1850: An Economy of Makeshifts.* Manchester: Manchester University Press, 2003.

Knights, Mark. *The Devil in Disguise: Deception, Delusion, and Fanaticism in the Early English Enlightenment.* Oxford: Oxford University Press, 2011.

Knott, John R. *Discourses of Martyrdom in English Literature, 1563–1694.* Cambridge: Cambridge University Press, 1993.

———. "John Foxe and the Joy of Suffering." *Sixteenth Century Journal* 27 (1996): 721–734.

Kugler, Anne. *Errant Plagiary: The Writing Life of Lady Sarah Cowper (1644–1720).* Stanford: Stanford University Press, 2002.

Kuriyama, Shigehisa. "The Forgotten Fear of Excrement." *Journal of Medieval and Early Modern Studies* 38 (2008): 413–442.

Laqueur, Thomas. *Making Sex: Body and Gender from the Greeks to Freud.* Cambridge, MA: Harvard University Press, 1990.

Lawrence, Susan C. *Charitable Knowledge: Hospital Pupils and Practitioners in Eighteenth-Century London.* Cambridge: Cambridge University Press, 1996.

LeJacq, Seth Stein. "The Bounds of Domestic Healing: Medical Recipes, Storytelling and Surgery in Early Modern England." *Social History of Medicine* 26 (2013): 1–18.

Leong, Elaine. "Collecting Knowledge for the Family: Recipes, Gender and Practical Knowledge in the Early Modern English Household." *Centaurus* 55 (2013): 81–103.

———. "Making Medicines in the Early Modern Household." *Bulletin of the History of Medicine* 82 (2008): 145–168.

Leong, Elaine, and Sara Pennell. "Recipe Collections and the Currency of Medical Knowledge in the Early Modern 'Medical Marketplace.'" In *Medicine and the Market in England and Its Colonies, c. 1450–c. 1850*, ed. Mark S. R. Jenner and Patrick Wallis, 133–152. Houndmills: Palgrave Macmillan, 2007.

Leong, Elaine, and Alisha Rankin, eds. *Secrets and Knowledge in Medicine and Science, 1500–1800*. Farnham: Ashgate, 2011.

Liliequist, Jonas, ed. *A History of Emotions, 1200–1800*. London: Pickering and Chatto, 2012.

Lindman, Janet Moore. "Acting the Manly Christian: White Evangelical Masculinity in Revolutionary Virginia." *William and Mary Quarterly* 57 (2000): 393–416.

———. *Bodies of Belief: Baptist Community in Early America*. Philadelphia: University of Pennsylvania Press, 2008.

Livingston, Julie. *Debility and the Moral Imagination in Botswana*. Bloomington: Indiana University Press, 2005.

Lorber, Judith. *Gender and the Social Construction of Illness*. Thousand Oaks: Sage Publications, 1997.

Louis-Courvoisier, Micheline, and Severine Pilloud. "Consulting by Letter in the Eighteenth Century: Mediating the Patient's View?" In *Cultural Approaches to the History of Medicine: Mediating Medicine in Early Modern and Modern Europe*, ed. Willem de Blecourt and Cornelie Usborne, 133–152. Houndmills: Palgrave Macmillan, 2004.

Lutz, Catherine, and Geoffrey M. White. "The Anthropology of Emotions." *Annual Review of Anthropology* 15 (1986): 405–436.

MacDonald, Michael. "*The Fearfull Estate of Francis Spira*: Narrative, Identity, and Emotion in Early Modern England." *Journal of British Studies* 31 (1992): 32–61.

———. *Mystical Bedlam: Madness, Anxiety, and Healing in Seventeenth-Century England*. Cambridge: Cambridge University Press, 1981.

Macfarlane, Alan. *The Family Life of Ralph Josselin, a Seventeenth-Century Clergyman: An Essay in Historical Anthropology.* New York: Norton, 1977.

Mack, Phyllis. *Heart Religion in the British Enlightenment: Gender and Emotion in Early Methodism.* Cambridge: Cambridge University Press, 2008.

Mann, Ronald D., ed. *The History of the Management of Pain: From Early Principles to Present Practice.* Carnforth: Parthenon, 1988.

Marshall, John. *John Locke, Toleration and Early Enlightenment Culture.* Cambridge: Cambridge University Press, 2006.

Martin, Emily. "The Egg and the Sperm: How Science Has Constructed a Romance Based on Stereotypical Male-Female Roles." *Signs* 16 (1991): 485–501.

———. *The Woman in the Body: A Cultural Analysis of Reproduction.* Boston: Beacon Press, 1987.

Mascuch, Michael. *Origins of the Individualist Self: Autobiography and Self-Identity in England, 1591–1791.* Cambridge: Polity Press, 1997.

Mayhew, Jenny. "Godly Beds of Pain: Pain in English Protestant Manuals (ca. 1550–1650)." In *The Sense of Suffering: Constructions of Physical Pain in Early Modern Culture,* ed. Jan Frans van Dijkhuizen and K. A. E. Enenkel, 299–322. Leiden: Brill, 2009.

McIntosh, Marjorie Keniston. *Working Women in English Society, 1300–1620.* Cambridge: Cambridge University Press, 2005.

Mendelson, Sara Heller. *The Mental World of Stuart Women: Three Studies.* Brighton: Harvester Press, 1987.

———. "Neighbourhood as Female Community in the Life of Anne Dormer." In *Women, Identities and Communities in Early Modern Europe,* ed. Susan Broomhall and Stephanie Tarbin, 153–164. Aldershot: Ashgate, 2008.

Mendelson, Sara Heller, and Patricia Crawford. *Women in Early Modern England, 1550–1720.* Oxford: Clarendon Press, 1998.

Mortimer, Ian. *The Dying and the Doctors: The Medical Revolution in Seventeenth-Century England.* Woodbridge: Boydell Press, 2009.

Moscoso, Javier. *Pain: A Cultural History.* Basingstoke: Palgrave Macmillan, 2012.

Mueller, Janel M. "Pain, Persecution, and the Construction of Selfhood in Foxe's *Acts and Monuments.*" In *Religion and Culture in Renaissance England,* ed. Claire McEachern and Debora Shuger, 161–187. Cambridge: Cambridge University Press, 1997.

Muldrew, Craig. "'A Mutual Assent of Her Mind'? Women, Debt Litigation and Contract in Early Modern England." *History Workshop Journal* 55 (2003): 47–71.

Munkhoff, Richelle. "Searchers of the Dead: Authority, Marginality, and the Interpretation of the Plague in England, 1574–1665." *Gender and History* 11 (1999): 1–29.

Mutschler, Ben. "The Province of Affliction: Illness in New England, 1690–1820." PhD diss., Columbia University, 2000.

Nance, Brian. "Wondrous Experience as Text: Valleriola and the *Observationes Medicinales.*" In *Textual Healing: Essays on Medieval and Early Modern Medicine*, ed. Elizabeth Lane Furdell, 101–118. Leiden: Brill, 2005.

Newton, Hannah. *The Sick Child in Early Modern England, 1580–1720.* Oxford: Oxford University Press, 2012.

Nussbaum, Felicity. *The Autobiographical Subject: Gender and Ideology in Eighteenth-Century England.* Baltimore: Johns Hopkins University Press, 1989.

Nutton, Vivian. "Pieter van Foreest and the Plagues of Europe: Some Observations on the *Observationes.*" In *Pieter van Foreest: Een Hollands Medicus in De Zestiende Eeuw*, ed. H. L. Houtzager, 25–40. Amsterdam: Rodopi, 1989.

O'Connor, Mary. "Interpreting Early Modern Woman Abuse: The Case of Anne Dormer." *Quidditas* 23 (2002): 44–67.

Ottaway, Susannah R. *The Decline of Life: Old Age in Eighteenth-Century England.* Cambridge: Cambridge University Press, 2004.

Outhwaite, R. B. "'Objects of Charity': Petitions to the London Foundling Hospital, 1768–72." *Eighteenth-Century Studies* 32 (1999): 497–510.

Palgrave, Mary E. *Mary Rich, Countess of Warwick (1625–1678).* London: J. M. Dent, 1901.

Park, Katharine. "The Organic Soul." In *The Cambridge History of Renaissance Philosophy*, ed. Charles B. Schmitt, Quentin Skinner, and Eckhard Kessler, 464–484. Cambridge: Cambridge University Press, 1988.

———. *Secrets of Women: Gender, Generation, and the Origins of Human Dissection.* New York: Zone Books, 2006.

Parsons, Talcott. *The Social System.* Glencoe: Free Press, 1951.

Paster, Gail Kern, Katherine Rowe, and Mary Floyd-Wilson, eds. *Reading the Early Modern Passions: Essays in the Cultural History of Emotion.* Philadelphia: University of Pennsylvania Press, 2004.

Payne, Lynda. *With Words and Knives: Learning Medical Dispassion in Early Modern England.* Aldershot: Ashgate, 2007.

Pelling, Margaret. "Appearance and Reality: Barber-Surgeons, the Body and Disease." In *London, 1500–1700: The Making of the Metropolis*, ed. A. L. Beier and Finlay Roger, 82–112. London: Longman, 1985.

———. *The Common Lot: Sickness, Medical Occupations and the Urban Poor in Early Modern England*. London: Longman, 1998.

———. "Compromised by Gender." In *The Task of Healing*, ed. Pelling and Hillary Marland, 101–133. Rotterdam: Erasmus, 1996.

———. *Medical Conflicts in Early Modern London: Patronage, Physicians, and Irregular Practitioners, 1550–1640*. Oxford: Clarendon Press, 2003.

Pelling, Margaret, and Charles Webster. "Medical Practitioners." In *Health, Medicine, and Mortality in the Sixteenth Century*, ed. Webster, 165–235. Cambridge: Cambridge University Press, 1979.

Pennell, Sara. "Perfecting Practice? Women, Manuscript Recipes and Knowledge in Early Modern England." In *Early Modern Women's Manuscript Writing*, ed. Victoria Burke and Jonathan Gibson, 237–258. Aldershot: Ashgate, 2004.

Pernick, Martin S. *A Calculus of Suffering: Pain, Professionalism, and Anesthesia in Nineteenth-Century America*. New York: Columbia University Press, 1985.

Petry, Yvonne. " 'Many Things Surpass Our Knowledge': An Early Modern Surgeon on Magic, Witchcraft and Demonic Possession." *Social History of Medicine* 25 (2012): 47–64.

Pollock, Linda A. "Anger and the Negotiation of Relationships in Early Modern England." *Historical Journal* 47, no. 3 (2004): 567–590.

———. "Childbearing and Female Bonding in Early Modern England." *Social History* 22 (1997): 286–306.

———. *With Faith and Physic: The Life of a Tudor Gentlewoman, Lady Grace Mildmay, 1552–1620*. London: Collins and Brown, 1993.

Pomata, Gianna. *Contracting a Cure: Patients, Healers, and the Law in Early Modern Bologna*. Baltimore: Johns Hopkins University Press, 1998.

———. "Observation Rising: Birth of an Epistemic Genre, ca. 1500–1650." In *Histories of Scientific Observation*, ed. Lorraine Daston and Elizabeth Lunbeck, 45–80. Chicago: Chicago University Press, 2011.

———. "*Praxis Historialis:* The Uses of *Historia* in Early Modern Medicine." In *Historia: Empiricism and Erudition in Early Modern Europe*, ed. Pomata and Nancy G. Siraisi, 105–146. Cambridge, MA: MIT Press, 2005.

———. "Sharing Cases: The Observationes in Early Modern Medicine." *Early Science and Medicine* 15 (2010): 193–236.

Porter, Roy. "Accidents in the Eighteenth Century." In *Accidents in History: Injuries, Fatalities and Social Relations*, ed. Roger Cooter and Bill Luckin, 90–106. Amsterdam: Rodopi, 1997.

————. *Health for Sale: Quackery in England, 1660–1850*. Manchester: Manchester University Press, 1989.

————. "Lay Medical Knowledge in the Eighteenth Century: The Evidence of the *Gentleman's Magazine*." *Medical History* 29 (1985): 138–168.

————. "The Patient's View: Doing Medical History from Below." *Theory and Society* 14 (1985): 175–198.

————. "Western Medicine and Pain: Historical Perspectives." In *Religion, Health and Suffering*, ed. John R. Hinnells and Porter, 364–380. London: Kegan Paul International, 1999.

————, ed. *The Medical History of Waters and Spas*. Medical History Supplement 10. London: Wellcome Institute for the History of Medicine, 1990.

————, ed. *Patients and Practitioners: Lay Perceptions of Medicine in Pre-industrial Society*. Cambridge: Cambridge University Press, 1985.

Porter, Roy, and Dorothy Porter. *In Sickness and in Health: The British Experience, 1650–1850*. New York: B. Blackwell, 1988.

————. *Patient's Progress: Doctors and Doctoring in Eighteenth-Century England*. Stanford: Stanford University Press, 1989.

Purkiss, Diane. "Women's Stories of Witchcraft in Early Modern England: The House, the Body, the Child." *Gender and History* 7 (1995): 408–432.

Rankin, Alisha. "Becoming an Expert Practitioner: Court Experimentalism and the Medical Skills of Anna of Saxony (1532–1585)." *Isis* 98 (2007): 23–53.

————. "Duchess, Heal Thyself: Elisabeth of Rochlitz and the Patient's Perspective in Early Modern Germany." *Bulletin of the History of Medicine* 82 (2008): 109–144.

————. *Panaceia's Daughters: Noblewomen as Healers in Early Modern Germany*. Chicago: University of Chicago Press, 2013.

Rey, Roselyne. *The History of Pain*. Trans. Louise Elliott Wallace, J. A. Cadden, and S. W. Cadden. Paris: La Découverte, 1993.

Robertson, Jean. *The Art of Letter Writing: An Essay on the Handbooks Published in England During the Sixteenth and Seventeenth Centuries*. Liverpool: University Press of Liverpool, 1942.

Rose, Mary Beth. "Gender, Genre, and History: Seventeenth-Century English Women and the Art of Autobiography." In *Women in the Middle Ages and the Renaissance*, ed. Rose, 245–278. Syracuse: Syracuse University Press, 1986.

Rosenwein, Barbara H. "Worrying About Emotions in History." *American Historical Review* 107 (2002): 821–845.

Rublack, Ulinka. "Fluxes: The Early Modern Body and the Emotions." *History Workshop Journal* 53 (2002): 1–16.

Sawyer, Ronald. "Patients, Healers, and Disease in the Southeast Midlands, 1597–1634." PhD diss., University of Wisconsin–Madison, 1986.

———. " 'Strangely Handled in All Her Lyms': Witchcraft and Healing in Early Modern England." *Journal of Social History* 22 (1988): 461–485.

Schiebinger, Londa. "Skeletons in the Closet: The First Illustrations of the Female Skeleton in Eighteenth-Century Anatomy." *Representations* 14 (1986): 42–82.

Schneider, Gary. *The Culture of Epistolarity: Vernacular Letters and Letter-Writing in Early Modern England, 1500–1700.* Newark: University of Delaware Press, 2005.

Scott, Joan W. "The Evidence of Experience." *Critical Inquiry* 17 (1991): 773–797.

Seaver, Paul S. *Wallington's World: A Puritan Artisan in Seventeenth-Century London.* Stanford: Stanford University Press, 1985.

Sharpe, Pamela. " 'The Bowels of Compation': A Labouring Family and the Law, c. 1790–1834." In *Chronicling Poverty: The Voices and Strategies of the English Poor, 1640–1840,* ed. Tim Hitchcock, Peter King, and Sharpe, 87–108. Houndmills: Macmillan Press, 1997.

———. "Survival Strategies and Stories: Poor Widows and Widowers in Early Industrial England." In *Widowhood in Medieval and Early Modern Europe,* ed. Sandra Cavallo and Lyndan Warner, 220–239. Harlow: Longman, 1999.

Shepard, Alexandra. "Manhood, Credit, and Patriarchy in Early Modern England, c. 1580–1640." *Past and Present* 167 (2000): 75–106.

———. "Manhood, Patriarchy, and Gender in Early Modern History." In *Masculinities, Childhood, Violence: Attending to Early Modern Women—and Men: Proceedings of the 2006 Symposium,* ed. Amy Leonard and Karen L. Nelson, 77–95. Newark: University of Delaware Press, 2011.

———. *Meanings of Manhood in Early Modern England.* Oxford: Oxford University Press, 2003.

Shoemaker, Robert B. *Gender in English Society, 1650–1850: The Emergence of Separate Spheres.* London: Longman, 1998.

Siena, Kevin. "The 'Foul Disease' and Privacy: The Effects of Venereal Disease and Patient Demand on the Medical Marketplace in Early Modern London." *Bulletin of the History of Medicine* 75 (2001): 199–224.

————. *Venereal Disease, Hospitals and the Urban Poor: London's "Foul Wards,"* *1600–1800*. Rochester: University of Rochester Press, 2004.

Silverman, Lisa. *Tortured Subjects: Pain, Truth, and the Body in Early Modern France*. Chicago: University of Chicago Press, 2001.

Slack, Paul. *The English Poor Law, 1531–1782*. Basingstoke: Macmillan Education, 1990.

————. *Poverty and Policy in Tudor and Stuart England*. London: Longman, 1988.

Smith, Lisa Wynne. " 'An Account of an Unaccountable Distemper': The Experience of Pain in Early Eighteenth-Century England and France." *Eighteenth-Century Studies* 41 (2008): 459–480.

————. "The Body Embarrassed? Rethinking the Leaky Male Body in Eighteenth-Century England and France." *Gender and History* 23 (2011): 26–46.

————. "Reassessing the Role of the Family: Women's Medical Care in Eighteenth-Century England." *Social History of Medicine* 16 (2003): 327–342.

————. "The Relative Duties of a Man: Domestic Medicine in England and France." *Journal of Family History* 31 (2006): 237–256.

————. "Women's Health Care in England and France (1650–1775)." PhD diss., University of Essex, 2001.

Smith-Rosenberg, Carroll. *Disorderly Conduct: Visions of Gender in Victorian America*. New York: Knopf, 1985.

Smith-Rosenberg, Carroll, and Charles E. Rosenberg. "The Female Animal: Medical and Biological Views of Woman and Her Role in Nineteenth-Century America." *Journal of American History* 60 (1973): 332–356.

Smyth, Adam. *Autobiography in Early Modern England*. Cambridge: Cambridge University Press, 2010.

Snell, K. D. M. *Annals of the Labouring Poor: Social Change and Agrarian England, 1660–1900*. Cambridge: Cambridge University Press, 1985.

Sokoll, Thomas. *Essex Pauper Letters, 1731–1837*. Oxford: Oxford University Press, 2001.

————. "Writing for Relief: Rhetoric in English Pauper Letters, 1800–1834." In *Being Poor in Modern Europe: Historical Perspectives, 1800–1940*, ed. Andreas Gestrich, Steven King, and Lutz Raphael, 91–111. Oxford: Peter Lang, 2006.

Solomon, Michael. *Fictions of Well-Being: Sickly Readers and Vernacular Medical Writing in Late Medieval and Early Modern Spain*. Philadelphia: University of Pennsylvania Press, 2010.

———. "Non-natural Love: Coitus, Desire and Hygiene in Medieval and Early Modern Spain." In *Emotions and Health, 1200–1700*, ed. Elena Carrera, 147–158. Leiden: Brill, 2013.

Stavreva, Kirilka. "Fighting Words: Witch-Speak in Late Elizabethan Docufiction." *Journal of Medieval and Early Modern Studies* 30 (2000): 309–338.

Stein, Claudia. *Negotiating the French Pox in Early Modern Germany*. Farnham: Ashgate, 2009.

Stephens, Isaac. " 'My Cheefest Work': The Making of the Spiritual Autobiography of Elizabeth Isham." *Midland History* 34 (2009): 181–203.

Stine, Jennifer. "Opening Closets: The Discovery of Household Medicine in Early Modern England." PhD diss., Stanford University, 1996.

Stolberg, Michael. *Experiencing Illness and the Sick Body in Early Modern Europe*. Basingstoke: Palgrave Macmillan, 2011.

Stowe, Steven. "Singleton's Tooth: Thoughts on the Form and Meaning of Antebellum Southern Family Correspondence." *Southern Review* 25 (1989): 323–333.

Sullivan, Erin. "The Watchful Spirit: Religious Anxieties Towards Sleep in the Notebooks of Nehemiah Wallington (1598–1658)." *Cultural History* 1 (2012): 14–35.

Sumich, Christi. *Divine Doctors and Dreadful Distempers: How Practicing Medicine Became a Respectable Profession*. Amsterdam: Rodpi, 2013.

Sweet, Rosemary, and Penelope Lane, eds. *Women and Urban Life in Eighteenth-Century England: On the Town*. Aldershot: Ashgate, 2003.

Tarter, Michele Lise. "Quaking in the Light." In *A Centre of Wonders: The Body in Early America*, ed. Janet Moore Lindman and Tarter, 145–162. Ithaca: Cornell University Press, 2001.

Thomas, Keith. *Religion and the Decline of Magic*. New York: Scribner, 1971.

Todd, Barbara J. " 'I Do No Injury by Not Loving': Katherine Austen, a Young Widow of London." In *Women and History: Voices of Early Modern England*, ed. Valerie Frith, 207–238. Concord: Irwin Publishing, 1997.

Todd, Margo. "Puritan Self-Fashioning: The Diary of Samuel Ward." *Journal of British Studies* 31 (1992): 236–264.

Tomalin, Claire. *Samuel Pepys: The Unequalled Self.* New York: A. A. Knopf, 2002.

van Dijkhuizen, Jan Frans. "Partakers of Pain: Religious Meanings of Pain in Early Modern England." In *The Sense of Suffering: Constructions of Physical Pain in Early Modern Culture,* ed. van Dijkhuizen and K. A. E. Enenkel, 189–220. Leiden: Brill, 2009.

van Dijkhuizen, Jan Frans, and K. A. E. Enenkel, eds. *The Sense of Suffering: Constructions of Physical Pain in Early Modern Culture.* Leiden: Brill, 2009.

Vickery, Amanda. *The Gentleman's Daughter: Women's Lives in Georgian England.* New Haven: Yale University Press, 1998.

Walker, Katherine. "A Gendered History of Pain in England, Circa 1620–1740." PhD diss., McMaster University, 2011.

Walsham, Alexandra. *Providence in Early Modern England.* Oxford: Oxford University Press, 1999.

Wear, Andrew. "Fear, Anxiety and the Plague in Early Modern England." In *Religion, Health and Suffering,* ed. John R. Hinnells and Roy Porter, 339–363. London: Kegan Paul International, 1999.

———. *Knowledge and Practice in English Medicine, 1550–1680.* Cambridge: Cambridge University Press, 2000.

———. "Puritan Perceptions of Illness in Seventeenth-Century England." In *Patients and Practitioners: Lay Perceptions of Medicine in Pre-industrial Society,* ed. Roy Porter, 55–99. Cambridge: Cambridge University Press, 1985.

Webster, Charles. *The Great Instauration: Science, Medicine, and Reform, 1626–1660.* Oxford: Peter Lang, 2002.

Weisser, Olivia. "Boils, Pushes, and Wheals: Reading Bumps on the Body in Early Modern England." *Social History of Medicine* 22 (2009): 321–339.

———. "Grieved and Disordered: Gender and Emotion in Early Modern Patient Narratives." *Journal of Medieval and Early Modern Studies* 43 (2013): 247–273.

Wiesner, Merry E. "*Wandervogels* and Women: Journeymen's Concepts of Masculinity in Early Modern Germany." *Journal of Social History* 24 (1991): 767–782.

Wilson, Adrian. "The Ceremony of Childbirth and Its Interpretation." In *Women as Mothers in Pre-industrial England,* ed. Valerie Fildes, 68–107. London: Routledge, 1990.

Withey, Alun. *Physick and the Family: Health, Medicine and Care in Wales, 1600–1750.* Manchester: Manchester University Press, 2011.

Wray, Ramona. "[Re]constructing the Past: The Diametric Lives of Mary Rich." In *Betraying Our Selves: Forms of Self-Representation in Early Modern English Texts,* ed. Henk Dragstra, Sheila Ottway, and Helen Wilcox, 148–165. New York: St. Martin's Press, 2000.

Yallop, Helen. *Age and Identity in Eighteenth-Century England.* London: Pickering and Chatto, 2013.

————. "Representing Aged Masculinity in Eighteenth-Century England: The 'Old Man' of Medical Advice." *Cultural and Social History* 10 (2013): 191–210.

Zahedieh, Nuala. *The Capital and the Colonies: London and the Atlantic Economy, 1660–1700.* Cambridge: Cambridge University Press, 2010.

Index

Page numbers in *italics* indicate illustrations.

Accidents/injuries, 168–169

Accomplish'd Ladies Delight, The (Woolley), 29, *30*

Actes and Monuments (Foxe), 133, *144*, 147, *148*. See also *Book of Martyrs* (Foxe)

Aging: effects of, 136; and masculinity, 11

Agues, 58–59, 172

Air: hot and cold, 22, 23, 170; impure, 22–23

Alcohol consumption, 23, 63–64, 139

Allestree, Richard, 10

Ambrose, Isaac, 76

Amputation, 19, 42, 126, *127*

Anatomy of Melancholy, The (Burton), 85

Anger, 23, 85

Animal spirits, 84, 85

Annesley, Arthur, 94, 106, 113, 126, 189

Anxiety, 86; financial, 82, 93–94; life event, 1–2

Apothecaries, 29–31, *31*, 33, 134, 169

Archer, Anne, 119

Archer, Isaac: biography of, 189; on deathbed suffering, 148–149, 150, 151; on mortality threat, 118, 119; natural remedies of, 26–27

Archer, John, 25–26

Arithmetic skills, 64–66

Armstrong, John, 24–25

Ars moriendi, 49, 73

Ascetics, and pain perception, 147

Ashburnham, Margaret, 39–40

Askew, Anne, 154

Astrological diaries, 59

Astrology, 58–59, 66, 79

Augustine's *Confessions*, 46–47, 68

Austen, Judith, 111

Austen, Katherine, 50–51, 57, 189

Bacon, Jane, 190

Baptista von Helmont, Johannes, 26

Barbers, medical services of, 34

Barbette, Paul, 35

Barrenness, 68

Beadle, John, 73

Beckett, William, 18

Becon, Thomas, 74

Behn, Aphra, 143

Beier, Lucinda, 8

Bile, in humoral body, 19, 20

Blindness, 104, 172

Blisters, 22

Blood: in humoral body, 19; menstruation, 24

Bloodletting, 24, 26, 27, 37, 41, 103, 104, 120, 138–139

Blundell, Nicholas, 125, 126, 190

Body, 184–185; approach to studying, 9–10; and emotional expression, 96; excretions from, 24, 26, 60–62; healers' physical examination of, 43–44; healthy, 12, 20, 60; humoral theory of, 1, 7, 19–21; perception over time, 14–15; rack imagery of pain, *144*, 144, 147; signs of divine grace, 68–70

Bonet, Théophile, 35

Book of Martyrs (Foxe), 133, 143, *144*, 147, *148*. See also *Actes and Monuments* (Foxe)
Boradale, Thomas, 167
Bowel movements, self-assessment of, 60–61
Bowle, John, 149
Boyle, Robert, 35
Breast cancer, 43
Breastfeeding, 20, 34, 91
Breast pain, 134
Bright, Timothie, 86, 96
Bunyan, John, 68
Burning at the stake, 147, *148*
Burrell, William, 125
Burton, Richard, 85

Calverley, Walter, 113, 190
Cannon, John, 153, 190
Carpenter, Richard, 142
Cary, Catherine, 24, 134, 137
Case notes, healers', 12, 34–44
Cataplasms, 27
Catherine of Braganza, Queen, 25
Catholicism, 133, 143, 156, 157
Chastity, 10
Chemical remedies, 26, 29, 39, 66, 139, 145
Childbirth: death in, 81, 141; pain of, 119, 120, 137, 140, 141, 143–144
Chirurgical and Anatomical Works (Barbette), 35
Choleric humor, 20, 21
Christ's redemption, pain as means of, 142–143
Church of England, 156
Clegg, James, 15, 24, 61, 67, 153, 169, 190
Clifford, Anne, 113, 190
Clifton, Lady Francis, 151–152
Cloughe, George and John, 176
Coe, William, 75, 190
Colbatch, John, 36, 127
Cold exposure, and illness causation, 1–2, 22, 23, 170
Colds, 21, 22, 50–51, 134, 145, 157
Coley, Henry, 66
Comber, Thomas, 92
Commonplace book, 13
Compassion, 106–107
Conduct manuals, 54
Confessions (St. Augustine), 46–47, 68
Contagions, 99–100

Convulsive fits, 25–26, 38–39, 40, 55, 90, 138
Conway, Anne, 51–52, 62, 191
Conway, Francis, 118
Cooper, Margaret, 104–105
Cordials, 17, 99
Corruption (putrefied matter), 20–21
Cottrell, Elizabeth, 151
Cowper, Sarah: biography of, 191; bodily sufferings of, 22, 40, 62, 74–75, 104, 116, 117, 160; on contagions, 99; devotional texts of, 76, 77; diary of, 12, 56–57, 183; on emotional responses, 94, 96; family neglect of, 110–111; on gluttony and health, 79; marital relations of, 105, 111; and martyrdom imagery, 143; mortality threat to, 122; others' suffering observed by, 57–58, 67; pain perception of, 136, 140, 151; sickbed visits to, 104–105, 108, 109–110, 115–116; speech and illness causation, 90
Cowper, William, 104, 105, 191
Crew, Samuel, 137
"Cucantellus's balsam," 28–29
Culpeper, Nicholas, 97
Cupping, 31, 34, 41
Curses, 90

Danby, Anne, 91–93
Danby, Catherine, 81
Darley, Francis, 119
Davies, Rowland, 117, 191
Dawson, Ann (Evans), 49–50, 192
Dead hand, as remedy for swelling, 98
Death: in childbirth, 81, 141; emotional response to, 94–95; funeral sermon, 76–77; pain as sign of, 119, 141–142; preparation for, 121; sickbed references to, 117–122
Deathbed: impious suffering, 77–78; insensibility to pain, 147–150; model of comportment, 49–50, 150–151; submission to God, 49, 73–74; witnesses at, 112
Death Made Comfortable (Kettlewell), 74, 75–76
Delaval, Elizabeth (Livingston), 25, 46, 79, 87, 191, 209n24
Devotional practices, 182; deathbed, 73–74; and gender, 71–72; illness as impediment, 70–71, 72–73, 79; meditation, 49, 50, 56,

68–69, 70, 73; prayer, 49, 50, 68–69, 70, 75–76; reading devotional texts, 47–48, 49, 68, 69, 71, 73–78; singing, 68; writing spiritual journal, 73

D'Ewes, Simonds, 192

Diaries: defined, 13; intended audience for, 13–14, 56; men's, 62–64, 78, 183; other people's illnesses described in, 49; published editions of, 206n32; spiritual journals, 13, 62, 73; suffering expressed in, 116–120; women's, 56–58, 62, 78, 183. *See also* Writing

Diet and illness causation: cold foods, 23; and emotions, 86; fruit consumption, 46–47, 79; and humoral theory of body, 21; impediment to devotional practices, 79; overeating, 24, 79. *See also* Drinks

Digby, Kenelm, 26

Disease. *See* Illness

Disfiguring illnesses, 174, 178

Divine Physician, The, 101

Domestic labor, 29, *30*, 54, 167

Dormer, Anne: biography of, 192; on deathbed suffering, 151; at husband's sickbed, 94; martyrdom imagery of, 145–147; pain perception of, 152–153; sickbed visits to, 108–109; spa visit of, 27–28, 32

Dormer, Robert, 94, 146

Douglas, John, 126–127

Dover, Tomas, 37

Drinks: alcoholic, 23, 63–64, 139; cold, 22, 23; cordials, 17, 99; "curdy," 24, 130; purging, 123; snail water, 55–56; spa water, 27–28, *29*, 32, 103, 119

Dropsy, 16–17, 39, 52–53, 98

Drunkenness, 63–64

Duden, Barbara, 8–9

Dugard, Lydia, 23, 98, 99, 192

Dugard, Samuel, 23, 98

Dunkirk distemper, 21

Economic status. *See* Socioeconomic status

Egerton, Elizabeth, 141, 192

Ego-literature, 13. *See also* Diaries; Writing

Emotions and illness causation, 184; anger, 23, 85; anxiety, 1–2, 86; fear, 23, 38, 41, 57, 84, 85–86, 87, 100, 171; financial concerns in, 82, 93–94; and gender, 10,

83, 93–103, 181; grief, 81–83, 85, 87–89, 93, 94–95, 107–108, 109; guilt, 157; jealousy, 101; joy, 85; as nonnatural, 23, 39; physiology of, 84–86; sadness, 23; scholarship on, 83–84; and sickbed visit, 106–107; social stimuli, 82; spoken word, 89–93; surprise, 23; sympathetic response in, 53, 81; terminology of, 84

Empirics: medical observations of, 36; remedies of, 32, *33*, 33

Enemas, 26, 122–123, 139

Evans, Ann (Dawson), 49–50, 192

Excretions, bodily, 24, 26, 60–62

Exercise, and illness causation, 23

Eye problems, 21, 115

Eyre, Adam, 192

Fanshawe, Ann, 87, 113, 128, 192

Fear: created by others' sufferings, 57; and illness causation, 23, 38, 41, 84, 85–86, 87, 100, 171; of mortality, 121–122

Feminine ideals, 9–10, 71

Fertility, humoral explanation of, 20

Fevers, 21, 22, 24, 52, 118, 172

Financial concerns: and illness causation, 82, 93–94; of pauper petitioners, 160, 162, 163–165, 174–176

Fissell, Mary, 9, 115

Fistulas, 172

Foley, Anne (North), 88–89

Fowles (empiric), 32

Foxe, John, 133, 143, *144*, 147, *148*

Freke, Elizabeth: biography of, 192–193; comparisons to others' suffering, 52–53, 56; family neglect of, 111–112; grief and illness causation, 88, 98; medical remedies of, 33, 114; near-fatal illness of, 118–119; social isolation of, 112–113; sufferings of, 62, 168

Freke, Percy, 111–112

Freke, Ralph, 111–112

Fruit, hazards of eating, 46–47

Funeral sermons, 76–77

Gawdy, Philip, 125

Gender: approach to studying, 3–4; and descriptions of suffering, 118, 181–182, 184; and devotional practices, 71–72; and emotion-induced illness, 10, 83, 93–103,

Gender (continued)
181, 184; feminine/masculine ideals, 9–10,
71; in healing trades, 33–34; in medical
encounter, 18; and pain perception, 41–43,
133, 152–156, 158; and self-assessment, 48,
62. *See also* Men; Women
Gossip and slander, 89, 91–93
Gout, 36, 113, 137, 155, 164
Gowing, Laura, 9, 91
Grace, divine: bodily sensations of, 68–70,
181–182; and fear of mortality, 122; and
pain, 156
Grace Abounding to the Chief of Sinners
(Bunyan), 68
Grave, Mary, 163–164, 175
Greatrakes, Valentine, 51
Grief-induced illness, 81–83, 85, 87–89, 93,
94–95, 107–108, 109
Guide to the Practical Physician, A (Bonet), 35
Guilt, 68, 157

Halkett, Anne, 193
Hamilton, David, 94
Harley, Brilliana, 12, 193
Harris, John, 86
Harrold, Edmund, 13, 34, 63–64, 65, 67,
79, 193
Harvey, William, 51
Hastings, Elizabeth, 55–56
Headaches, 22, 51, 69, 70, 137, 141, 149,
172
Healer-patient interaction. *See* Medical
encounters
Heart, and emotions, 85, 86
Heat exposure, and illness causation, 22,
23, 170
Hemorrhoids, 33, 117, 125
Henbane, 140
Heywood, Oliver, 144–145, 149, 193
Hooke, Robert, 15, 193
Hooper, John, 147, *148*
Houghton, Margaret, 76
Humoral theory of body, 1, 7, 19–21

Ibbetson, Samuel, 82, 93
Illness: agues, 58–59, 172; colds, 21, 22,
50–51, 134, 145, 157; common ailments,
181; convulsive fits, 25–26, 38–39, 40, 55,
90, 138; corruption (putrefied matter),
20–21; as cultural exchange, 2–3; dropsy,
16–17, 39, 52–53, 98; duration of, 113–115;
fevers, 21, 22, 24, 52, 118, 172; gout, 36,
113, 137, 155, 164; headaches, 22, 51, 69,
70, 137, 141, 149, 172; hemorrhoids, 33,
117, 125; kidney stones, 61, 129–132, *131*;
occupational injuries/illness, 168–170,
172–173; of pauper petitioners, 160,
171–172, 182, 200; reproductive
disorders, 8, 33; rheumatic disorder, 40;
scrofula (king's evil), 170; sex-specific,
180–181; smallpox, 24–25, 44, 85–86, 87;
St. Anthony's fire, 104; swelling, 22, 85,
98, 170; toothache, 153; venereal disease,
33, 37, 145, 177. *See also* Nonnatural
causes of illness; Pain; Remedies; Sickbed
Imagination, 85, 97
*Instruction of a Christen (Christian)
Woman* (Vives), 54
Ireton, Henry, 135, 136
Isham, Elizabeth, 193–194

Jeake, Samuel, 21, 58–60, 62, 64, 66–67, 78,
79, 143, 194
Jealousy, 101
Job, as model of suffering, 76
Jogues, Isaac, 142, 143
Jolly, Thomas, 194
Jones, Katherine (Lady Ranelagh), 34–35,
196
Josselin, Ralph, 194
*Journal or Diary of a Thankful Christian,
The* (Beadle), 73
Joy, 85

Kettlewell, John, 74, 75–76
Kidney stones, 61, 129–132, *131*, 135
King, Edmund, medical records of, 34–35
King's evil (scrofula), 170
Kirton, Joshua, 93
Knyvett, Thomas, 108
Kyrk, Samuel, 93

Lacroze (master at Eton), 41
Lactation, 20, 34, 61, 96
Lameness, 171, 172
Lane, Betty, 157
Laudanum, 17, 18, 140
Laxatives, 26, 27

Leong, Elaine, 33
Letter writing, 12, 14, 98–99
Life-cycle poverty, 162
Lister, Joseph, 17–18, 121–122, 194
Livingston, Elizabeth (Delaval), 25, 46, 79, 87, 191, 209n24
Llewellyn, Peter, 43–44
Lowe, Roger, 64, 95, 114, 194
Low-status patients. *See* Pauper petitioners

MacDonald, Michael, 83–84
Magic, belief in, 25, 182
Manchester, Lady, 49
Marriage: grief at husband's death, 87, 98, 107, 109; grievances of, 105, 109, 111, 146; and infidelity, 157; martyrdom imagery of, 145–147; and sickbed neglect, 111–112; wedding day illness, 1–2, 3–4
Marten, John, 177–178
Martindale, Adam, 194
Martyrdom imagery, 133, 143–150, *144*, *146*, *148*, 182
Masculine ideals, 9–10
Mathematical skills, 64–66
Mayne, John, 65
Medical care: by empirics, 32, *33*; healing trades, 33–34; by mountebanks, 16; varieties of practitioners, 32; witchcraft and magic, 25. *See also* Medical encounters; Remedies; Surgeons and surgery
Medical encounters: approach to studying, 8; compensation and fees, 34; and gender, 18, 41–42; negotiations with family and friends, 123, 126–127; patients' authority in, 2, 16–18; patients' contradictory assessments in, 18–19; with pauper petitioners, 176–178; physical examinations, 43–44, 45; records of, 34–35
Medical knowledge, women's, 54–56, 135
Medical observations, 19; by alternative practitioners, 36; historical background, 35–36; of patients' physical descriptions, 18, 39–42, 45; of patients' self treatment, 38–39; of physical examination, 43–44
Meditation, 49, 50, 56, 68, 70, 71, 73
Melancholic humor, 20
Men: devotional practice of, 71; emotional responses of, 94–95, 100–101, 103; financial anxiety of, 82, 93–94; grief of, 93; in

healing trades, 34; and masculine ideals, 9–10; mathematical skills of, 64–65; pain perception of, 153–154; self-writing of, 62–64, 66; work/occupations, 66, 113–114, 166
Menstruation, 20, 24, 61, 96, 134
Mercury treatment, for venereal disease, 37, 145
Middling-status patients, 6, 133, 153, 169
Midwives, 33
Mildmay, Humphrey, 153–154
Mimetic suffering, 99, 181
Ministers/vicars: funeral sermons, 76–77; physical effect of work on, 169; and sickbed visits of, 114
Miscarriage, 97
Molins, James, 126
Moore, Giles, 34, 194
More, Henry, 51, 117
Morris, Claver, 195
Mort, Thomas, 59
Mortality. *See* Death; Deathbed
Mountebanks, 16

Napier, Richard, 83–84
Natural remedies, 26
Natural spirits, 84–85
Nettleton, Grace, 149–150
Nonnatural causes of illness, 21–22, 84, 160, 170; air, 22–23; diet (*see* Diet and illness causation); emotions (*see* Emotions and illness causation); exercise, 23; in modern era, 183–184; retention/excretion, 24, 26; sleep, 23
North, Anne (Foley), 88–89
North, Anne (Montagu), 195
North, Dudley, 88, 195
North, Elizabeth (Paston), 56, 195
North, Roger, 88–89

Observations. *See* Medical observations; Self-assessment
Obstructions, purging, 30–32, 39, 63, 66, 86, 123–124
Occupations. *See* Work/occupations
Ointments, 27, 134, 139
Opium, 17, 140
Oroonoko (Behn), 143
Overeating, 24, 79

Packe, Susannah, 55
Pain: acceptance of, 12, 147, 150; approach
    to studying, 132–133; of childbirth, 119,
    120, 137, 140, 141, 143–144; as disorder,
    137–139; and gender, 41–43, 133, 152–156,
    158; martyrdom imagery of, 133, 143–150,
    144, 148; and mortality, 119, 141–142;
    patients' description/evaluation of, 39–41,
    129–130, 134, 135–137; redemptive,
    142–143; remedies for, 28–29, 41, 134,
    139–140; social performance of, 152–153
Paracelsus, 26
Park, Katharine, 97
Parker, Hephzibah, 48, 138
Parsons, Talcott, 2
Pascal, Blaise, 142
Passions and illness causation. *See* Emotions
    and illness causation
Passions of the Minde, The (Wright), 107
Paston, Elizabeth (North), 56, 195
Paston, Katherine, 24
Patient-healer interaction. *See* Medical
    encounters
Patient self-assessment. *See* Self-assessment
Patrick, Simon, 76
Pauper petitioners: accidents/injuries to,
    168–170, 172–173; bodily complaints of,
    160, 171–172, 182, 200, 238n25; deferential
    language of, 165; duration of disability,
    173–174; economic needs of, 160, 162,
    163–165, 174–176, 182; explanation of
    illness, 160, 163, 170–171, 182; gruesome/
    disfiguring illnesses of, 174, 178; letters for
    parish relief, 6–7, 159, *160*, 161–162, *162*;
    manhood characterizations of, 11, 166–167;
    medical testimony on behalf of, 176–178;
    moral worth emphasis of, 165–166, 167,
    178–179; occupations of, 173, 201; social
    supports of, 159, 182–183
Pelling, Margaret, 171
Pepys, Elizabeth, 123, 157
Pepys, Samuel, 2, 43, 78, *130*, 143; biography
    of, 195–196; bodily function documented
    by, 59–60, 67, 132; diary keeping of, 13,
    62–63, 66; emotional responses of, 95, 97,
    100–101; on illness causation, 22, 169;
    kidney stone surgery of, 131–132;
    mathematical skills of, 64–65; pain
    perception of, 129–130, 136, 153;

purgative remedy for, 122–124; sickbed
    stays, 113; spiritual attitudes of, 156–158
Petiver, James, 33
Petty, William, 42
Phlegm, in humoral body, 19–20
Physicians. *See* Medical care; Medical
    encounters; Surgeons and surgery
Physick (purgatives), 30–32, 39, 63, 66,
    123–124, 138
Physiology of emotions, 84–86
Pimples, humoral explanations for, 21
Pity, 106–107, 116, 126, 177
Plasters, 26–27
Pledger, Elias, 169, 196
Poley, Elizabeth, 99
Poor. *See* Pauper petitioners
Poor law, 159, *160*, 161, 162, 167–168
Porter, Dorothy, 8, 105
Porter, Roy, 8, 105
Poultices, 26–27
Powell, Walter, 63
Prayer: as devotional practice, 49, 50, 68,
    70, 75–76; in sickbed visit, 107
Protestants: and body-soul connection, 71;
    and pain perception, 140; persecution of,
    133, 143, 147, 154; personal writing of,
    5–6; and word of God, 89–90. *See also*
    Religion and illness
Providence, 6, 67–68, 120, 122
Psychological disorders, 84
Punishment, divine, 12, 21, 140, 157
Purgatives, 30–32, 39, 61, 63, 66, 86,
    123–124, 134, 138, 139
Puritans, 5–6
Putrefied matter, retention/secretion of,
    24, 26

Quack remedies, 32, *33*
Quarter Sessions, pauper petitions to, 162
Quickening, 68

Rack imagery of pain, *144*, 144, 147
Ranelagh, Viscountess (Katherine Jones),
    34–35, 196
Reading, devotional, 47–48, 49, 68, 69, 71,
    73–78
Reason, 85
Recipes, recipe books, 55, 125–126
Redemption, Christ's, 142–143

Religion and illness: approach to studying, 5–6; Catholicism, 143, 156, 157; and charms, 89–90; death and salvation, 49, 121–122; divine grace, 68–69, 122, 156, 181–182; divine punishment, 12, 21, 140, 157; and emotional restraint, 101; indulgence and sin, 46–47; martyrdom imagery, 133; models of suffering, 49–50, 76, 79; and providence, 6, 67–68, 120, 122; and redemptive pain, 142–143; during sickbed confinement, 114–115. *See also* Devotional practices; Ministers/vicars; Protestants

Remedies: from apothecaries, 29–30, 31, 134; bloodletting, 24, 26, 37, 41, 103, 104, 120, 138–139; charms, 89–90; chemical, 26, 29, 39, 66, 139, 145; cordials, 17, 99; cupping, 31, 34; domestic/commercial practices in, 33; emetics/laxatives, 26; enemas, 26, 122–123, 139; evacuative, 26; financial concerns in, 44; homemade, 29; laudanum, 17, 18, 140; medical observations on, 36; of mountebanks, 15; natural, 26–27; ointments, 27, 134, 139; opiates, 140; for pain, 28–29, 41, 134, 139–140; purgatives (physick), 30–32, 39, 61, 63, 66, 86, 123–124, 134, 138, 139; quack, 32, 33; recipes for, 55–56, 125–126; rhubarb, 26, 61; snuff, 40; spa baths, 32; spa waters, 27–28, 28, 32, 103, 124–125, 134; sympathetic cures, 25–26, 97–98; topical, 26–27, 38, 39, 134; and trade expansion, 7; for venereal infection, 37–38, 145

Reproductive ailments, 8, 33

Retention of wastes, and illness causation, 24

Rheum, 22, 40

Rheumatic disorder, 40

Rheumatism, 137

Rhubarb, 26, 61

Rich, Charles, 69, 77–78, 90–91, 109, 196

Rich, Mary (Countess of Warwick), 50, 122; biography of, 196; devotional practices of, 69–71, 72–73; grief and illness causation, 87, 98, 109; and impious suffering, 77–78, 79; marital relations of, 77–78, 90–91, 109; and martyrdom imagery, 143; as model of piety, 76–77; and mortality of others, 49; sickbed visits of, 106–107; spoken words and illness causation, 90–91, 98

Royal Society, 67

Rule and Exercises of Holy Dying (Taylor), 141

Ryder, Dudley: biography of, 196; diary of, 63; emotional responses of, 94–95, 100; and masculine ideal, 11; pain perception of, 153; remedies tried by, 28–32; sickbed visit by, 116

Ryder, Hugh, 19, 38

Sadness, 23

St. Anthony's fire, 104

St. John, Dorothy, 27

Saints, and pain, 147

Salmon, William, 16–17, 18, 36, 41, 149

Salvation, 49, 121–122, 147

Sanguine humor, 19

Savage, Sarah, 121, 196

Scott, Joan, 4

Scourge of Venus and Mercury, The (Sintelaer), 145, 146

Scrofula (king's evil), 170

Seasonal shifts, health impact of, 24

Self-assessment: astrological computation in, 58–59, 66, 79; of bodily excretions, 60–62; comparisons to others' experiences, 48, 51–53, 56–58, 62, 136; contradictory to healer, 18–19; and gender, 48, 62; humoral framework for, 1–2, 3–4, 19–21; mathematical skills in, 64–66; medical knowledge in, 54–56, 134–135; and natural world, 66–67; of nonnatural causes, 21–24, 84; prior experiences in, 59–60, 130; and supernatural, 24–25

Self-treatment, 26–27, 28–32, 38–39, 61

Self-writing. *See* Diaries; Writing

Sermons, funeral, 76–77

Sexuality: and chastity, 10; and infidelity, 101; quantification of, 64; and slander, 91

Shakerley, Jane, 4, 23, 114

Shepard, Alexandra, 11

Shirley, Mary, 116–117

Sickbed: and church attendance, 114; death references/fear of mortality, 117–122; extreme suffering described, 116–117; social isolation of, 112–113; time frame of, 113–115; and work responsibilities, 113–114. *See also* Deathbed; Pain; Remedies; Sickbed visit

Sickbed visit: expectations and norms of, 105–106, 109–110; false front during, 115–116; feigned suffering during, 116; health benefits of, 107–108, 127–128; negative effects of, 108–109; neglect of family and friends, 11, 110–112; pity and compassion in, 94, 106–107; social dynamics of, 106; from vicar, 114

Sickness. *See* Illness

Sick role, 105

Siena, Kevin, 19

Single women, 10–11

Sintelaer, John, 37–38, 145, *146*

Slander-induced illness, 91–93

Sleep, and illness causation, 23

Sloane, Hans, 39–40, 60, 62

Smaley, Roger, 159–160, *160*, 161

Smallpox, 24–25, 44, 85–86, 87

Snail water, 55–56

Snuff, 40

Social interaction and illness: in modern era, 184; negotiation of medical encounters, 123, 126–127; and pain perception, 152–153; of pauper petitioners, 159, 182–183; sickbed isolation, 112–113; *See also* Emotions and illness causation; Sickbed visit

Socioeconomic status: approach to studying, 6–7; and cost of treatment, 44; low-status (*see* Pauper petitioners); middling-status, 6, 133, 153, 169; upper-status, 42, 114, 133, 155–156, 169; and work/occupations, 114, 168–169

Soul, 85

Spa baths, 32

Spa towns, 124–125

Spa water, drinking, 27–28, *28*, 32, 103, 119, 124–125, 134

Speech-induced illness, 89–93

Spencer, Dorothy, 197

Spirits, 25, 31, 40, 60, 74, 81, 82, 84–85, 107–108, 117, 119, 127, 138, 139

Spirituality and illness. *See* Religion and illness

Spiritual journal, 13, 62, 73

Stockton, Owen, 121, 197

Stout, William, 153, 197

Stowe, Stephen, 14

Sudorifics, 26

Supernatural explanations of illness causation, 24–25, 182

Surgeons and surgery, *124*; amputation, 19, 42, 126, 127; barbers as, 34; kidney stone removal, *131*, 131–132; medical observations of, 36, 45; negotiation with family and friends, 126–127; pain tolerance considerations of, 42–43; and pauper petitioners, 176–178; physical evaluations of, 43–44, 45; remedies prescribed by, 122–123, 126; tumor removal, 43

Surprise, 23

Sweats, 20, 22, 23, 26, 60

Swelling, 22, 85, 98, 170

Sycke Mans Salue, The (Becon), 73, 74

Sympathetic cures, 25–26, 97–98

Sympathetic suffering, 53, 81, 99

Taylor, Jeremy, 74, 75, 141

Tears, 86, 94, 96, 107

Temperament, humoral terms for, 19–20

Temperature changes, and illness causation, 22, 23, 170

Thoresby, Ralph, 59, 64, 66, 67, 77, *83*; biography of, 197; fear and illness causation, 100; grief and illness causation, 82, 93; and martyrdom imagery, 143; and pain and mortality, 141; sickbed of, 114, 115

Thornton, Alice: biography of, 197; on deathbed suffering, 150–151; diary of, 4, 13; fear and illness causation, 85–86, 87; grief and illness causation, 81–83, 87, 96–97, 101; and near-fatal illnesses, 119–120; pain perception of, 143–144, 152; sickbed of, 113; slander and illness causation, 91–93; wedding day illness of, 1–2, 3–4

Time frame, sickbed, 113–115

Tomalin, Claire, 63

Toothache, 153

Topical remedies, 26–27, 38, 39, 134

Trade, in medicinal ingredients, 7

Treatise of Melancholie (Bright), 86, 96

Treatment. *See* Medical care; Medical encounters; Remedies; Surgeons and surgery

Trumbull, Elizabeth, 87–88, 125, 146

Tudor, Mary (Queen), 133, 143

Tunbridge Wells, *28*

Tyldesley, Thomas, 63, 154, 155–156, 197–198

Tylston, Katherine, 102, 198

Upper-status patients, 42, 114, 133, 155–156, 169

Uterine disorders, 33

Venereal disease, 33, 37, 145, 177

Vexing words, 91

Vision, 97

Vives, Juan Luis, 54

Walker, Anthony, 76–77

Walkington, Thomas, 85

Wallington, Nehemiah, 47, 198

Walsham, Alexandra, 5

Wandesford, Alice, 150–151, 154

Warwick, Countess of. *See* Rich, Mary

Waters, Ned, 34

Way to the Tree of Life, A (White), 71

Weckherlin, George, 125, 136–137, 198

Weeping, 86, 94, 96, 107

Westover, John, medical records of, 34

White, John, 71

Widows, 10–11, 175

Willet, Deb, 157

Willis, Thomas, 43, 51

Wiseman, Richard, 41, 42, 43

Witchcraft, 13, 25, 90, 182

Women: autonomy of, 10–11; bodies of, 10, 96; breastfeeding/lactation, 20, 34, 61; in caregiver roles, 34, 53; childbirth, 119, 120, 137, 140; devotional practices of, 71–72; diaries of, 56–58, 62; domestic labor of, 29, *30*, 54, 167; emotional responses of, 95–100, 103; feminine ideals, 9–10, 71; homemade remedies of, 29; lactation, 20, 34, 61, 96; mathematical skills of, 65–66; medical knowledge of, 54–56, 135; medical practitioners, 33, 43; menstruation, 20, 24, 61, 96, 134; miscarriage, 1, 97; pain perception of, 42–43, 152–153, 154–155, 158; physical examination of, 43–44; reproductive disorders of, 8, 33; self-assessments of, 48, 61–62; widows, 10–11, 175; work/occupations of, 53, 54, 65, 114, 173. *See also* Gender; Marriage

Wood, Margaret, 168–169

Woolley, Hannah, 29, *30*

Work/occupations: healing trades, 33–34; injuries/illness associated with, 169–170, 172–173, 182; mathematical skills in, 64–66; men's, 66, 113–114, 166; and pain, 155–156; of pauper petitioners, 166, 173, 201; women's, 29, *30*, 53–54, 167, 173

Wounds, artificial, 26

Wright, Thomas, 107

Wrinkles, humoral explanation of, 20

Writing: approach to studying, 4–5; biases in, 12–13; genres of self-writing, 4, 12–14; letters of pauper petitioners, 6–7, 159, *160*, 161–162, *162*; letter writing, 12, 14, 98–99; recipe books, 55, 125–126; and religious beliefs, 5–6. *See also* Diaries; Medical observations

Writing practices, 4